HIGHLIGHTS IN SKIN CANCER

Edited by **Pierre Vereecken**

Highlights in Skin Cancer
http://dx.doi.org/10.5772/46072
Edited by Pierre Vereecken

Contributors

Rohinton S Tarapore, Burhan Engin, Laurence Coiffard, Marian Dmochowski, Justyna Gornowicz-Porowska, Paweł Pietkiewicz, Monika Bowszyc-Dmochowska, Lisa Passantino, Max Costa, Mary Matsui, Cintia Andrade, Natalia Inada, Dora Ramirez, Vanderlei Bagnato, Cristina Kurachi, Pierre Vereecken, Carolyn Heckman, Susan Darlow, Teja Munshi, Clifford Perlis, Małgorzata Juszko-Piekut, Terrence Jerald Piva, Rethika Ravi

Published by InTech

Janeza Trdine 9, 51000 Rijeka, Croatia

Publishing Process Manager Danijela Duric
Technical Editor InTech DTP team
Cover InTech Design team

Additional hard copies can be obtained from orders@intechopen.com

Highlights in Skin Cancer, Edited by Pierre Vereecken
p. cm.
ISBN 978-953-51-1073-6

For EU product safety concerns:
IN TECH d.o.o., Prolaz Marije Krucifikse Kozulić 3, 51000 Rijeka, Croatia,
info@intechopen.com or visit our website at intechopen.com.

Meet the editor

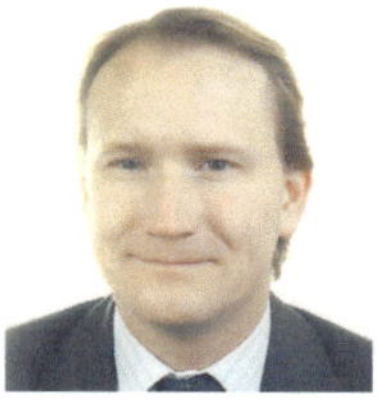

After studying medicine at the Université Libre de Bruxelles completed in 1991 with the highest grade (La Plus Grande Distinction), Dr. Pierre Vereecken becomes Medical Officer and works in Germany in the framework of the Belgian Forces in Germany (1991-1995). During this period he takes six months as a United Nations peacekeeper Officer in the former Yugoslavia, particularly in Central Bosnia. Back to Belgium, he specializes in both Dermatology (1999) and Oncology (2001), and manages to follow various additional training in Belgium and abroad, particularly in France and the United States, in Dermatology, Oncology, and Aesthetics. In 2008, Dr. Pierre Vereecken receives his PhD degree, the highest academic degree, after the presentation of a research work focused on the biology of melanoma, including the study of metastatic process and the role of galectins as a marker of tumor progression.
Head of Academic Services (CHU-Brugmann 2005-2009, Cliniques Universitaires Saint-Luc 2010-2011), and ensuring a triple academic mission, namely clinical, teaching and research, Dr. Pierre Vereecken has always been attentive to offer his patients a quality medicine.
Dr. Pierre Vereecken is the author or coauthor of more then 100 national and international publications and editor or coauthor of more than 10 books.
Member of numerous national and international scientific societies among which the European Academy of Dermatology and Venereology (EADV) and the European Organisation for Research and Treatment of Cancer (EORTC)
Today, Dr. Pierre Vereecken is deeply devoted to his patients, while maintaining scientific rigor, guaranteeing the best care. He provides different courses and presentations in various organizations (education, professional associations and regulatory authorities, ...). He works in the largest private hospital network in Belgium, the CHIREC and in private practice. Dr. Pierre Vereecken founded in 2012 Cliderm (Clinics in Dermatology), multifunctional structure dedicated to clinical dermatology and dermatological research and the European Institute for Dermatology Practice and Research (EIDPR).

Contents

Preface

Since the middle of the 20th century, the incidence of skin cancers such as malignant melanoma is increasing most in the Caucasian population, doubling every 10 years to reach the current rate of 10-15 new cases per year per 100,000 inhabitants. Epidemiological models suggest that prediction is that now a person out of 75 is likely to develop a melanoma in his lifetime. Cutaneous carcinomas are also more frequent.

Along with the increased incidence, increased mortality secondary to melanoma was observed in the second half of the twentieth century, followed by a stabilization probably related to efforts in primary and secondary prevention. Therapeutic advances in this area have been quite limited until recently , despite the enthusiasm generated by clinical trials of immunotherapy, and encourage further efforts to organize prevention and screening compaigns.

Prevention and detection of skin cancer and melanoma in particular are important public health goals in order to decrease the impact of these frequent tumours in young patients. These objectives require particularly strong solidarity between GPs and dermatologists, both in firstline for the evaluation of the skin of patients and to detect their risk factors.

Despite the fact that new recent progress in skincancer treatment have been described, and that new targeted molecules or new therapeutic procedures help our patients, new insights regarding skin biology are also needed to develop new strategies. Moreover interactions between dermatologists and oncologists are mandatory: many targeted therapies developed to treat systemic malignancies have shown important efficacy for the treatment of both cutaneous malignancies and non-malignant skin disease, such as Hedgehog inhibition for basal cell carcinoma and Rituximab for Pemphigus Vulgaris.

This Highlights in Skincancer written by leading experts in their field synthesize common skincancer topics in clinics and research. It is not a guide intended to be a comprehensive and exhaustive review of all the aspects of dermato-oncology but really a companion that should help the clinicians and researchers to find important and specialized information in this field. It is also an awareness of the close collaboration that must exist between dermatologists and medical oncologists in the management of our patients.

Pierre Vereecken, MD, PhD
Cliderm, European Institute for Dermatology Practice and Research,
Chirec Cancer Institute, Brussels, Belgium

Chapter 1

Incidence of Melanoma and Non-Melanoma Skin Cancer in the Inhabitants of the Upper Silesia, Poland

Małgorzata Juszko-Piekut, Aleksandra Moździerz, Zofia Kołosza, Magdalena Królikowska-Jerużalska, Paulina Wawro-Bielecka, Grażyna Kowalska-Ziomek, Dorota Olczyk and Jerzy Stojko

Additional information is available at the end of the chapter

http://dx.doi.org/10.5772/55239

1. Introduction

In recent years, non-melanoma incidence rate has been ranked in the 4th place, and cutaneous melanoma has not been recorded in the first ten places among the most frequent cancers in the inhabitants of the Upper Silesia. Despite high incidence rates, the prognoses of the skin cancers are good, thus the cancer mortality is ranked lower than in the first ten places [1-3]. The authors of the study have already presented epidemiological analyses of the incidence of those cancers [4-7]. Thus the aim of the present study was to continue the evaluation of the incidence rates of non-melanoma skin cancers in the inhabitants of the Upper Silesia in 1999-2007.

The Upper Silesia Industrial Area, occupying the central part of Silesia, has been the most industrial and most ecologically degraded area of Poland. Called the Silesia Agglomeration, it is the biggest urban and industrial agglomeration in the country assembling a number of big cities and industrial areas surrounding them. This affects the landscape and living conditions of habitants. Here, the main source of pollution is the industry, especially mining and energy industries. Heavy industry, underdeveloped as well as underinvested, emits enormous amount of the particulate matter and gases into the atmosphere [8].

Moreover, it was the most populated area of Poland where there were 393 inhabitants per 1km^2.

2. Materials and methods

In a retrospective epidemiological analysis, we evaluated the statistical data of the non-melanoma skin cancer (C44 according to the 10th revision of ICD) and the cutaneous melanoma (C43) in the residents of the Upper Silesia, an administrative region established by the Local Government Reorganization Act of 1998 (effective 1 January 1999). The incidence data were obtained from the Department of Epidemiology and Silesia Cancer Registry, Maria Sklodowska-Curie Memorial Cancer Center and Institute of Oncology, Gliwice Branch. The non-melanoma and melanoma incidence were estimated by calculating both, age-specific and crude rates, and the standardized incidence rates (per the population of 100 000) with the use of a direct method and "the world's population" as a standard [9].

The cumulative risk was also calculated. The cumulative risk is the risk which an individual would have of developing the skin non-melanoma and melanoma from birth to age74 years if no other causes of death were in operation. Moreover, melanoma and non-melanoma skin cancer incidence rates were estimated according to the lesion distribution over the body. The following distribution was included into the study: the head and neck, trunk, arms and legs.

3. Results

Both non-melanoma and melanoma skin cancers belong to the group of cancers typical for the elderly, which can be also observed in the population of Silesia, a region in Poland (Figure 1). Incidence rates are of fundamental importance for the evaluation of a skin cancer risk due to growing effectiveness of treatment, which is related to early diagnosis, and the skin cancer's frequent recurrence.

In the Upper Silesia, continuous progression of melanoma as well as non-melanocytic skin cancers is observed. One in 60 males and one in 80 females runs a risk of developing the skin cancer till the age of 75 years. During the discussed period, i.e. 1999-2007, 4202 cases of cancer were recorded in men, and the standardized incidence rate was 14.96/100 000. The average age of the analyzed male population was 66.7 years, whereas it was 67.8 in the female population. Incidence rates increased systematically with age in both populations, and an increase in the rates was quite strong in older age groups. When compared to young males, young females developed the cancer more frequently, especially those aged 15–39 years. 4389 cases of skin cancer were recorded in women, and the standardized incidence rate was 10.94/100 000. The sex ratio was 1.37 for men due to higher incidence rates in men aged 50 years and more, and the difference increased with age (Table 1), (Figure 2).

http://dx.doi.org/10.5772/55239

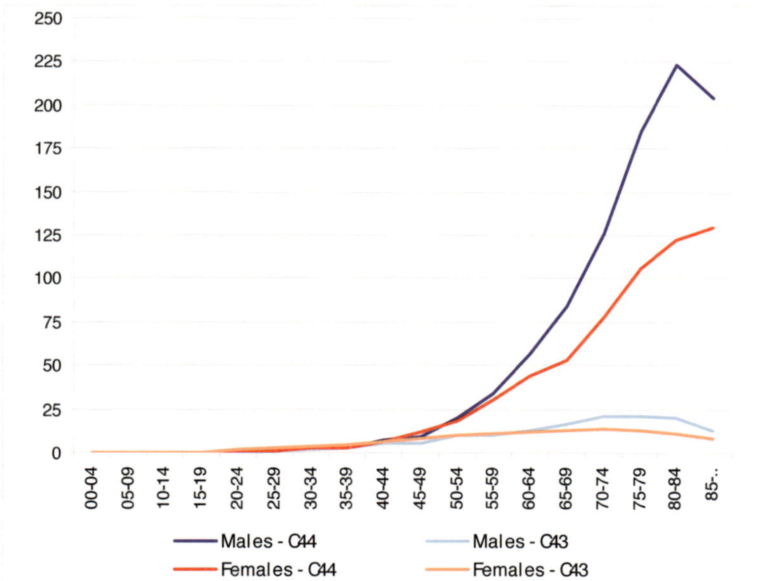

Figure 1. Age-specific incidence rates for non-melanoma cancer (C44) and melanoma (C43) of the skin by sex, Upper Silesia, 1999–2007.

	Males		Females	
Age (years)	**N**	**Rate**	**N**	**Rate**
0-4	0	0.00	0	0.00
5- 9	1	0.09	0	0.00
10-14	1	0.07	1	0.07
15-19	4	0.23	4	0.24
20-24	3	0.17	11	0.63
25-29	14	0.86	20	1.24
30-34	28	1.92	33	2.30
35-39	34	2.36	45	3.15
40-44	119	7.28	105	6.36
45-49	157	9.00	213	11.76
50-54	306	19.75	309	18.68
55-59	391	33.73	384	29.90
60-64	540	56.45	487	43.94
65-69	688	83.57	549	53.14
70-74	751	125.56	685	77.43

	Males		Females	
Age (years)	N	Rate	N	Rate
75-79	650	185.56	721	106.04
80-84	342	223.51	476	122.62
85+	173	204.64	346	129.19
N		4202		4389
Crude rate		20.39		19.97
ASR		14.96		10.94
Cumulative		0.02%		0.01%
Median age				
Mean age				
Sex ratio				

N – number of cases

Crude rate – cases per 100 000

ASR – age standardized rate (World Standard Population)

Cumulative – cumulative risk (0-74 years)

Table 1. Age-specific, crude and age-standardized incidence rates of non-melanoma skin cancer (C44) among men and women in Upper Silesia, 1999-2007.

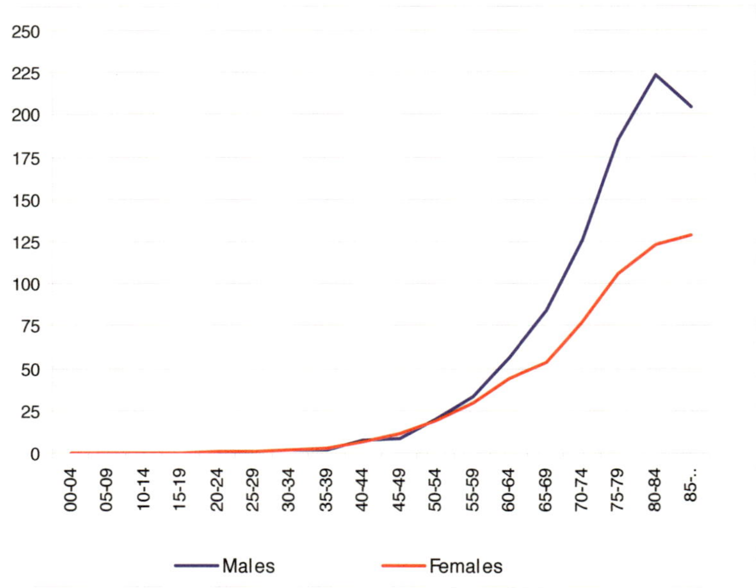

Figure 2. Age-specific incidence rates for non-melanoma skin cancer in males and females, Upper Silesia, 1999–2007.

Cutaneous melanoma is significantly less frequent in comparison with non-melanoma skin cancers, and the same is observed in Silesia. In this area, recorded malignant melanoma incidence rates are approximately 4 times lower in men and 3 times lower in women than non-melanoma incidence rates (Table 1, 2), (Figure 1). During the period of our studies, there were 1072 cases of cutaneous melanoma diagnosed in men, and 1282 in women. An average age of the analyzed males was 57.3 years, whereas it was 55.5 in women, thus the age was lower than in the case of non-melanoma cancer patients. The standardized incidence rates for the Silesian population were $3.88/10^5$ and $4.02/10^5$ for males and females, respectively. Sex ratio was 0.96 for females, thus women run a slightly bigger risk of developing melanoma than men. Young adult and middle aged females are diagnosed with melanoma more frequently than males. Correspondingly to nonmelanocytic skin cancers, the cancer growth rate is bigger in men than in women, however men older than 60 years develop melanoma more frequently, and the difference increases with aging of the population (Table 2), (Figure 1, 3).

	Males		Females	
Age (years)	**N**	**Rate**	**N**	**Rate**
0-4	0	0.00	0	0.00
5- 9	1	0.09	0	0.00
10-14	0	0.00	2	0.15
15-19	7	0.41	5	0.30
20-24	16	0.90	29	1.67
25-29	19	1.16	45	2.80
30-34	27	1.85	53	3.69
35-39	45	3.12	61	4.26
40-44	86	5.26	104	6.230
45-49	101	5.79	143	7.89
50-54	150	9.68	172	10.40
55-59	118	10.18	135	10.51
60-64	126	13.17	133	12.00
65-69	137	16.64	130	12.58
70-74	124	20.73	122	13.79
75-79	73	20.84	84	12.35
80-84	31	20.26	41	10.56
85+	11	13.01	23	8.59
N		1072		1282
Crude rate		5.20		5.83
ASR		3.88		4.02
Cumulative		0.00%		0.00%
Median age				

	Males		Females	
Age (years)	N	Rate	N	Rate
Mean age				
Sex ratio				

N – number of cases

Crude rate – cases per 100 000

ASR – age standardized rate (World Standard Population)

Cumulative – cumulative risk (0-74 years)

Table 2. Age-specific, crude and age-standardized incidence rates of cutaneous melanoma (C43) among men and women in Upper Silesia, 1999-2007.

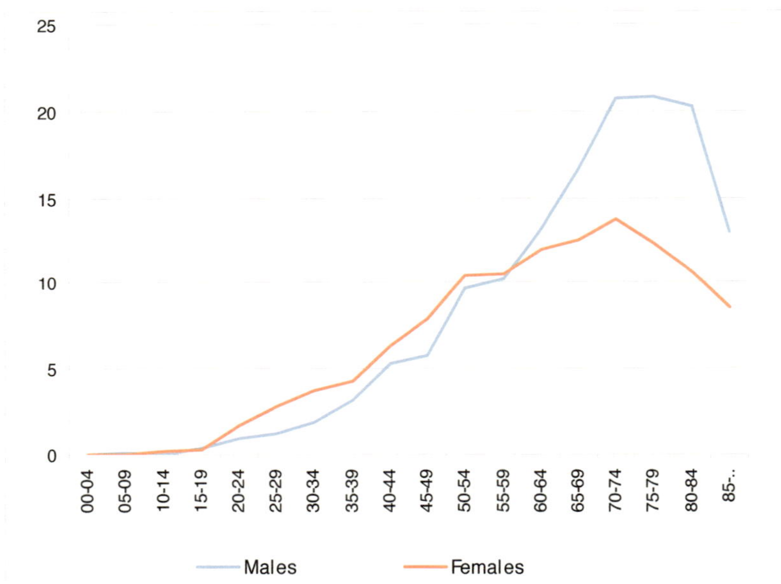

Figure 3. Age-specific incidence rates for cutaneous melanoma in males and females, Upper Silesia, 1999–2007.

Cutaneous melanoma affects mainly young adults. Our collected data show that in people younger than 40 years there are 10.7% of cases of cancer in men and 15.2 % in women. Just to compare, we can say that for non-melanoma skin cancers the percentage was 2% and 2.6% for men and women, respectively, whereas the incident cases of all cancers for all those age groups are 4.1% and 5.6% for men and women, respectively. The results suggest that there are 2 epidemiology reference groups of a melanoma incidence rate for the young and old subgroups, which corresponds to the observations from other parts of Europe [10-15].

When the incidence rates for non-melanomatous skin cancers were compared in relation to the part of the patient's body affected by neoplastic lesions, it was concluded that there were statistically significant differences between males and females, namely more men developed cancers in all studied cancer sites. Such results were most evidently observed for arms (sex ratio M:F 1.86) and trunk (sex ratio M:F 1.71) (Table 3), (Figure 4, 5).

	Males		Females		Sex ratio	
	N	ASR	N	ASR		95% CI
overall	**4202**	**14.96**	**4383**	**10.94**	**1.37**	**1.31-1.43**
Head & neck (C44.0-4)	3124	11.13	3402	8.43	1.32	1.25-1.39
Lip & eyelid (C44.0-1)	429	1.51	562	1.48		
external ear (C44.2)	376	1.34	98	0.24		
face (C44.3)	2035	7.26	2517	6.15		
Scalp & neck (C44.4)	284	1.01	225	0.56		
trunk (C44.5)	432	1.54	327	0.90	**1.71**	**1.47-1.99**
arms (C44.6)	185	0.67	142	0.36	**1.86**	**1.47-2.35**
legs (C43.7)	187	0.66	227	0.54	1.23	1.01-1.51
unspecified (C44.8-9)	247	0.97	291	0.71		

N – number of cases

ASR – age standardized rate (World Standard Population)

Table 3. Site-specific rate ratios of non-melanoma skin cancer (C44) in Upper Silesia, 1999-2007.

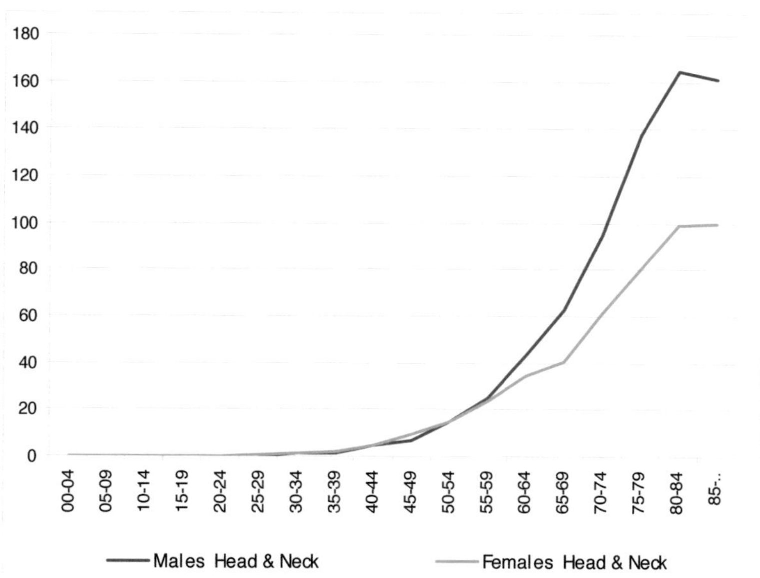

Figure 4. Incidence rates of non-melanoma skin cancer for head and neck in males and females by 5-year age groups, Upper Silesia, 1999-2007.

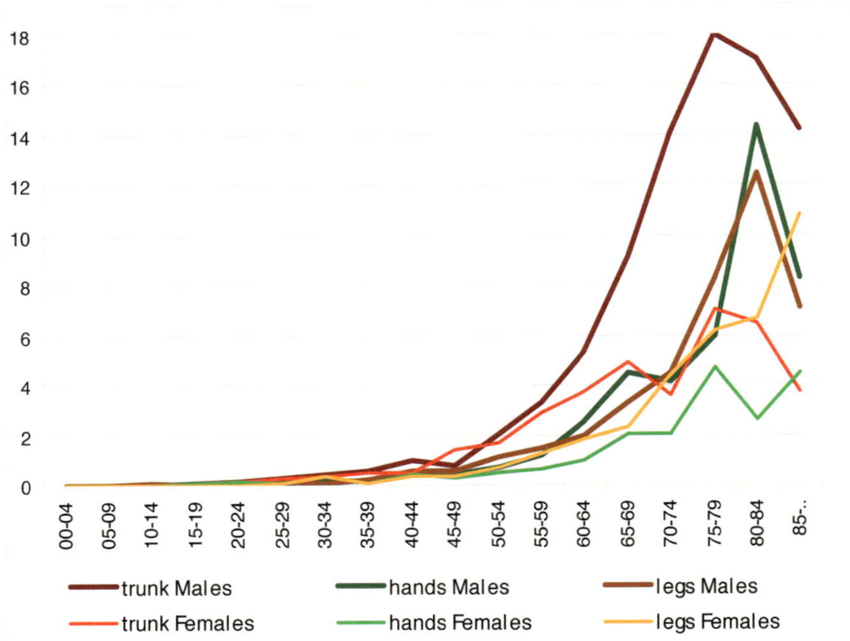

Figure 5. Incidence rates of non-melanoma skin cancer in males and females by 5-year age groups and anatomic site except head and neck, Upper Silesia, 1999-2007.

The majority of the lesions was localized on the head and neck (C44.0-C44.4), i.e. 74% of all neoplastic lesions in men and 78% in women. Most of the lesions were on the face (C 44.3), i.e. 48% and 57% in men and women, respectively. The standardized incidence rate for this cancer site (head and neck) was 11.13/100 000 in men and 8.43/100 000 in women. When compared to female patients, the incidence rates of the skin cancer localized on the head and neck are growing in males aged over 50 years, and the rates are two times higher in those aged more than 75 years, whereas among younger generations more lesions were recorded in young females (Table 3), (Figure 4).

The sites of neoplastic lesions in females were ranked in the following order: trunk (C44.5), legs (C44.7) and arms (C 44.6), whereas in males they were on the trunk (C44.5), arms (C44.6) and legs (C44.7). The analysis showed that young females developed skin cancers of such localizations more frequently than males. Higher incidence rates for males than for females were recorded for the lesions on the trunk, legs and arms in patients older than 35. A strong increase was recorded for patients older than 50, and the trend persisted until old age. To sum up, it can be observed that the incidence rates related to the cancer sites are systematically increasing with age in both populations (Table 3), (Figure 5).

A specific cancer site of melanoma is sex dependent. In males, the most commonly affected body part is the trunk (especially neoplastic lesions in elderly men), whereas they are legs in females, which is also observed in the inhabitants of Silesia (Table 4), (Figure 6, 7). Among all the cases of melanoma diagnosed in male inhabitants of the Upper Silesia, most of the lesions,

	Males		Females		Sex ratio	
	N	ASR	N	ASR		95% CI
overall	**1072**	**3.88**	**1282**	**4.02**	**0.96**	0.89-1.05
Head & neck (C43.0-4)	151	0.54	180	0.52	1.03	0.82-1.29
Lip & eyelid (C43.0-1)	23	0.08	25	0.07		
external ear (C43.2)	15	0.05	16	0.05		
face (C43.3)	57	0.20	106	0.29		
Scalp & neck (C43.4)	56	0.21	33	0.12		
trunk (C43.5)	511	1.85	305	1.00	**1.85**	**1.60-2.14**
arms (C43.6)	147	0.53	225	0.72	0.74	0.60-0.91
legs (C43.7)	161	0.59	494	1.55	**0.38**	**0.32-0.45**
unspecified (C43.8-9)	102	0.37	78	0.23		

N – number of cases

ASR – age standardized rate (World Standard Population)

Table 4. Site-specific rate ratios of cutaneous melanoma (C43) in Upper Silesia, 1999-2007.

namely 48%, were on the trunk (C43.5). Such neoplastic lesions are equally frequent in women until they are aged 50 years, but in older patients the female incidence rates decreased, whereas the male rates increased strongly. In cancer patients aged 65-79 years, the male incidence rates for the trunk were 4 times higher than the female ones. In older men, the main cancer site is the trunk.

In females, in 38% of cases, the lower limbs were affected by cancer (C43.7), and a strong increase in the incidence rate was recorded for women aged 40-79 years. Such cancer site is 3 times more frequent in females than in males. We should emphasize that young females develop the skin cancer more frequently than young men, and the highest incidence rate for melanoma on legs were recorded for women aged 65-79 years. What is more, female incidence rates of melanoma for such a site are higher than male ones until old age. The incidence rate decreased in both population in the oldest age groups.

Arms are a frequent site of melanoma both in males and females (C43.6). In the group of patients younger than 70 years, higher incidence rates are recorded for females, whereas in those older than 70 years the incidence rates are 2 times higher in men than in women. The incidence rates increased systematically with age in both populations (Table 3, 4), (Figure 6, 7).

Summing up, until 50 years of age the body parts affected by melanomas are ranked in the following order in women: legs, trunk, arms, head and neck, whereas the order is the trunk,

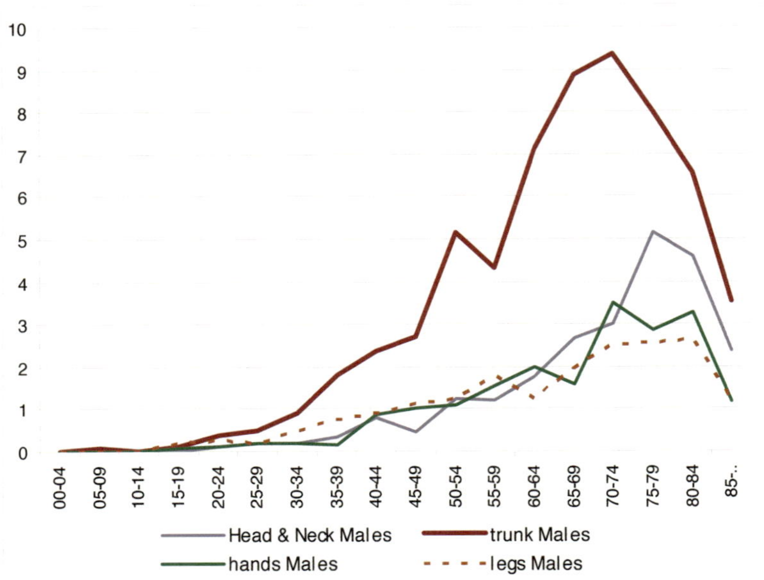

Figure 6. Incidence rates of cutaneous melanoma in males by 5-year age groups and anatomic site, Upper Silesia, 1999-2007.

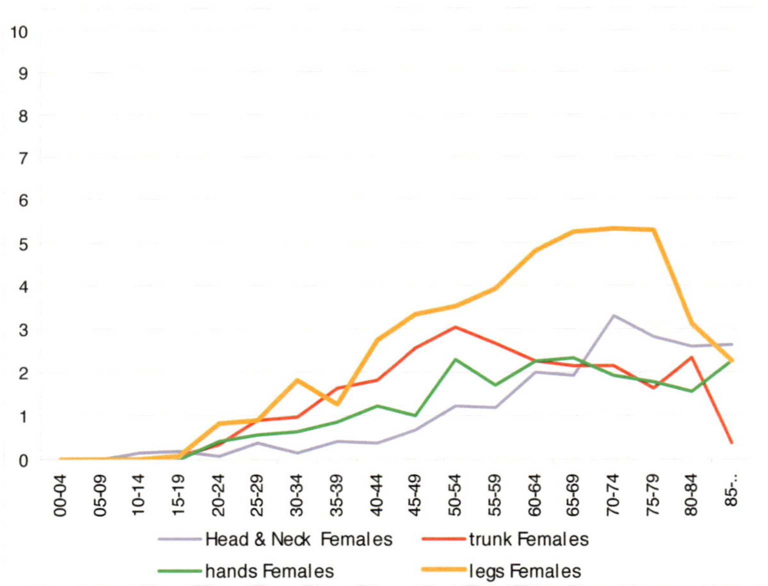

Figure 7. Incidence rates of cutaneous melanoma in females by 5-year age groups and anatomic site, Upper Silesia, 1999-2007.

legs, arms, head and neck in men. At this age, the risk of developing melanomas in all parts of the body (except the torso) is higher for women than for men. On the other hand, in patients over 50 years of age the rate of melanomas increases with age on legs and decreases for the trunk in women, but in men the rate increases for the trunk, however melanoma develops more slowly on legs.

When both types of skin cancers are compared, we can notice that the rates increase systematically with age. The incidence rate of non-melanoma skin cancer, in comparison with melanoma, is 4 times higher in men and 2.5 times higher in women. The distribution of age-specific incidence rates indicates a strong increase in melanoma rates in patients until 40 years of age. Yet over 40 years of age, namely with aging of the population, a strong increase in the rates of non-melanoma skin cancers can be observed. In the oldest age groups of men and women, the incidence rate is approximately 12 times higher than for melanoma.

The analyzed skin cancers differ in terms of the ratios of affected body parts. Huge disproportions between non-melanoma skin cancer and melanoma are recorded for the face. In men, non-melanoma skin cancers on the face comprise 48% of all skin cancers, whereas melanoma comprises 5%, while in women, it is 57% in case of non-malignant skin cancers and 8% for melanoma.

4. Discussion

Malignant neoplasms of the skin constitute the most numerous group of human malignancies, especially among representatives of a Caucasian race in the subtropical region. The two main groups of the skin cancer are non-melanomas and malignant melanoma.

The skin cancer incidence rates(C44,C43) are continually increasing in the world population [10-21]. In Poland, an increasing trend has also been recorded for all age groups since the 1970s, and according to the estimations this upward trend will continue in future [19]. A systematic increase in the rates is also observed in the Silesian population [2,3,20]. In 2009, all skin cancers, including melanoma, constituted above 8% of all malignant neoplasms in male and female inhabitants of Silesia. We can compare it with the values recorded for Poland, namely 8% of cases in men and 9% in women [18]. The results presented in the tables 1 and 2 indicate that a risk of non-melanomas and melanoma in young and middle aged adults is higher for females, whereas it is higher for men in the other age groups, especially in those aged over 50 years. In the years 1999-2003, an increased incidence rate was recorded for both skin cancer types in men aged 55 years. Both skin cancer types are more frequent in young women than in men, however the skin cancer growth rate in the population of middle aged adults is higher for men, and the difference increases with age. Similar situation has been observed in all regions of Poland [18,19], in Europe, and in the world population [10,16].

Standardized incidence rates of skin cancers were higher in the years 1999-2007 than the published values referring to the earlier periods [4-7,17]. In 1999-2003, the male standardized incidence rate of non-melanoma skin cancer was 13.50, whereas it was 9.70 for women. The incidence rate was 14.0 and 10.2 for men and women, respectively, in the years 1999-2005 [6]. During the analyzed period, i.e. 1999-2007, the value of male incidence rate increased up to

14.96, whereas the female rate reached a value of 10.94. In the years 1999–2003, an average annual non-melanoma incidence rate increased by 4.2% in men and by 4.8% in women. The sex ratio M:F was 1.1, but it increased to 1.37 during the presently studied period, which indicates a bigger risk of non-melanoma skin cancer for men than for women. In the first studied period, one in 68 male inhabitants of the Upper Silesia and one in 91 female ones could develop non-melanoma skin cancer, whereas in the years 1999-2005 one in 62 men and one in 87 women could be affected. The risk of developing the cancer until the age 74 years was still increasing, and in the years 1999-2007 one in 60 men and one in 80 women could develop non-melanoma skin cancer. On the other hand, one in 227 men and one in 232 women could develop malignant melanoma over this studied period.

In Silesia, cutaneous melanoma is diagnosed in men 4 and in women 2.5 times less frequently than non-melanomas, and this ratio is similar in the rest of Europe [10,14]. However, a slightly higher risk of cancer is recorded for men younger than 74 years than for women. Over a quite long period of time, an upward trend have been observed for both sexes. The results of our previous analyses in the years 1985-1989:1990-1994:1995-1998 show that incidence rates were increasing systematically.

In men, the consecutive incidence rates were 1.92, 2.69, and 2.86, while a cumulative risk was 0.20%, 0.32%,and 0.33% [17]. In the following years, a further progression of cancer was recorded, namely, in1999-2003 the incidence rate was 3.53 and the risk was 0.40% [4]. In the years 1999-2007, the highest incidence rate and the biggest cumulative risk were recorded, i.e. 3.88 and 0.44%, respectively, for men.

In the years 1985-1989:1990-1994:1995-1998, the following female incidence rates were registered:2.13, 2.56, and 3.11, while a cumulative risk was 0.21%, 0.26%, and 0.32% [17]. In 1999-2003, the incidence rate increased to 3.72, whereas a risk of cutaneous melanoma was 0.4% for women, which indicates that both sexes ran a similar risk of developing the cancer over this period of time [4,21].

In the previous years, men ran a slightly higher risk of cancer than women, though women developed the skin cancer more frequently, and such a trend is also observed at present. In the analyzed period of time, a standardized rate per 100 000 was also high for women, i.e. 4.02. The sex ratio M:F was 0.96 and it was unfavorable for women like in the previous years. To compare, the sex ratio M:F was 0.97 in the 1985-1998, and 0.95 in 1999-2003. This trend is similar to the one observed in Germany in the 1990s, where the incidence rates were equal for both sexes. However, cutaneous melanoma incidence rate recorded in Australia is higher for men [22].

In comparison to the age of non-melanoma patients (men 66.7; women 67.8), an average age suggests that malignant melanoma affects younger population in Silesia (men 57.3; women 55.5). It is worrying that the incidence rates are increasing for both sexes in all age groups in Silesia (C44 and C43). What is more, the age of afflicted persons is decreasing, especially in women, which is in agreement with observed world trends [6,22-24]. Additionally, the values of male and female incidence rates of non-melanoma skin cancers are getting equal in older age groups, whereas cutaneous melanoma rates are reaching similar values in younger age groups. This might indicate that in future more cases of non-melanoma skin cancers will be diagnosed in older women, and more younger men will develop melanoma.

When the non-melanoma and melanoma incidence rates are compared, it can be observed that in the Silesian population, people younger than 40 years developed mainly cutaneous melanoma. In people older than 40 years, there is a strong increase in the non-melanoma incidence rate with aging of the population. Both in the oldest male and female age groups, non-melanoma incidence rate is approximately 12 times higher than melanoma incidence rate.

The number of epidemiological studies on the non-melanoma and melanoma incidence and mortality rates in the inhabitants of the Upper Silesia is more than modest. In this area of Poland, the etiology of those cancers was poorly defined, since very first publications on the non-melanoma incidence and mortality rates in the inhabitants of the Upper Silesia pertained to the years 1985–1993. During that period, the ratio of histologically confirmed non-melanoma skin cancers held rather steady. The standardized rate for the Silesia was 6.3 per 100,000, and it was 6.4 per 100,000 in the cities. The carcinomas were recorded in males aged 10-15 years, and they were diagnosed until a very old age with evident increase in the incidence rate from 35 to 39 years of age [5,21].

Melanoma and non-melanoma skin cancers (NMSC) are now the most common types of cancer in white populations. Both cancers show an increasing incidence rate worldwide, but a stable or decreasing mortality rate. The rising incidence rates of NMSC may be caused by a combination of increased sun exposure or exposure to ultraviolet (UV) light, higher levels of outdoor activities, changes in clothing style, increased longevity, ozone depletion, genetics and immune suppression in some cases. A dose-dependent increase in the risk of squamous cell carcinoma (SCC) of the skin was found to be associated with exposure to psoralen and UVA irradiation. Intensive UV exposure in childhood and adolescence was a causative factor of basal cell carcinoma (BCC), whereas early chronic UV exposure was considered the cause of SCC [22]. In Poland, UVI (ultraviolet index) rarely exceeds 7, i.e. a value indicating a high UV radiation intensity [25].

An increase in incidence rates of skin cancers can also be caused by frequency of other risk factors such as oncogenic viruses or immunosuppressive drugs [26-28]. Other factors favorable for developing the skin cancer are post-burn scars, excessive keratosis, cutaneous horn, leukoplakia, xerodermapigmentosum (XP), nevoid basal cell carcinoma syndrome, and Bowen's disease (squamous cell carcinoma in situ). Immunological mechanisms may be involved in the pathogenesis of melanoma. Genetic predisposition is associated with about 10% of cases, and a number of genes whose mutations are a direct cause of cancer. The best known genes associated with familial melanoma include CDK4 (12q14), P16 (9p21) and CMM1 (1p36) [22,29-31].

The incidence of cutaneous melanoma is most rapidly increasing among all cancer rates in white populations. Its incidence is closely associated with constitutive skin color, and depends on a geographical zone. The highest incidence rates have been reported in Queensland, Australia, with 56 new cases per 100,000 men and 43 per 100,000 women per year. Mortality rates of melanoma have stabilized in the USA, Australia and also in European countries. Neoplastic lesion thickness is the most important prognostic factor for the primary melanoma. For the last two decades, thin melanomas have been diagnosed more frequently. Epidemiological studies have confirmed the hypothesis that the majority of all melanoma cases are caused, at least in part, by excessive exposure to sunlight. Unlike squamous cell carcinoma, a melanoma risk does not seem to be associated with cumulative, but rather intermittent exposure to sunlight [22,32].

The basal cell carcinoma incidence rate increases linearly with the UV intensity. The increase in the incidence rate is proportional to the distant to the equator, and a squamous cell carcinoma incidence rate is doubled with decreasing latitude by every 8-10 degrees. On the equator, UV dose per unit of time is by 30% higher than in the south of the United States, and by 200% higher than in Europe, and in the northern part of the US [27,33-35]. An increase in the intensity of UV radiation that reaches the earth surface is explained by continuous and significant reduction of the ozone layer [31,36,37]. In Australia, Brazil and the USA, the skin cancer incidence rates are higher than in Northern, Central and Eastern Europe since there the sun exposure is proportionally higher than in Europe [38].

Non-melanoma skin cancers (NMSC) are the most common cancers diagnosed in the United States. Over 1 million new cases of basal and squamous cell carcinomas of the skin are diagnosed annually, and the exposure to UV radiation is a leading risk factor [39]. The ultraviolet (UV) band of the solar radiation is often divided into three sub-bands, namely, UV-C (wavelengths less than 280 nm); UV-B (280-320 nm), and UV-A (32-400 nm) when considering the biological effects. The atmosphere blocks the Sun's output of UV-C range (highly dangerous for plants and animals). UV radiation at the Earth's surface consists mostly of UV-A and UV-B. Ozone absorbs much of the UV-B radiation but this absorption weakens as a wavelength of 320 nm is approached. Life on the Earth is particularly affected by this part of the solar spectrum. An overexposure to UV-B radiation causes skin reddening and reduction of vitamin-D synthesis (result of a short-term overexposure), and the more serious skin cancer developing after long-term overexposure. Yet higher skin cancer incidence rates are recorded in Brazil, and they are related to a higher UVI as well as higher ozone concentration in the air. The UVI has strong seasonal variability in regions and parts of the year [38]. It can also be observed in Silesia, since the mountainous part of this region (i.e. Bielsko-Biała region) has higher non-melanomas and melanoma incidence rates than other regions of Silesia [4,5].

In Silesia, increased rates are recorded for women and men, however squamous skin carcinoma is more frequent in men [5]. The most common non-melanoma is basal cell carcinoma (BCC) diagnosed in 80% of cases, and squamous cell carcinoma, which originates in the malpighian layer, and is developed by 20% of patients. Our previously published studies showed that in the years 1999-2005, the ratio of basal cell carcinoma to squamous cell carcinoma was 4:1 and 7:1 for the male and female populations, respectively [6]. This can be related to the fact that men more frequently work outdoors and practice outdoor sports. Non-melanoma skin cancers, which are almost 100% curable, may occur in people who are overexposed for very long periods of time, like farmers, or construction workers and postal workers, street peddlers and other informal workers in cities [40].

The incidence rate may also be related to the exposure to other occupational factors, e.g. employment in industry. Silesia is the most industrialized region of Poland, where intensive development of industry began in the 19th century and continued in the 20th century.

http://dx.doi.org/10.5772/55239

Arsenic and its inorganic compounds is one of the factors that play a special role in the pathogenesis of skin cancers related to the industrial exposure[41,42]. In Slovakia, for instance, in the Prievidza region, elevated concentration of arsenic in the air and soil near the power plant where coal is used for heating, increased the incidence rate of skin cancers [43]. Special attention should be paid to this factor in the Upper Silesia since there are several power plants, thermal-electric power plants and coking plants in which coal is used. Additionally, skin cancer development is induced by groundwater or drugs contaminated by arsenic [26,27,42,44-46].

In the 1970s, there was an increase in the number of people who spent their vacations in the sunny areas of Europe and Northern Africa. Nowadays, India or Central America have also become vacation destination. People also tend to spend their weekends in the nearby mountainous region of Bielsko-Biała. What is more, suntan has been regarded as the symbol of social status, which imposes taking additional doses of UV radiation in solar salons, especially during those seasons when there is little sunshine in our climate zone.

The malignant melanoma incidence rate is sex and age dependent [22,26]. In countries where the malignant melanoma incidence rate is low, the rate is usually higher for women than for men, whereas a different trend is observed in the USA. When compared to men, American women younger than 40 years run a slightly bigger risk of skin cancer, while in persons over 40 years the proportion changes and the risk is higher for men. The differences are getting bigger with aging of the population [17,23].

The shape of age-related incidence curve for the inhabitants of the Upper Silesia is similar to the one for the US population, however a significant increase in the male incidence rate is recorded in those aged 50 years [23]. Our studies indicate that a male incidence rate has clearly increased in older age groups over the years [4,5,17], and in the nearest future the incidence rate in male inhabitants of the Upper Silesia may increase especially for elderly males. It can also be concluded that soon the age of the population in which more men than women will be affected by the skin cancer will decrease.

The fact that melanoma and non-melanoma skin cancers are more frequently diagnosed in inhabitants of regions with intensive insolation can suggest that a total UV dose may have a significant effect on developing skin cancers, which was also confirmed by our analyses. The mountainous Bielsko-Biała region with low air pollution and high UV radiation had the highest melanoma incidence rate in the whole Upper Silesia [4,5].

The highest risk of developing cutaneous melanoma occurs due to occasional solar exposure, which can be called recreational one. This especially applies to childhood years and repeated sunburns. It was established that as much as 80% of total solar exposure in a lifetime falls on the first 18 years. Multivariate analysis shows that in individuals who suffered from repeated sunburns when they were younger than 18 years, the risk of developing the cancer increases almost 6.5 times [2-5,17,21,47,48]. Nowadays, it is agreed that suffering from sunburns in childhood, especially before the age of 12 years, is a significant risk factor of cutaneous melanoma [22,47]. In children with sunburns, a decrease in 7-dehydrocholesterol level, converted into vitamin D3 in the skin, was recorded even 14 months after sunburn. Correspondingly, low levels of an active form of vitamin D3 was diagnosed in malignant melanoma patients [49,50].

Skin cancers are neoplastic lesions typical for elderly people. However, cutaneous melanoma is disproportionally more frequently diagnosed in young adults. Cutaneous melanoma is assumed to occur after 20-40 years since the exposure to a risk factor, e.g. ultraviolet (UV) radiation. Thus, the incidence rates of cohorts consisting of the inhabitants of the Upper Silesia from 1978 and 1998, respectively, were compared. After 20 years, a significant increase in the number of neoplastic lesions could be seen among the people who were young then [17].

Numerous studies suggest that solar exposure is not the only but a highly probable environmental risk factor in developing malignant melanoma, especially in the population where cutaneous melanotic nevi ('moles') do not occur. Solar exposure may play varied roles in etiology of malignant melanoma [6,32,51,52]. UV radiation is a significant carcinogenic factor in people but only one of about 60 risk factors recognized by WHO [53]. It was observed that in people with diagnosed elastosis, the mortality rate due to malignant melanoma was half of the rate recorded in individuals who were not afflicted by the disease.

The positive influence of sunlight is related to its role in the synthesis of the vitamin D3 in human body. A direct reaction which occurs in the skin after UVB exposure is the synthesis of inactive form of the vitamin D3, i.e. cholecalciferol, into an active form, i.e. 1.25- dihydroxyvitamin, which has a diversified, beneficial effect on cells since it induces apoptosis in many disease processes. The vitamin D3 inhibits proliferation and induces differentiation of melanoma cells. The ability to convert provitamin into an active form of the vitamin D3 is highly impaired in the residents of northern latitudes. Populations living far from the equator may suffer from vitamin D3 deficiency during winter months [54]. Consequently, a low level of 1.25-dihydroxyvitamin is detected in malignant melanoma patients' serum. The opinion that sunlight might have a healthful effect on certain types of cancers has been around for a few decades [53]. When compared to the southern states inhabitants, increased mortality rates were reported for leading cancer types including breast, prostate and colon cancers in individuals of Caucasian race who inhibit northern states of the USA [55]. In 1990, the vitamin D3 was mentioned as a factor which could explain the differences in geographic distribution of the mortality rates [56]. In individuals who regularly spend some time outdoors, the vitamin D3 deficiency decreases. Thus, this hypothesis may elucidate not entirely expected protective effects of sunscreens [57]. High SPF value of sunscreen products can fully block the vitamin D3 synthesis in the skin, which is undesirable. Sun tanning serves as a protection against sunlight since melanin granules absorb the sunlight and, to some extent, neutralize the negative effect of UBV, e.g. by promoting degradation of connective tissue due to the damage of collagen fibers and elastin, or inducing DNA mutation which can result in neoplastic transformation [49-51].

This is consistent with the observations that people working outdoors with certain intervals run lower risk of developing malignant melanoma localized in the skin exposed to UV radiation than people who work indoors [58-60]. Continuous sun exposure may reduce a risk of sunburns, which are a known etiologic factors of malignant melanoma. What is more, smaller vitamin D3 deficiency in individuals who are regularly exposed to sunlight can serve as another explanation for low malignant melanoma incidence rate values [54]. However, it is only an assumption which should be confirmed by further studies, since all the effects of vitamin D and its receptors are not completely known.

The worldwide incidence trends are reflected by the skin cancer incidence rates in the Upper Silesia, namely, the highest rates are recorded in older age groups, which may result from the accumulating of risk factors over time and a continuous increase of life span. Our results show that there are 2 different groups of epidemiological factors of malignant melanoma for young and old age subgroups, which was also observed by other authors [12].

Distribution of non-melanomas (head and neck) and malignant melanoma (trunk) correspond to the worldwide trends, too [22,47,48,61]. Longer exposure to sunlight may be a causative factor of skin cancers developed on the head, neck, trunk and lower limbs [17,50].

Basal cell carcinoma (BCC), which is the most common among non-melanomas and constitutes 75%-86% of all cases, occurs on the head and neck a slightly more frequently in men [62,63]. In the Upper Silesia in 1999-2003, one in 107 men ran a risk of BCC, whereas one in 68 men could develop all types of skin cancer [4]. In the years 1999-2007, in comparison with 1999-2003, both populations ran a significantly higher risk of developing non-melanoma skin cancer in all cancer sites. Still, most neoplastic lesions were on the patients' head and neck. When compared to an earlier period, the incidence rate for this cancer site, i.e. the head and neck (C44.0-4), increased especially in men. A standardized incidence rate was 9.60 per 100,000 in 1999-2003, while it was 11.13 per 100,000 in 1999-2007. The same trend but a slower rate was recorded in women. Still, the sex ratio is unfavorable for men, and resembles the one in the years 1999-2003. Over these years, the female incidence rate increased from 7.36 to 8.43, but men ran a higher risk of neoplastic lesions on the head and neck than women. Corresponding results were obtained for the neoplastic lesions on the trunk (C44.5) and legs (44.7), but the disproportion between sex ratios was getting bigger in comparison with 1999-2003,and in men the ratio increased for neoplastic lesions on the trunk, whereas it decreased for arms and legs.

In the whole area of the Upper Silesia, a continuous increase in malignant melanoma incidence rate can be observed. The growth rate for this cancer in people older than 50 years is higher for men than for women, and the difference is increasing with age. A specific cancer site is age and sex dependent. More frequently, neoplastic lesions on the trunk and lower limbs are typical for older age groups, while an increase in malignant melanoma incidence rate for the head and neck (80%) characterizes the oldest age groups [21].

In the younger population, i.e. among persons younger than 50 years, cutaneous melanoma develops most frequently on the body parts continually exposed to the sun such as arms and legs, and on the neck and face in those older than 50 years [17,21,64]. Corresponding observations were made for the inhabitants of the Upper Silesia. The analysis of melanoma incidence rate related to the affected body parts indicates that neoplastic lesions in elderly men were most frequently on the trunk, while in women older than 20 years, cutaneous melanoma affected lower limbs and the trunk. In older age groups, especially in men, malignant melanoma incidence rate increased for the head and neck as well as for arms.

In the years 1999-2007, both men and women ran the same risk of malignant melanoma on the head and neck (C43.0-4), whereas in 1985-1998 the sex ratio M:F was 1.25, thus the risk of developing cancer at such a site decreased in men. In the years 1999-2003, neoplastic lesions on the face (C 43.3) were 2 times more frequent in women than in men. However in 1999-2007, such huge differences were not recorded, which resulted from an increased incidence rate in men but a decreased rate in women.

In men, most frequently malignant melanoma affected the trunk. As early as in 1985-1998, the sex ratio M:F for the trunk (C43.5) was 1.58 and was unfavorable for men, and increased significantly in the following years (1999-2003) up to 1.60. The differences between sexes were getting bigger [17,21]. In here presented analysis of the years 1999-2007, the ratio was 1.85, which indicates that the disproportions between sexes for this cancer site were increasing. When we compared the years 1995-1998 and 1985-1989, we noticeda 2-fold increase in the number of neoplastic lesions on the trunk in men.

Additionally, the sex ratio was unfavorable for women when the results for neoplastic lesions on legs (C43.7) were analyzed. This trend has prevailed in the Upper Silesia for years. In the above mentioned periods of time, the sex ratio M:F was ranked as follows: 0.47, 0.41, 0.38. In the years 1999-2007, the female incidence rate of malignant melanoma on lower limbs was almost 3 times higher than in men, in 1999-2003 it was 2.5 times higher, whereas it was 2 times higher in 1985-1999. In comparison to men, more young women developed malignant melanoma on legs. After the comparison of the previous analyzed periods, we could observe that incidence rates of those cancer sites increased in both sexes. The highest relative increase in female incidence rate was registered for arms (C43.6), was also recorded during the past years [7]. The values of female standardized incidence rate were as follows: 0.37 in 1985-1999, 0.63 in 1999-2003, and 0.72 in 1999-2007 [18,23]. The differences between cancer sites in both sexes may result from the differences in the way they dress, which suggests that there are variations in time of UV exposure of body parts

However, the UV radiation dose inducing skin cancer in humans is still unknown.

The development of all nevi types, including dysplastic nevi, is related to skin pigmentation degree and malignant melanoma is most frequent in white people. For instance, in Argentina, in the population of Cordoba with high values of malignant melanoma incidence rates, the risk of developing the cancer increases over 2 times if grandparents were Europeans and over 5 times in individuals of fair skin and eyes [5].

The risk also increases with the number of melanotic nevi ('moles'). Adults have 15-20 moles on average and their location can be varied, i.e. they can occur on the scalp or places exposed to solar radiation. Developing malignant melanoma in solarium clients is also related to a large number of moles and the neoplastic lesions are most frequently located on the trunk [17]. In general, solarium clients are young people, predominantly young women. Thus, indoor tanning can also contribute to the increase in the number of the lesions on the trunk in female inhabitants of the Upper Silesia.

The number of detected dysplastic nevi significantly decreases in people who consumed small quantities of food but of large vitamin D, α- and β-carotene, cryptoksantin and lute in content.

Although this is directly related to the skin response to repeated exposure to UV radiation, supplementation of the above listed components does not bring the required effect [26].

Extensive case-control studies of the population of the Silesia would be necessary to establish which environmental risk factors play an essential role in developing cutaneous malignant melanoma. Due to the increase in the values of malignant melanoma incidence rates, also in the inhabitants of the Upper Silesia, appropriate health education and prophylactic strategies related to solar exposure have to be implemented.

Slip-Slop-Slap was the iconic and internationally recognized sun protection campaign prominent in Australia during the 1980s. Launched by Cancer Council Victoria in 1981, the Slip! Slop! Slap! campaign features a singing, dancing Sid Seagull encouraging people to reduce sun exposure and protect themselves against an increased risk of skin cancer [65,66]. Sid had Australians slipping on long sleeved clothing, slopping on sunscreen and slapping on a hat. This successful program was funded by public donations. The health campaign was extended in later years by the Sun Smart to encourage the use of sunglasses and shade. That is: Slip on a shirt, Slop on the 30+ sunscreen, Slap on a hat, Seek shade or shelter, Slide on some sunnies. - "Slip, Slop, Slap, Seek, Slide". By this stage, however, the skin cancer aware message of the campaign had successfully been absorbed into the Australian psyche. Slip, Slop, Slap was also used in New Zealand, where the mascot is a lobster, voiced by Ants from What Now. Some Canadian cities have also started their own Slip-Slop-Slap campaigns.

The campaign is considered one of the most successful and recognizable health campaigns in Australia, but despite its popularity and success, Australia has the highest incidence of skin cancer in the world. Each year in Australia, various forms of skin cancer are diagnosed in more than 300 thousand people, about 1,600 people die from malignant melanoma.

The American Cancer Society recommends the following:

- Slip on a shirt with sleeves.
- Slop on sunscreen (at least an SPF 15) and remember to reapply.
- Slap on a hat with a brim wide enough to shade your face, ears, and neck.
- Sunglasses to protect your eyelids from UV damage and your eyes from getting cataracts [67].

Appropriate cancer screening programs and doctors' training should also be introduced, which would facilitate early detection and proper care of patients with melanotic nevi characterized by high risk of developing malignant melanoma. Such implementations have brought satisfactory results in Australia and Scandinavian countries.

5. Conclusion

Due to the increase in the values of malignant melanoma incidence rates in the inhabitants of the Upper Silesia, it is necessary to implement health education and prophylactic strategies related to solar exposure. What is more, it would be advisable to sensitize doctors to attentively observe patients' skin lesions.

Author details

Małgorzata Juszko-Piekut[1], Aleksandra Moździerz[1], Zofia Kołosza[2], Magdalena Królikowska-Jerużalska[1], Paulina Wawro-Bielecka[1], Grażyna Kowalska-Ziomek[3], Dorota Olczyk[1] and Jerzy Stojko[1]

*Address all correspondence to: amozdzierz@sum.edu.pl

1 Medical University of Silesia in Katowice, School of Pharmacy, Department of Hygiene, Bioanalysis and Environmental Studies, Poland

2 Cancer Epidemiology Department, Maria Skłodowska-Curie Memorial Cancer Center and Institute of Oncology, Gliwice, Poland

3 Medical University of Silesia in Zabrze, Division and Department of Histology and Embryology, Poland

References

[1] Silesia Cancer Registry (Śląski Rejestr Nowotworów) Available at: http://www.rejestrslaski.io.gliwice.pl/

[2] Kołosza Z, Banasik TR, Zemła BFP: Cancer in the Silesia Voivodeship In 2004. (Nowotwory złośliwe w województwie śląskim w 2004 roku). Maria Skłodowska-Curie Memorial Cancer Center and Institute of Oncology. Regional Silesia Cancer Registry, Cancer Epidemiology Department, Gliwice 2006.

[3] Kołosza Z, Banasik TR, Zemła BFP: Cancer in the Silesia Voivodeship in 2007. (Nowotwory złośliwe w województwie śląskim w 2007 roku). Maria Skłodowska-Curie Memorial Cancer Center and Institute of Oncology. Regional Silesia Cancer Registry, Cancer Epidemiology Department, Gliwice 2009.

[4] Juszko-Piekut M, Kołosza Z, Moździerz A, Stojko J, Olczyk D: Incidence of melanoma malignum and non-melanoma cancer of the skin in male inhabitants of Silesian Voivodeship (including two subregions of diverse UV exposure) in 1999-2003. Polish J. Environ. Stud. 2006; 15, (2B):1175-1181.

[5] Juszko-Piekut M, Kołosza Z, Moździerz A, Zenła B, Stojko J, Morawiec T: Nonmelanoma skin cancer incidence in the inhabitants of the Bielsko-Biala subregion of the Silesian Voivodeship. Polish J. Environ. Stud. 2007; 16, (5C):206-209.

[6] Juszko-Piekut M, Kołosza Z, Moździerz A, Zemła BFP: Incidence of non-melanoma skin cancer in the population of the Silesian Voivodeship (including industrial subregions central and Rybnicko-Jastrzębski) in the years 1999-2005. (Zachorowalność na nieczerniakowate nowotwory złośliwe skóry populacji przemysłowych podregionów województwa śląskiego (region centralny i rybnicko jastrzębski) w latach 1999-2005). Medycyna Środowiskowa 2007; 10,2:46-53.

[7] Juszko-Piekut M, Kołosza Z, Moździerz A, Zemła BFP, Stojko J: The incidence of malignant nonmelanoma skin cancer In the inhabitants of the silesian voivodeship. Family Medicine& Primary Care Review 2008, 10,4:1286-1289.

[8] Moździerz A, Juszko-Piekut M, Kołosza Z, Stojko J, Olczyk D, Morawiec T: Comparative study of certain pollutant concentrations in the former Katowice voivodeship (1991-1998 and 1983-1990). Polish J. Environ. Stud. 2007; 16,5C Pt.2: 399-404.

[9] Jensen OM, Parkin DM, MacLennan R, Muir CS, Skeet RG: Cancer Registration: Principles and methods. IARC Scientific Publications No. 95 Lyon, France 1991.

[10] Curado MP, Edwards B., Shin HR, Storm H, Ferlay J, Heanue M, Boyle P: Cancer Incidence in Five Continents 2007, Vol. IX IARC Scientific Publications No 160, Lyon, IARC.

[11] Grande F: Epidemiology of cutaneous melanoma: descriptive data in France and Europe. Ann. Dermatol. Venereol. 2005, 132:975-82.

[12] Nørgaard C, Glud M, Gniadecki R: Are all melanomas dangerous? Acta Derm. Venereol. 2011,91(5):499-503.

[13] Erickson C, Driscoll MS: Melanoma epidemic: Facts and controversies. Clin. Dermatol. 2010; 28(3):281-6.

[14] Hollestein LM, van den Akker SA, Nijsten T, Karin-Kos HE, Coebergh JW, de Vries E: Trends of cutaneous melanoma in The Netherlands: increasing incidence rates among all Breslow thickness categories and rising mortality rates since 1989. Ann. Oncol. 2012; 23(2):524-30.

[15] Barbarić J, Znaor A: Incidence and mortality trends of melanoma in Croatia. Croat. Med. J. 2012; 53(2):135-40.

[16] American Cancer Society. Cancer Facts and Figures 2011. Available at: http://www.cancer.org/Research/CancerFactsFigures/CancerFactsFigures/cancer-facts-figures-2011

[17] Juszko-Piekut M, Kołosza Z, Moździerz A: Epidemiological analysis of cutaneous malignant melanoma incidence in the population of Upper Silesia. Polish J. Environ. Stud. 2004; 13, suppl II:181-187.

[18] Didkowska I, Wojciechowska U, Zatoński W: Cancer In Poland In 2009. (Nowotwory złośliwe w Polsce w 2009.), Maria Skłodowska-Curie Memorial Cancer Center, De-

partment od Epidemiology and Cancer Prevention, Polish National Cancer Registry, Warszawa 2011.

[19] Didkowska I, Wojciechowska U, Zatoński W: Prediction of cancer incidence and mortality In Poland up to the year 2025. (Prognozy zachorowalności i umieralności na nowotwory złośliwe w Polsce do 2025 roku.), Maria Skłodowska-Curie Memorial Cancer Center, Department od Epidemiology and Cancer Prevention, Polish National Cancer Registry, Warszawa 2009.

[20] Kołosza Z, Banasik TR, Zemła BFP: Cancer in the Silesia Voivodeship in 2003. (Nowotwory złośliwe w województwie śląskim w 2003 roku). Maria Skłodowska-Curie Memorial Cancer Center and Institute of Oncology. Regional Silesia Cancer Registry, Cancer Epidemiology Department, Gliwice 2006.

[21] Juszko-Piekut M, Moździerz A, Kolosza Z, Olczyk D, Zemła BFP, Stojko J: Incidence of cutaneous malignant melanoma in the population of Upper Silesia in the years 1999–2003 Hygiene and environmental determinants of health. (Higieniczno-środowiskowe uwarunkowania zdrowia) / Red.: I. Jackowska, M. Iskra, A. Borzęcki, K. Sztanke. Lublin, Department of Hygiene, Medical University of Lublin, 2012 (Katedra i Zakład Higieny Uniwersytetu Medycznego w Lublinie, 2012)*(work in print).*

[22] Leiter U, Garbe C: Epidemiology of melanoma and nonmelanoma skin cancer – the role of sunlight. Adv. Exp. Med. Biol. 2008; 624,89-103.

[23] Diepgen TL, Mahler V: The epidemiology of skin cancer. Br. J. Dermatol. 2002; 146,61:1-6.

[24] Levi F, Te VC, Randimbison L, La Vecchia C: Trends in incidence of various morphologies of malignant melanoma in Vaud and Neuchatel, Switzerland. Melanoma Res. 2005;15:73–5.

[25] Krzyścin JW, Jarosławski J, Sobolewski P: On an improvement of UV index forecast: UV index diagnosis and forecast for Belsk, Poland, in Spring/Summer 1999. J. Atmosfheric Solar Terresrial Physics 2001; 63:1593-1600.

[26] Braun-Falco O, Plewig G, Wolff HH, Burgdorf W: Dermatologia. Tom II. Gliński W, Wolska H, Zaborowski P. red. wyd. pol. Wydawnictwo Czelej, Lublin 2004.

[27] Zak-Prelich M, Narbutt J, Sysa-Jędrzejowska A: Environmental Risc Factors Predisponing to the Development of Basal Cell Carcinoma. Dermatologic Surgery 2004; 30,2,(2):248-252.

[28] Adami J, Gabel H, Lindelof B, Ekstrom K, Rydh B, Glimelius B, Ekbom A, Adami HO, Granath F: Cancer risk fallowing organ transplantation: a nationwide cohort study in Sweden. Br J Cancer 2003; 89(7):1221-1227.

[29] Ping XL, Ratner D, Zhang H, Wu XL, Zhang MJ, Chen FF, Silvers DN, Peacocke M, Tsou HC: PTCH mutations in squamous cell carcinoma of the skin. J. Invest. Dermatol. 2001; 116:614-6.

[30] Ling G, Ahmadian A, Persson A, Undén AB, Afink G, Williams C, Uhlén M, Toftgård R, Lundeberg J, Pontén F: PATCHED and *p53* gene alterations in sporadic and hereditary basal cell cancer. Oncogene 2001; 20:7770-8.

[31] Fabbrocini G, Triassi M, Mauriello MC, Torre G, Annunziata MC, De Vita V, Pastore F, D'Arco V, Monfrecola G: Epidemiology of skin cancer: Role of some environmental factors. Cancers 2010; 2:1980-1989.

[32] Shirley SH, Grimm EA, Kusewitt DF: Ultraviolet radiation and the slug transcription factor induce proinflammatory and immunomodulatory mediator expression in melanocytes. Journal of Skin Cancer, 2012; Article ID 410925.

[33] Holick MF: Vitamin D deficiency. N. Engl. J. Med. 2007; 357:266-281.

[34] Athas WF, Hunt WC, Key CR: Changes in nonmelanoma skin cancer incidence between 1977-1978 and 1998-1999 in Northcentral New Mexick. Cancer Epidemiol. Biomarkers Prev. 2003; 12(10):1105-1108.

[35] Nestor MS: The incidence of nonmelanoma skin cancer and actinic keratoses in South Florida. J. Clin. Aesthet. Dermatol. 2012; 5(4):20-24.

[36] Salmon PJ, Chan, WC, Griffin J McKenzie R, Rademaker M: Extremely high levels of melanoma In Tauranaga, New Zealand: Possible causes and comparisons with Australia and the northern hemisphere. Australes J. Dermatol. 2007; 48,208-216.

[37] Van der Leun JC, Piacentini RD, de Gruijl FR: Climate change and human skin cancer. Photochem. Photobiol. Sci. 2008; 7,730-733.

[38] Correa MP, Dubuisson P, Plana-Fattori A: An overview of the ultraviolet index and the skin cancer cases in Brazil. Photochemistry and Photobiology 2003; 78,(1):49-54.

[39] Jemal A, Thomas A, Murray T, Thun M: Cancer statistics. 2002. CA Cancer J. Clin. 2002; 52:23-47.

[40] Lewis E.C, Mayer JA, Slymen D: Postal workers' occupational and leisure-time sun safety behaviors (United States). Cancer Causes&Control, 2006; 17, 2,181

[41] Karagas MR, Stukel TA, Morris JS, Tosteson TD: Skin cancer risk in relation to toenail arsenic concentrations in US population-based case-control study. AJE 2001; 153, 6: 559-565.

[42] IARC Working Group on the Evaluation of carcinogenic risk to humans. Some drinking-water disinfectants and contaminats, including arsenic. IARC Monogr. Eval. Carcinog. Risk Hum. 2004;84,269-477.

[43] Pesch B, Unfried K, Jakubis P, Jakubis M: Risk Factors for nonmelanoma skin cancer in Previdza district, Slovakia. Przegląd Epidemiologiczny 2002; 56: 281-294.

[44] Beane Freeman BLE, Dennis LK, Lynch ChF, Thorne PS, Just CL: Toenail arsenic content and coetaneous melanoma in Iowa. Am. J .Epidemiol. 2004;160:679-687.

[45] Chouhan S, Flora SJ: Arsenic and fluoride: two major ground water pollutants. Indian J. Exp. Biol. 2010; 48,666-678.

[46] Yu HS, Liao WT, Chain CY: Arsenic carcinogenesis In the skin. J. Biomed. Sci. 2006; 13, 657-666.

[47] Chang YM, Barrett JH, Bishop DT, Armstrong BK, Bataille V, Bergman W, et al.: Sun exposure and melanoma risk at different latitudes: a pooled analysis of 5700 cases and 7216 controls. Int. J. Epidemiol. 2009;38:814–30.

[48] Bataille V, Winnett A, Sasieni P, Swerdlow A, Newton Bishop JA, Cuzick J: Exposure to the Sun and sunbeds and the risk of cutaneous melanoma in the UK: a case-control study. Eur. J. Cancer. 2004; 40:429-435.

[49] Maguire-Eisen M, Rothman K, Demierre MF: The ABCs of Sun Protection for Children. Dermatology Nursing 2005; 17, 6:419-433.

[50] Trzmiel DA, Wyględowska–Kania ME, Lis AD, Pierzchała EK, Brzezińska–Wcisło LA: Contemporary views on the treatment of melanoma. (Współczesne spojrzenia na leczenie czerniaka złośliwego) Wiad. Lek. 2002; LV, 9-10:608-615.

[51] Lazovich DA, Sweeny C, Weinstock MA, Berwick M: A prospective study of pigmentation, sun exposure, and risk of cutaneous malignant melanoma in women. J Natl. Cancer Inst. 2004; 96(4):335-339.

[52] Brewster AM, Alberg AJ, Strickland PT, Hoffman SC, Helzlsouer K: XPD polymorphism and risk of subsequent cancer in individuals with nonmelanoma skin cancer. Cancer Epidemiol. Biomarkers Prev. 2004 13,(8).

[53] World Health Organization; Available at: http://www.who.int/en/

[54] Egan KM, Sosman JA, Blot WJ: Sunlight and reduced risk of cancer: Is the real story vitamin D? J. Natl. Cancer Inst. 2005; 97(3):161-163.

[55] Tangpricha V, Pearce EN, Chen TC, Holick MF: Vitamin D insufficiency among free-living healthy young adults. Am. J. M. 2002; 112(8):659-662.

[56] Devesa SS, Grauman DJ, Blot WJ, Pennello GA, Hoover RN, Fraumeni JFl: Atlas of cancer mortality in the United States: 1950 to 1994. Washington, DC: US Govt Print Off; 1999 [NIH Publ No. (NIH) 99-4564].

[57] Garland FC, Garland CF, Gorham ED, Young JF: Geographic variation in breast cancer mortality in the United States: a hypothesis involving exposure to solar radiation. Prev. Med. 1990; 19(6):14-22.

[58] Dennis LK, Beane Freeman LE, VanBeek MJ: Sunscreen use and the risk for melanoma: a quantitative review. Ann. Intern. Med. 2003; 139(12):966-978.

[59] Słoma-Kuczyńska J, Bilski B: Primary prevention in wolkers exposed to ultrafiolet radiation and radiation-related risk. (Profilaktyka pierwszorzędowa u pracowników

narażonych na promieniowanie nadfioletowe pochodzenia słonecznego oraz ryzyko związane z tym czynnikiem) Med. Pracy 2004; 55(3):283-287.

[60] Zemła BFP, Kołosza Z, Banasik TR: Atlas zachorowalności i umieralności na nowotwory złośliwe w obrębie województwa katowickiego w latach 1985-1993. Maria Skłodowska-Curie Memorial Cancer Center and Institute of Oncology. Regional Silesia Cancer Registry, Cancer Epidemiology Department, Gliwice 1999.

[61] Berwick M, Amstrong BK, Ben-Porat L, Fine J, Kricker A, Eberle C, Barnhill R: Sun exposure and mortality from melanoma. J. Natl. Cancer Inst. 2005, 97(3):195-199.

[62] Le Marchand L, Saltzman BS, Hankin JH, Wilkens LR, Franke AA, Morris SJ, Kolonel LN: Sun exposure, diet, and melanoma In Hawaii Caucasians. Am. J. Epidemiol. 2006; 164:232-245.

[63] Weber RS, Geoffrey LR, Garden AS et al.: Aggressive basal and squamous cell skin cancer of the head and neck. In: Head and neck cancer. A multi-disciplinary approach. Harrison LB, Sessions RB, Hong Wki. Lippincott-Raven Publ. Philadelphia 1999;669-704.

[64] Wathkinson JC, Gaze MN, Wilson JA: Tumors of the skin and ear. In: Stell and Maran's head and neck surgery. Butterworth-Heinemann. Oxford 200; 409-440.

[65] Available at: http://www.sunsmart.com.au/news_and_media/media_campaigns/a_history_of_sunsmart_media_campaigns

[66] Lunn S: Sun worshippers need a slap of reality. The Australian. Available at: http://www.cancer.org.au/cancersmartlifestyle/SunSmart/Campaignsandevents/SlipSlopSlapSeekSlide.htm

[67] Yoder L.H. Be sun safe! Understand skin cancer prevention and detection. Medsurg Nursing. 14,4,254-256, 2005.

Chapter 2

Serum Markers in Clinical Management of Malignant Melanoma

Pierre Vereecken

Additional information is available at the end of the chapter

http://dx.doi.org/10.5772/55530

1. Introduction

The incidence of cutaneous malignant melanoma (CMM) is increasing in the Western world, despite the implementation of prevention campaigns for several years. Early detection, targeted at-risk populations helps to identify patients with beginning melanoma lesions, but despite these efforts, many patients - often young,- present with thicker tumors (with a higher Breslow, over 1mm - Breslow is a measurement in mm of the vertical thickness of the primary tumor-). [1]

A late diagnosis is also often associated with a greater Breslow thickness index and a greater risk for invasion of regional lymph nodes (stage III), or distant metastatic lesions (stage IV) [2]. CMM usually progresses from an in situ proliferation in a radial growth pattern. Then appears the vertical growth phase which is a major event for the dissemination of cells, as it allows cells to migrate deeper into the dermis, the lymphatic vessels and blood flow.

In the seventh revision of the American Joint Committee on Cancer (AJCC) staging for melanoma (2009), patients can be divided into four stages: stage I and II disease (local) stage III (locoregional disease) and stage IV (metastatic disease). In this ranking, the only serum marker that was built for clinical use is the lactate dehydrogenase (LDH) as the serum LDH was confirmed in multivariate analysis to be an independent predictor even after taking into account site and number of metastases [2]. The value of LDH is still often discussed in local/ locoregional conditions.

Surgery is the mainstay of treatment of melanoma. The major concern after diagnostic excision of the primary lesion is whether CMM has already metastasized or not. Indeed many arguments emphasize that early detection of melanoma metastases may improve the prognosis of

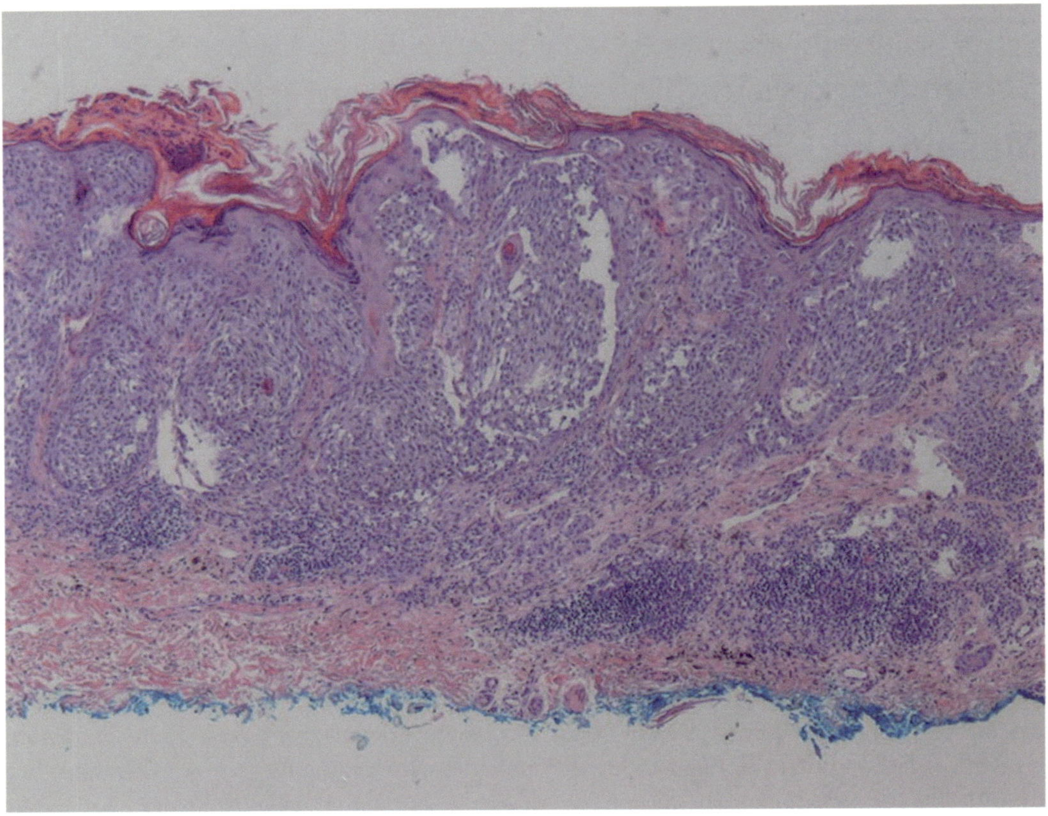

Figure 1. Breslow index measures in mm the thickness of the lesion

patients, at least for some of them. To date, no marker for early detection of melanoma metastases is unanimously recognized.

A melanoma patient around high risk (high risk of recurrence) can be defined as a patient with a 50% risk of relapse within up to 10 years, despite optimal initial surgical treatment. These high-risk patients should be carefully monitored and treated if possible with adjuvant therapeutic strategies. Interferon-α and, more recently, ipilimumab have been proposed as adjuvant therapies, but their effect on survival is still a matter of debate. To date, no predictive marker of response has been described.

The metastatic process involves the spread of cancer cells in locoregional or distant anatomic sites via the lymphatics and / or blood flow. In the case of melanoma, circulating cells can find a suitable microenvironment in the sentinel node (the first lymph drainage lymph node area), other lymph nodes or distant organs (lymph nodes, liver, lungs, brain, bone).

In fact, the understanding of the biology and mechanism of metastatic cascade provides new molecular targets and can help us to discover new biomarkers. Biomarkers can be divided into diagnostic markers for disease detection and prognostic and predictive markers, which should predict response to treatment. Cancer biomarkers consist of many molecular structures such as proteins, peptides, DNA, mRNA. Interest is the fact that these markers can be found in the tissues, cells and / or body fluids. Also viable melanoma cells can also be found in the peripheral blood of melanoma patients. We limit ourselves in this article to the description of serum molecular markers in CMM.

The ideal biomarker should be a molecule easily detectable in the serum of a patient who presents a growing tumor. The biomarker should have a sufficient sensitivity and specificity to minimize false negatives and false positives. Sensitivity refers to the proportion of patients with confirmed disease who have a positive test for a biomarker, whereas specificity can be defined as the proportion of healthy individuals with a negative test. Previous studies have shown that many molecules that may be involved in oncogenesis and cancer spread can be found in the serum of cancer patients in particular patients with melanoma, but their sensitivity and / or specificity are still debatable. These molecules can be produced and secreted or excreted into the bloodstream directly by melanoma cells or indirectly by destruction of melanoma cells by chemotherapy, immunotherapy or combination therapy [3].

Below, we detail the most important molecules in serum that have been described as a biomarker for CMM.

2. Main serum markers in CMM

2.1. Lactate Dehydrogenase (LDH)

As mentioned above, this enzyme has been considered as the main serum prognostic parameter in patients with metastatic melanoma (AJCC stages III and IV). Numerous studies have validated LDH as the factor most predictive of patient outcome, and this independently and statistically significant. This led to a stratification of the AJCC :patients with metastatic melanoma with high levels of LDH are designated as M1c whatever the site of metastasis [2].

Note, however, that Hamberg stated that in a series of 53 patients with stage IV AJCC melanoma only 38% had elevated LDH, suggesting that elevated LDH is not the ideal marker for this condition [4]. Moreover, in a multivariate analysis of 64 patients with AJCC stage IV melanoma Hauschild has failed to demonstrate the independent prognostic value of LDH [5]. It should be recalled that the LDH assay can be falsely positive due to hemolysis and other factors, including hepatitis.

However, Weide et al also insist in a study of 855 patients on the prognostic value of LDH [6].

2.2. C-Reactive Protein (CRP)

CRP is a nonspecific inflammatory parameter that may have a role in the detection of melanoma progression. This protein is produced by hepatocytes as acute phase response of nonspecific inflammatory processes.

Elevated serum CRP was associated with a poor prognosis in various cancers. Deichmann et al. analyzed the prognostic significance of CRP compared to the LDH patients AJCC stage IV

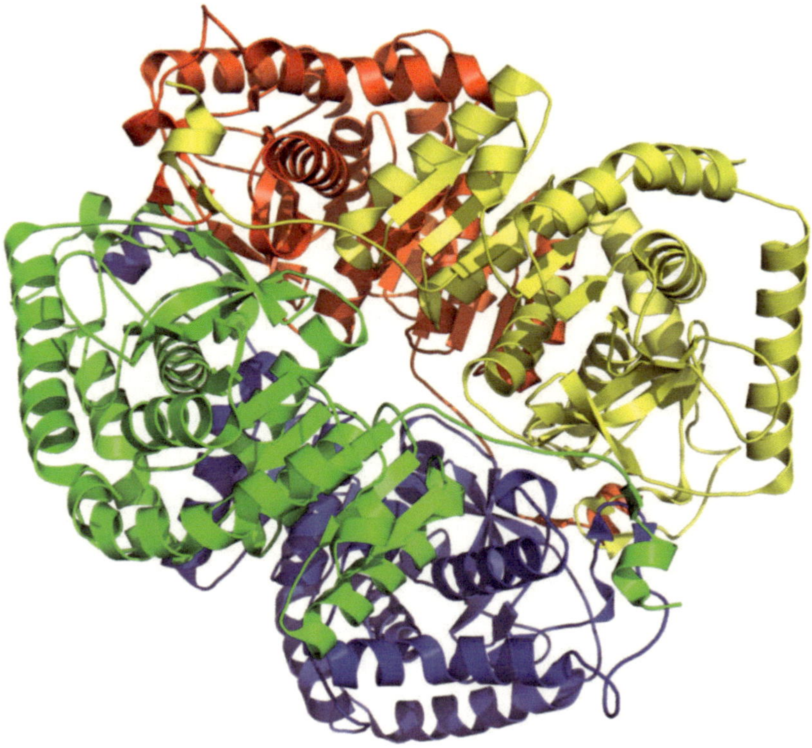

Figure 2. LDH is a tetrameric enzymle and consists of several sub-units M and H, encoded by two different genes (Chromosome 11 and 12)

melanoma. With a definition of a threshold 3mg/dL, the identification of a stage IV can be done with a sensitivity of 76.9% and a specificity of 90.4%. In another prospective study of 67 patients, Deichmann found that CRP was the only prognostic factor even reliable [7-9]. These results are debated.

2.3. S100-β proteins (S100B)

Serum S100B is described as more related to the tumor burden and thus reflects both the clinical stage and tumor progression (the higher the rate of serum S100B, the greater the tumor burden). It may therefore be used to monitor the effectiveness of therapy whatever the type of treatment (surgical, chemotherapy, immunotherapy). Retsas et al. have suggested the use of S100B instead of LDH in the classification system of the AJCC while other authors consider that S100B has no added value when comparing the sensitivity and specificity of the CRP and LDH [10]. For some, S100B has probably become the most useful marker in clinical practice, but it interest seems to be limited to advanced stages III and IV [11]. In stages I and II S100B provides no independent prognostic information.

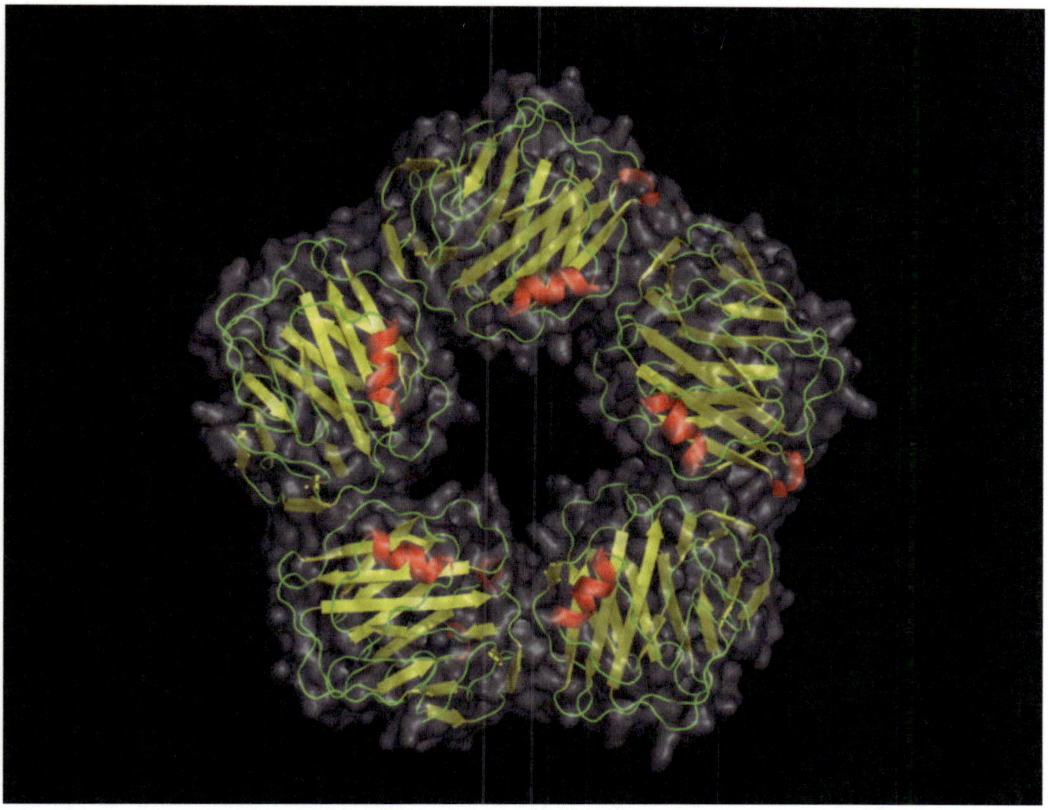

Figure 3. Molecular structure of CRP, five sub-units each comprising 206 amino acids. The gene responsible for its synthesis is located on chromosome 1.

Moreover, it must be remembered that S100B is not specific to melanoma and its serum levels may be elevated in healthy subjects, patients with cancer of non-melanoma skin, neurological disorders, tumors of the nervous system central, and even in various gastrointestinal cancers, and patients infected with HIV.

2.4. Melanoma Inhibiting Activity (MIA)

The roles of this protein are multiple among them modulation of cell growth and cell adhesion. MIA rates are higher in the group of patients relapsing after initial surgery. Some authors consider that the sensitivity of the two molecules S100B and MIA is equal. For other authors, MIA is superior to LDH and CRP. In children and pregnant women (after week 38), MIA is increased and serum levels should be avoided in these two groups [12].

2.5. Galectin-3

Gal-3 has been described to be overexpressed in malignant melanocytic lesions and its concentration in the serum of patients with melanoma is increased by the joint action of

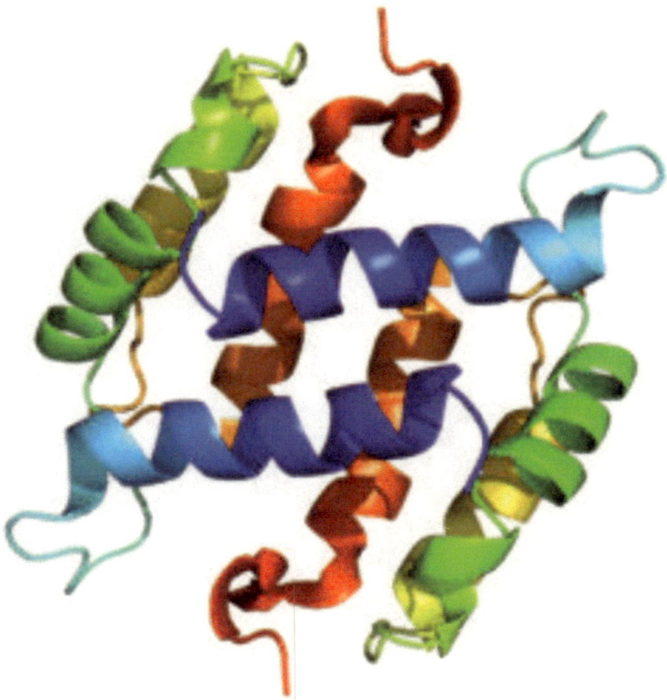

Figure 4. S100B is a 21-kD dimeric protein, consists of two β subunits. This protein is a member of a family of 19 protein and was first isolated from bovine brain in the mid sixties. S100B is expressed by glial cells and melanocytes and is produced by brain tumors and melanomas. The roles of S100B are probably multiple and underestimated.

melanoma cells and inflammatory cells. Gal-3 plays an important role in cell proliferation, cell differentiation, cell adhesion, cell migration, angiogenesis and metastasis. Thus, Gal-3 deserves special attention. Clarification of the role of extracellular Gal-3 should help us to understand the significance of elevated serum levels of this molecule in patients with advanced melanoma [13].

3. Other molecules and molecular approaches

3.1. Melanoma Associated Antigens (MAA)

Malignant transformation of melanocytes is associated to changes in gene definition. This leads to the expression of melanoma associated antigens molecules called (MAA), which are more or less specifically associated with the malignant phenotype (Table 1). In fact sometimes these MAA can also be expressed in normal melanocytes. MAA play an important role in triggering the immune response agains melanoma cells. These antigens were mainly identified by immunological approaches, including in vitro and in vivo reactions and serological tests. These antigens can be defined by their ability to interact with T cells or B and peptides derived from

http://dx.doi.org/10.5772/55530

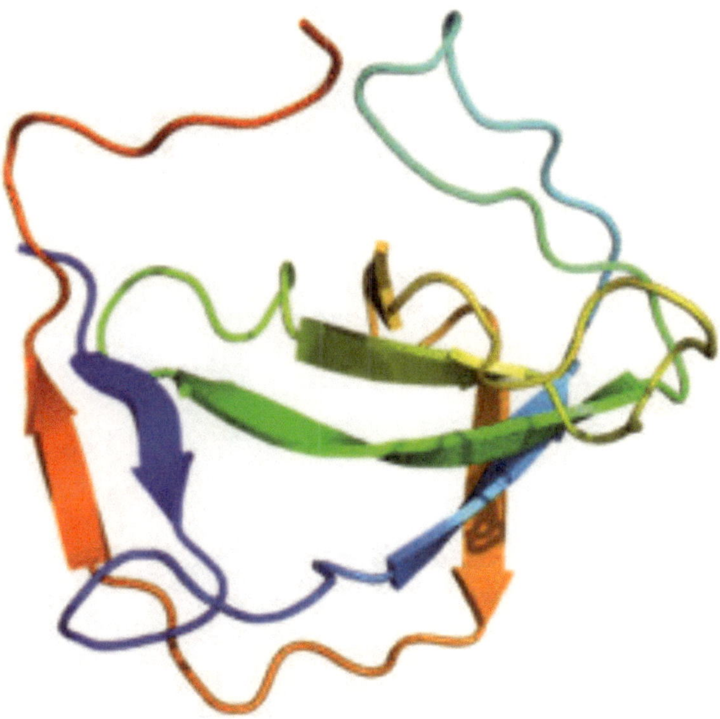

Figure 5. MIA is a 12kDa soluble protein, whose role has been characterized as an inhibitor of cell autocrine growth. It can be expressed by melanoma cells and chondrocytes.

these antigens have been used to induce or maintain a specific immune response. Mage-1 was the first identified MAA and now belongs to a large family of at least 12 antigens differentially expressed by benign and malignant melanocytic cells. Immune responses to these genes can be used as markers of progression and / or immunological response.

Tyrosinase RT-PCR detection in patients with melanoma is correlated with a higher risk of relapse (55% of these patients have a clinical relapse), but the specificity of this technique has yet to be optimized [15, 16]. When combined with a dosage of S-100, Domingo-Domenech showed that tyrosinase RT-PCR adds valuable prognostic information in patients with S-100 <0.15μg / l, although the team showed that S-100 had a higher predictive value. Curry et al. suggested that RT-PCR detection of tyrosinase can be useful to determine a subgroup of patients with an increased risk of metastases [17].

Profiling of autoantibodies associated with certain MAA was different by Sabel et al as potentially useful to select patients with melanoma who should benefit from the research of a sentinel node.

These results have yet to be validated [18].

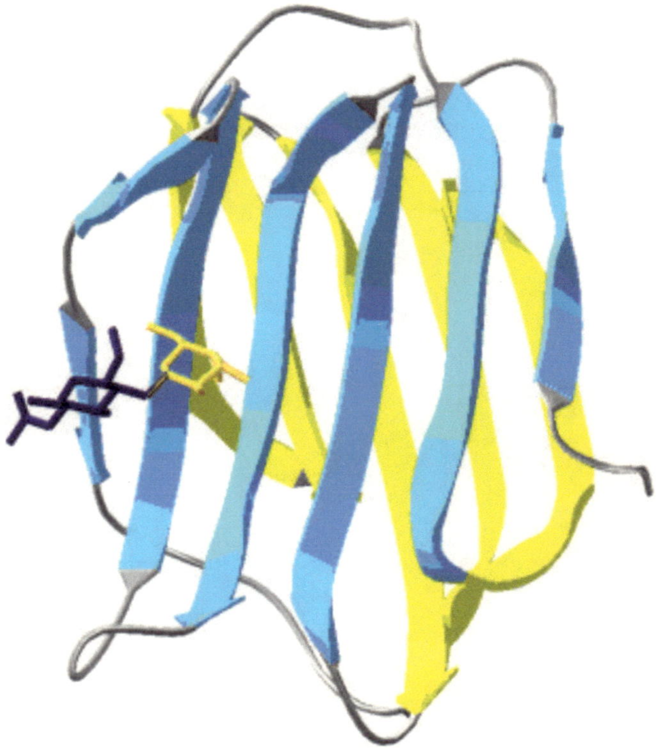

Figure 6. Galectin-3 is a member of the family of lectins that can bind to β-galactoside residues. Many members of the galectin family are differentially expressed in cancer. Gal-3 is a molecule that contains an NH2-terminal domain, a COOH-terminal domain.

3.2. Melanine metabolites

5-S-cysteinyl dopa (5SCD) is a precursor of phaeomelanin and is produced by melanocytes and melanoma cells, as a product of the binding of a molecule named dopaquinone and highly reactive with cysteine. 5SCD is detectable in the urine and serum of melanoma patients and correlates with disease progression. In patients with progressive disease, the level of 5SCD can rise before the onset of clinical signs. A comparative report stated that with the LDH and S100B, 5SCD has an interesting value even if the authors of this report concluded that S100B could be considered as the most sensitive of the three markers. Due to the effect of UV exposure on melanin, the use of this 5SCD as a biomarker may be limited in Caucasians, whereas its use in other populations, particularly in Japan, would be more reliable. In addition, patients with metastatic but non-pigmented melanoma lesions do not usually have elevated serum 5SCD. 3,4-dihydroxyphenylalanine (L-DOPA) is the first metabolite involved in melanogenesis and its plasma levels were also correlated with melanoma progression and tumor burden, as well as the ratio of plasma L-dopa / L tyrosine-which represents an index of the activity of tyrosinase and tyrosine hydroxylase. Stoitchkov et al. showed that the latter ratio has predictive value, especially in patients with stage III, and advocated the use of multiple biomarkers [19].

http://dx.doi.org/10.5772/55530

Antigen	HLA restriction
Oncospermatogonal antigens	
MAGE-A1	A*01, A*03, A*24, A*28, B*3701, B*53, Cw*0201, Cw*0301, Cw*1601
MAGE-A2	A*0201, B*3701
MAGE-A3	A*01, A*02, A*2402, B*3701, B*44, DR*11
MAGE-4	A*0201
MAGE-A6	A*3402, B*3701
MAGE-A10	A*0201
MAGE-A12	A*0201
MAGE-B1	A*0201
MAGE-B2	A*0201
BAGE	Cw*1601
GAGE-1	Cw*6
LAGE-1	A*0201
PRAME	A*24
NY-ESO-1	A*02, A*31
DAM-6	A*02
Melanocytic differentiation antigens	
Tyrosinase	A*01, A*0201, A*2402, B*44, DRβ1*0401
MART-1/Melan-A	A*0201, A*02, B*4501
Gp100	A*0201, A*03, A*0301, A*1101, A*2402, C*0802, DRβ1*0401
TRP-1	A*31
TRP-2	A*31, A*33, A*0201, C*0802, A*68011
MC1R	A*0201
Mutated antigens	
MUM-1	B*44
CDK4	A*02
B-catenin	A*24
P15	A*24
GnT-V	A*02
TPI	DRβ1*0101
Annexin II	DRβ1*0401
CDC27	DRβ1*0401
Oncogene-derived antigens	
HER2/Neu	A*0201

Table 1. Melanoma associated antigens (adapté de Visser et al. [14]).

3.3. Matrix Metalloproteinases (MMP)

MMPs are a family of 24 structurally related endopeptidases. These zinc-dependent enzymes are defined by their own substrates and can lyse components of the extracellular matrix (ECM) (eg, collagen type IV, which is a major component of the basement membrane by gelatinases such as MMP-2 and MMP-9) and play a role in angiogenesis and the renewal of the ECM. MMPs can also cleave different molecules such as other proteinases, proteinase inhibitors, growth factors, adhesion molecules and thereby modulate the inflammatory response, the process of tumor growth, tumor invasion and metastasis.

A balance between MMPs and tissue inhibitors of metalloproteinases (TIMP) can be broken by upregulation of MMP and TIMP downregulation, this is shown in malignant phenotype.

Another important role, angiogenesis, has been attributed to MMP, which could allow a therapeutic target possible. Batimastat (BB-94, a synthetic broad-spectrum inhibitor of metalloproteinases), for example, has shown efficacy for inhibiting angiogenesis of liver metastases in a mouse model.

MMP overexpression has been reported in melanoma progression, and elevated serum MMP, ie MMP-1 and MMP-3, have been correlated with poor survival [20].

3.4. Cytokins, chimiokins and their réceptors [21]

Chemokines are small polypeptides signaling can bind to and activate G protein-coupled receptors, a family of seven transmembrane molecules. Multiple roles have been attributed to these chemokines, and are involved in tumor transformation and metastatic process. The differential expression of these chemokines and their receptors may explain the organ specificity of metastases.

Melanoma cells expressing the chemokine CXCL8, also known as interleukin-8 (IL-8) have been described and a report showed that serum levels of IL-8 are associated with tumor burden and a poor prognosis. This track is interesting and could be exploited for therapeutic purposes. In vivo studies have indeed shown that anti-IL8 humanized antibodies are able to reduce tumor growth and angiogenesis.

A recent study of 29 serum cytokines assayed simultaneously in 179 melanoma patients (versus 378 control individuals, healthy) showed a profile of specific serum cytokines in patients compared to controls: higher serum concentrations of interleukin (IL)-1alpha, IL-1beta, IL-6, IL-8, IL-12p40, IL-13, G-CSF, MCP-1, MIP-1alpha, MIP-1 beta, IFN-alpha, TNF-alpha, EGF, VEGF and TNF receptor II. [22, 23, 24].

3.5. Growth and angiogenic factors

Angiogenesis is an important step in tumor growth as it ensures the supply of oxygen and substrates to tumor cells. This process is in fact the result of complex interactions between pro-angiogenic factors and anti-angiogenic released by tumor cells, endothelial, epithelial, mesothelial cells and leukocytes. Vascular Endothelial Growth Factor (VEGF) has been described as a potent mitogen for endothelial cells and its expression, which can be increased in hypoxic conditions, was also correlated with tumor progression and poor prognosis.

Different VEGF have been described, but none has been reported as an independent prognostic factor. At most a few studies have correlated the presence / absence of certain molecules in very specific situations, eg serum VEGF-C is decreased in patients with metastatic cutaneous metastases [25].

An imbalance in the ratio of serum angiopoietin 1 and angiopoietin 2 than could, according et al Gardizi sign a metastatic progression. [26]

3.6. Cell surface and adhesion molecules

3.6.1. Integrins

Integrins are cell components that ensure adhesion to other cells, ECM, or other proteins. Other important roles are played by integrins such as the transmission of information between the extra-and intracellular space, and angiogenesis.

Integrins are heterodimeric receptors consisting of two subunits α and β,. On the basis of their common subunit, heterodimers can be classified αv, β1 β2 integrins. The main integrins involved in the progression of melanoma include avß3 (vitronectin receptor and fibronectin), α2β1 (collagen), α4β1 (fibronectin) and α6β1 (laminin).

Some reports have shown that increased serum concentrations of β integrins were associated with shorter survival. The clinical impact of this has not yet been defined.

3.6.2. CD44

CD44 is a transmembrane glycoprotein surface, originally described as a lymphocyte receptor. CD44 is a cell surface receptor for hyaluronic acid, While some studies have highlighted its role in tumor invasion and metastasis, it is clear that no study has identified a prognostic value for serum CD44.

3.6.3. ICAM-1

ICAM-1 is a new intercellular adhesion molecule, located in the cell membranes of leukocytes and endothelial cells. ICAM-1 is a ligand of LFA-1 (lymphocyte function-associated antigen-1) in T cells, B cells, macrophages, and neutrophils. Leukocyte migration is facilitated by the binding ICAM-1/LFA-1. One study showed that serum ICAM-1 is increased in patients with metastatic but has no independent prognostic value in multivariate analysis [27].

3.7. Others

Ever, new publications emerge with new molecular perspectives (protein profiling, micro-RNAs dosage,...).

Luo et al showed in well constructed paper that isoenzymes of aldehyde dehydrogenase 1A (ALDH) appear as stem cell markers of melanoma, but their presence in serum and their prognostic significance has yet to be defined [28].

Adhesion molecule type 1 related to carcinoembryonic antigen (CEACAM 1) has also recently been shown as a promising biomarker by an Israeli team: measuring the serum in a retrospective study is correlated with metastatic progression and survival patients with melanoma [29].

The utility of serum DNA of mutated BRAF gene has also recently been presented as a prognostic factor and predictor of response to biochetherapies. This would probably be very useful for patients treated with vemurafenib. These results need to be confirmed [30].

4. Discussion

Cancer is a major cause of morbidity and mortality in our society. It shows a huge price and has many devastating effects. Melanoma is a tragic example of these realities.

The prognosis of melanoma is closely linked to early diagnosis. Current treatments have limited effectiveness, and surgery remains the mainstay of treatment. Better treatments are certainly necessary, even with the arrival of molecules such as ipilimumab or vemurafenib that enable new perspectives for our patients with metastatic disease.

In the past, the only prognostic factor in melanoma patients has been limited to histology (tumor thickness) and the location of the primary tumor. These parameters are important, but were supplemented by numerous clinical variables, pathological and biological, particularly in patients with advanced melanoma. Recently, the use of serum markers, alone or in combination, has been proposed to refine the prognosis of a patient in order to ensure proper tracking and predicting the potential benefits of therapy. More specific or nonspecific markers of melanoma can be measured in the serum of patients, and in most cases, these markers are directly correlated with the tumor mass.

Among these biomarkers, LDH and S100B serum biomarkers appear with an independent prognostic value, although disputed by some. In advanced melanoma, their dosage is probably more accurate and sensitive than CRP levels (LDH and CRP are obviously more accessible and measured) as shown by some studies, but not ideal. Even if the LDH is incorporated into the new AJCC classification, for some authors, S100B is superior in terms of prognostic value [31].

To a lesser extent due to poor sensitivity or lower specificity, CRP, MIA, and Gal-3 can also be considered as interesting biomarkers. The dosages of new other molecules should be included in future prospective clinical protocols, distinguishing their prognostic value (patient outcome) and predictive value (response to treatment).

Storage conditions of serum should also be made clear in all the articles as they have a major influence on results and therefore conclusions. This suggests that a standard methodology should be set in order to compare the published studies [32].

http://dx.doi.org/10.5772/55530

Research into new biomarkers in melanoma is important issue because i twill lead to better understand the biology of this tumor, and thus it improve patient monitoring, early detection and treatment of secondary lesions and open new perspectives for targeted therapies. Multiple molecular changes of melanoma progression are currently intensively studied.

Author details

Pierre Vereecken*

Address all correspondence to: dr.vereecken@dermatologist.be

CLIDERM (Clinics in Dermatology), European Insititute for Dermatology Practice and Research (EIDPR), CHIREC et CHIREC CANCER INSTITUTE, Brussels, Belgium

References

[1] Garbe, C, Peris, K, Hauschild, A, Saiag, P, Middleton, M, Spatz, A, Grob, J. J, Malhevy, J, Newton-bishop, J, Stratigos, A, Pehamberger, H, & Eggermont, A. M. Diagnosis and treatment of melanoma. European consensus-based interdisciplinary guideline-Update 2012. Eur J Cancer (2012). , 48(15), 2375-90.

[2] Balch, C. M, Gershenwald, J. E, Soong, S. J, Thompson, J. F, Atkins, M. B, Byrd, D. R, Buzaid, A. C, Cochran, A. J, Coit, D. G, Ding, S, Eggermont, A. M, Flaherty, K. T, Gimotty, P. A, Kirkwood, J. M, Mcmasters, K. M, Mihm, M. C, Morton, D. L, Ross, M. I, Sober, A. J, & Sondak, V. K. Final version of (2009). AJCC melanoma staging and c lassification. J Clin Onclo 2009 ; , 27(36), 6199-206.

[3] Palmer, S. R, Erickson, L. A, Ichetovkin, I, Knauer, D. J, & Markovic, S. N. Circulating serologic and molecular biomarkers in malignant melanoma. Mayo Clin Proc (2011). , 86(10), 981-90.

[4] Hamberg, A. P, & Korse, C. M. Bonfrer JMG, De Gast GC. Serum S100B is suitable for prediction and monitoring of response to chemoimmunotherapy in metastatic malignant melanoma. *Melanoma Research*. (2003). PubMed], 13(1), 45-49.

[5] Hauschild, A, Michaelsen, J, Brenner, W, et al. Prognostic significance of serum S100B detection compared with routine blood parameters in advanced metastatic melanoma patients. *Melanoma Research*. (1999). PubMed], 9(2), 155-161.

[6] Weide, B, Elsässer, M, Büttner, P, Pflugfelder, A, Leiter, U, Eigentler, T. K, Bauer, J, Witte, M, Meier, F, & Garbe, C. Serum Markers lactate dehydrogenase and S100B predict independently disease outcome in melanoma patients with distant metastasis. Br J Cancer (2012). , 107(3), 422-8.

[7] Deichmann, M, Benner, A, Kuner, N, Wacker, J, Waldmann, V, & Näher, H. Are responses to therapy of metastasized malignant melanoma reflected by decreasing serum values of S100β or melanoma inhibitory activity (MIA)? *Melanoma Research.* (2001). PubMed], 11(3), 291-296.

[8] Deichmann, M, Benner, A, Bock, M, et al. S100-beta, melanoma-inhibiting activity, and lactate dehydrogenase discriminate progressive from nonprogressive American joint committee on cancer stage IV melanoma. *Journal of Clinical Oncology.* (1999). PubMed], 17(6), 1891-1896.

[9] Deichmann, M, Kahle, B, Moser, K, Wacker, J, & Wüst, K. Diagnosing melanoma patients entering American joint committee on cancer stage IV, C-reactive protein in serum is superior to lactate dehydrogenase. *British Journal of Cancer.* (2004). PMC free article] [PubMed], 91(4), 699-702.

[10] Retsas, S, Henry, K, & Mohammed, M. Q. MacRae K. Prognostic factors of cutaneous melanoma and a new staging system proposed by the American Joint Committee on Cancer (AJCC): validation in a cohort of 1284 patients. *European Journal of Cancer.* (2002). PubMed], 38(4), 511-516.

[11] Kruijff, S, & Hoekstra, H. J. The current status of S100-B as a biomarker in melanoma. Eur J Surg Oncol (2012). , 38(4), 281-5.

[12] Bosserhoff, A. K, Küster, H, & Hein, R. Elevated MIA levels in the serum of pregnant women and of children. *Clinical and Experimental Dermatology.* (2004). PubMed], 29(6), 628-629.

[13] Vereecken, P, Awada, A, Suciu, S, Castro, G, Morandini, R, Litinska, A, Lienard, D, Ezzedine, K, Ghanem, G, & Heenen, M. Evaluation of the prognostic significance of serum Galectin-3 in American Joint Committee on Cancer Stage III and stage IV melanoma patients. Melanoma Res (2009). , 19(5), 316-20.

[14] Visser, M, Velders, M. P, Rudolf, M. P, & Kast, W. M. Molecular characterization of melanoma-derived antigens. In: Nickoloff BJ, editor. *Melanoma: Methods and Protocols.* 1st edition. Totowa, NJ, USA: Humana; (2001). Methods in Molecular Medicine)., 61

[15] Sonesson, B, Eide, S, Ringborg, U, Rorsman, H, & Rosengren, E. Tyrosinase activity in the serum of patients with malignant melanoma. *Melanoma Research.* (1995). PubMed], 5(2), 113-116.

[16] Tsao, H, Nadiminti, U, Sober, A. J, & Bigby, M. A meta-analysis of reverse transcriptase-polymerase chain reaction for tyrosinase mRNA as a marker for circulating tumor cells in cutaneous melanoma. *Archives of Dermatology.* (2001). PubMed], 137(3), 325-330.

[17] Curry, B. J, Myers, K, & Hersey, P. MART-1 is expressed less frequently on circulating melanoma cells in patients who develop distant compared with locoregional metastases. *Journal of Clinical Oncology.* (1999). PubMed], 17(8), 2562-2571.

[18] Sabel, M. S, Liu, Y, Griffith, K. A, He, J, Xie, X, & Lubman, D. M. Clinical utility of serum autoatntibodies detected by protein microarray in melanoma. Int J Proteomics (2011).

[19] Stoitchkov, K, Letellier, S, Garnier, J. P, Bousquet, B, Tsankov, N, Morel, P, & Ghanem, G. Le Bricon T. Evaluation of the serum L-dopa/L-tyrosine ratio as a melanoma marker. Melanoma Res (2003). , 13(6), 587-93.

[20] Nikkola, J, Vihinen, P, Vuoristo, M. S, Kellokumpu-lehtinen, P, Kähäri, V. M, & Pyrhönen, S. High serum levels of matrix metalloproteinase-9 and matrix metalloproteinase-1 are associated with rapid progression in patients with metastatic melanoma. Clin Cancer Res (2005). , 11(14), 5158-66.

[21] Neagu, M. The immune system- a hidden treasure for biomarker discovery in cutaneous melanoma. Adv Clin Chem (2012). , 89-140.

[22] Yurkovetsky, Z. R, Kirkwood, J. M, Edington, H. D, et al. Multiplex analysis of serum cytokines in melanoma patients treated with interferon-alpha2b. *Clinical Cancer Research*. (2007). PubMed], 13(8), 2422-2428.

[23] Boyano, M. D, Garcia-vazquez, M. D, Lopez-michelena, T, et al. Soluble interleukin-2 receptor, intercellular adhesion molecule-1 and interleukin-10 serum levels in patients with melanoma. *British Journal of Cancer*. (2000). PMC free article] [PubMed], 83(7), 847-852.

[24] Vuoristo, M. S, Laine, S, Huhtala, H, et al. Serum adhesion molecules and interleukin-2 receptor as markers of tumour load and prognosis in advanced cutaneous melanoma. *European Journal of Cancer*. (2001). PubMed], 37(13), 1629-1634.

[25] Vihinen, P. P, Hilli, J, Vuoristo, M. S, Syrjänen, K. J, Kähäri, V. M, & Pyrhönen, S. O. Serum VEGF-C is associated with metastatic site in patients with malignant melanoma. *Acta Oncologica*. (2007). PubMed], 46(5), 678-684.

[26] Gardizi, M, Kurschat, C, Riese, A, Hahn, M, Krieg, T, Mauch, C, & Kurschat, P. A decreased ratio between serum levels of the antagonistic angiopoietins 1 and 2 indicates tumour progression of malignant melanoma. Arch Dermatol Res (2012). , 304(5), 397-400.

[27] Hasegawa, M, Takata, M, Hatta, N, Wakamatsu, K, Ito, S, & Takehara, K. Simultaneous measurement of serum 5-S-cysteinyldopa, circulating intercellular adhesion molecule-1 and soluble interleukin-2 receptor levels in Japanese patients with malignant melanoma. *Melanoma Research*. (1997). PubMed], 7(3), 243-251.

[28] Luo, Y, Dallaglio, K, Chen, Y, Robinson, W. A, Robinson, S. E, Mc Carter, M. D, Wang, J, Gonzalez, R, Thompson, D. C, Norris, D. A, Roop, D. R, Vasiliou, V, & Fujita, M. ALDHA1 isoenzymes are markers of human melanoma stem cells and potential therapeutic targets. Stem Cells (2012). , 2100-13.

[29] Sapoznik, S, Faranseh, S, Ortenberg, R, Hamburger, T, Barak, V, Peretz, T, Schachter, J, Markel, G, & Lotern, M. Serum CEACAM-1 correlates with disease progression and survival in malignant melanoma patients. Clin Dev Immunol (2012).

[30] Shinozaki, M, Day, O, Kitago, S. J, Amersi, M, Kuo, F, Kim, C, & Wang, J. HJ, Hoon DSB. Utility of circulating B-RAF DNA mutation in serum for monitoring melanoma patients receiving biochemotherapy. Clin Cancer Res (2007). , 13(7), 2068-74.

[31] Bouwhuis, M. G, Suciu, S, Kruit, W, Sales, F, Stoitchkov, K, Patel, P, Cocuyt, V, Thomas, J, Liénard, D, Eggermont, A. M, & Ghanem, G. Prognostic value of serial blood S100B dterminations in stage IIB-III melanoma patients : a corollary study for the EORTC trial 18952. Eur J Cancer (2011). , 47(3), 361-8.

[32] Butterfield, L. H, Potter, D. M, & Kirkwood, J. M. Multiplex serum biomarkers assessments : technical and biostatistical issues. J Transl Med (2011). Oct 11 ; 9 : 173.

Chapter 3

An Overview of Important Genetic Aspects in Melanoma

Rohinton S. Tarapore

Additional information is available at the end of the chapter

http://dx.doi.org/10.5772/55257

1. Introduction

Cancer of the skin is the most common form of malignancy in humans and is divided into two categories – non-malignant skin cancer and cutaneous melanoma. Non-melanoma skin cancer (basal cell and small cell carcinoma) make up a vast majority of skin cancers. According to data from National Cancer Institute (NCI) in 2012, more than 2 million new cases of non-melanomas will be identified with less than a 1000 deaths. Despite according for only 4% of all cases, melanoma is the deadliest of skin cancers resulting in over 79% of skin cancer deaths [1]. In the United States, melanoma is the fifth most common cancer in men and the sixth most common in women. In 2011, 70,230 new melanoma cases were identified with 8,790 deaths. The median age of diagnosis is between 45-55; although 25% of melanomas occur in individuals over 40 years.

2. Types of skin cancer

a. Basal Cell Carcinoma (BCC): This is the most common form of skin cancer and accounts for more than 90% of all skin cancers in the United States. BCC causes damage by growing and invading the surrounding tissue and usually does not metastasize to other parts of the body. Intermittent sun exposure (especially early in life), age and light colored skin are important factors in the development of BCC. Approximately a fifth of BCCs, develop in regions that are not sun-exposed such as chest, arms, neck, back and scalp [2]. Weakening of the immune system on account of the disease or immune-suppressive drugs is known to promote the risk of developing BCCs. Usually BCC begins as a small, dome-shaped bump and is covered by small superficial blood vessels called telangiectases and its texture is often shiny and translucent. Hereditary predisposition to BCC [3,4] occurs among individuals with albinism and Xeroderma Pigmentosum. These disorders can be linked to either instability of the skin or diminished pigmentation.

b. Squamous Cell Carcinoma (SCC): This cancer begins in the squamous cells that form the surface of the skin, lining of hollow organs of the respiratory and digestive tracts. The earliest form of SCC is called as actinic keratosis (AK) [2] that appear as rough, red bumps on the scalp, face, ears and back of the hands. The rate at which the bumps (keratosis) invade deeper in the skin to become fully developed squamous cell carcinoma is estimated to be 10-20% over a 10 year period. Actinic keratinosis that becomes thicker and more tender could increase the possibility of getting transformed to an invasive squamous cell carcinoma phenotype. The most important risk factor is sun exposure. Lesions appear after years of sun damage in the forehead, cheeks as well as the backs of hands. Other minor factors like exposure to hydrocarbons, arsenic, heat or X-rays could predispose to SCCs. Unlike BCC, SCCs can metastasize to other parts but are easy to treat.

c. Melanoma: This is the cancer of the melanocytes, the "skin-color producing cells" of the body. An estimated 132,000 new cases of melanoma occur worldwide every year [5,6,7] with approximately 65,161 deaths according to estimates from the World Health Organization (WHO). The high mortality rate of melanoma is remarkably high considering the fact that melanoma is nearly always curable in its early stages; the high mortality rate can be attributed to late diagnosis in which the cancer spreads to other parts of the body [5]. Melanoma incidence has increased more rapidly than that of any other cancer, yet our ability to treat disseminated disease has been lagging [8,9,10]. The predicted 1 year survival for Stage IV melanoma ranges between 41% to 59% [11]. At a very early point in the progression of melanoma, the cancer gains metastatic potential.

3. Risk factors

There are multiple risk factors that contribute to escalating incidence of melanomas in humans (Table 1). Ultraviolet (UV) radiation especially UVA (315-400 nm) and UVB (280-315 nm) from sunlight is an important contributing factor for melanoma progression. A study by Glanz et al [5,12] revealed that 90% of all melanomas are attributed to exposure to ultraviolet radiation.

The damaging effects of UV radiation (UVR) is on account of direct cellular damage and alterations in immunologic functions. UVR causes DNA damage (by formation of pyrimidine dimers), gene mutations, oxidative stress, immunosuppressive and inflammatory responses. All these effects play an important role in photoaging of the skin and predispose to skin cancer [13]. UVR creates mutations in p53, a key tumor suppressor gene that plays an important role in DNA repair and apoptosis. Thus if p53 is mutated, the cells lose the DNA repair process leading to the deregulation of apoptosis, expression of mutated keratinocytes and initiation of skin cancer [13,14]. Darker skinned individuals have lower incidence of cutaneous melanoma primarily as a result of increased epidermal melanin. Studies indicate that epidermal melanin in African-American individuals filters twice as much UVB radiation than in Caucasians. This

http://dx.doi.org/10.5772/55257

is on account of the larger, more melanized melanosomes located in the epidermis of dark skin individuals that absorb and scatter more light energy than the smaller, less melanized melanosomes of white skin. The incidence rate of skin cancer (both melanoma and non-melanoma) has increased significantly in the last decade [15]; particularly among young women. For most individuals, exposure to UVR from the sun is the main source of skin cancer. Nonetheless, some individuals are exposed to high UV doses through artificial sources – sunbeds and sunlamps used for tanning purposes. Indoor tanning is widespread in most developed countries in Northern Europe, Australia and the United States [16]. Intense early sunburns and blistering sunburns are closely associated with melanoma development [17,18, 19]. Statistics indicate that one severe childhood sunburn is associated with a two-fold increase in melanoma risk [20]. Chronic UV exposure results in increased skin aging, wrinkles, uneven skin pigmentation, loss of elasticity and a distribution in the skin barrier function [21]. Chronic UVR exposure is an important risk factor in the development of actinic keratosis (precursor of SCCs).

Ultraviolet (UV radiation)
UVA
UVB
Genetic syndromes
Xeroderma pigmentosum
Oculocutaneous albinism
Basal cell nevus syndrome
Ionizing radiation
X-rays
Other risk factors
Artificial UV radiation (tanning)
Smoking
Color of skin (having fair skin, especially with blue or hazel eyes)
History of precursor lesions
Chronically injured or non-healing wounds
Working outdoors
Increasing age

Table 1. Risk factors for skin cancer [1-8]

Candidate Gene	Protein	Location on chromosome	Stage of melanoma	References
Gene losses *PTEN*	Pten	10q	Primary & metastatic	[135,136,137]
CDKN2A	p16Ink4a/p14Arf	9p	Primary & metastatic	[135,136]
ITGB3BP	Beta-3-endonexin	1p31	Uveal	[138]
Gene amplification *BRAF*	Braf	7q21.3	Cutaneous	[135]
CCND1	cyclinD1	11q13	Acral	[136]
CDK4	cdk4	12q14	Acral & mucosal	[136]
CDH2	N-cadherin	18q	Uveal & metastatic	[137,139]
c-MYC	c-myc	8q23	Ocular, primary & metastatic	[135,137,140,141]
MITF	Mitf	3p14	Cutaneous, metastatic	[142,143]

Table 2. Chromosomal aberrations involving important genes found in melanoma

4. Roadway to melanoma

Malignant melanomas arise from epidermal melanocytes or the melanocyte precursor cell which are derived from the neural crest and migrate to the skin and hair follicles [22]. Melanoma initiation and progression is accompanied by a series of histological changes. The five distinct changes are: 1) nevus – benign lesion characterized by an increased number of nested melanocytes; 2) dysplastic nevus – which is characterized by random, discontinuous and atypical melanocytes; 3) radial-growth phase (RGP) melanoma where the cells acquire the ability to proliferate intraepidermally; 4) vertical growth phase (VGP) melanoma – characterized by melanoma cells acquiring the ability to penetrate through the basement membrane (BM) into underlying dermis and subcutaneous tissue; and 5) metastatic melanoma – characterized by the spread of melanoma cells to other areas of the skin and other organs. The most critical event in melanoma progression is the RGP-VGP transition which involves the escape from keratinocyte mediated growth control. This is consistent with tumor thickness being a strong predictor of metastatic disease and adverse clinical outcome [23].

Gene	Protein	Function	Commentary	References
Up-regulation *ATM*	ATM kinase	Cell cycle control, DNA damage response	Melanocytic infiltration	[135,136,137]
CDH2	N-cadherin	Cell-cell adhesion	Melanoma invasiveness	[144,145]
MMP-1, 2	Metallo proteinases -1, 2	Degradation of ECM	Tumor progression	[146]
SPP1	Osteopontin	Inductor of MMP	Risk of metastasis	[144,147]
SPARC	Osteonectin	Angiogenesis	Tumor progression	[144]
WNT5A	Wnt5a	Cell signaling	Melanoma invasiveness	[125,148]
CKS2	Cdc28/cdk1 protein kinase subunit 2	Cell cycle control	Poor prognosis	[147]
EIF2gamma	EIF2γ	DNA translation	Tumor progression	[149]
PCNA	PCNA	Cofactor DNA polymerase	Genome destabilization	[150]
Down Regulation *CDH1*	E-cadherin	Cell-cell adhesion	Tumor progression	[144,145,147]
CDH3	P-cadherin	Cell-cell adhesion	Tumor progression	[145,151]
CDH10	Cadherin-10	Cell-cell adhesion	High risk of metastasis	[144]
DSC1	Desmocollin-1	Desmosomal component	Loss of cell adhesion	[137,139,179]

Table 3. Genetic expression signatures associated with the progression of melanomas [24]

Acquisition of somatic mutations in key regulatory genes is the driving force behind the initiation and progression of melanoma development. For the past few decades numerous research teams around the world have researched on melanoma genetics leading to an overwhelming body of information.

5. Susceptibility genes

Approximately 8-12% of all melanomas are familial – occurring in individuals with a history of familial melanoma [24]. Two genes have been found to be associated with high penetrance susceptibility – CDKN2A and CDK4. Using linkage analysis of families with high melanoma incidences, the first melanoma incidence susceptibility gene, CDK2N2A was identified at chromosome 9p21 [25,26]. The gene CDKN2A encodes two unrelated proteins – $p16^{Ink4A}$ and $p14^{Arf}$. These proteins are tumor suppressors involved in cell cycle regulation. Numerous studies indicate that $p16^{Ink4A}$ inhibits G1 cyclin dependent kinase (cdk4/cdkb) mediated phosphorylation of retinoblastoma protein (pRB) resulting in cell cycle progression arrest through G1-S; while p14 favors apoptosis and blocks oncogenic transformation by stabilizing p53 levels through the inhibition of Mdm2-mediated p53 ubiquitination [27,28,29,30]. Loss of p16 promotes hyper-phosphorylation of pRb resulting in its inactivation while the loss of p14 inactivates p53 — leading to unrestricted cell cycle progression. Germline mutations in CDKN2A have been found in 40% of families with 3 or more family members affected by melanoma [31]. Not all individuals carrying germline CDKN2A mutations develop mutations. Individuals with large numbers of pigment lesions or nevi have familial atypical mole-melanoma syndrome (FAMS) are associated with increased risk to developing melanoma [32,33].

The other melanoma susceptibility gene, CDK4 is located at chromosome 12q14 [34,35,36]. Mutations in CDK4 abrogate binding of cdk4 to p16 have been associated with melanoma pathogenesis [32]. This is evidence that links the entire p16^{Ink4A}-cdk4/cdk6-pRb pathway to melanoma indicating that hereditary retinoblastoma patients with germline inactivation of retinoblastoma (Rb1) are predisposed to melanoma [37,38].

6. Acquired genetic alterations in melanoma

Understanding the regulating pathways involved in melanoma development and progression has advanced significantly in recent years. The discovery of genetic alterations that aids in the formation of various cancers has aided in the development of numerous molecularly targeted therapies for individuals with metastatic disease [39,40,41]. These genes are known to be key molecular driver in melanoma; >70% cases harbor activating mutations in these genes. The molecule that is most commonly found to be mutated in melanomas is BRAF (~50% of all cancers) followed by NRAS (20%) and c-kit (1%) [42,43,44]. Melanoma is the result of complex changes in multiple signaling pathways affecting growth, cell mobility, metabolism and the ability to escape cell death progression. The Ras-Raf-Mek-Erk pathway followed by PI3K/Akt pathway is constitutively activated in a significant number of melanoma tumors.

7. The Ras-Raf-Mek-Erk

In 2002, a breakthrough study found that Braf to be mutated in a large percentage of melanomas – triggering new studies that focus on MAPK (mitogen activated protein kinase) signaling in melanomas. Braf is mutated in upto 82% of cutaneous nevi [45,46], 66% of primary melanomas [44] and 40-68% of metastatic melanomas [47,48]. A specific mutation substitution of valine with glutamic acid at residue 600 (BRAF V600E), account for 90% + BRAF mutation. Raf, a downstream effector of RAS is a serine-threonine specific protein kinase that activates Mek, which inturn activates Erk. Humans have 3 Raf genes: A-raf, B-raf and C-raf. The occurrence of mutation in Nras or Braf is 80-90% of all melanomas suggests that constitutive activation of extracellular signal regulated protein kinase (Ras-Raf-Mek-Erk). Most Ras mutations are present in codon 61 of N-Ras with K-Ras and H-

Ras mutations being relatively rare [49,50]. Constitutive activation of Ras-Raf-Mek-Erk cascade has been shown to contribute to tumorigenesis by inhibiting apoptosis and increasing cell proliferation, tumor invasion and metastasis. Activated Erk plays a pivotal role in cell proliferation by controlling the G1- to S-phase transition by negative regulation of p27 inhibition and upregulation of c-myc activity [51,52]. Inhibition of Erk activity is associated with G1 cell cycle arrest by upregulation of p21 and reduced phosphorylation [52]. Activated Erk is also known to stimulate cell proliferation by increasing the transcription and stability of c-Jun which is mediated by CREB (cyclic adenosine monophosphate responsive element-binding) and Gsk-3β (glycogen synthase kinase-3beta) respectively [53]. Erk is also believed to increase proliferation by inhibiting differentiation. Constitutively active Erk limits differentiation in melanoma by targeting MITF (microphthalmia-associated transcription factor) for degradation [54,55,56]. The activated Erk pathway enhances melanoma specific survival by differentially regulating RSK-mediated phosphorylation and inactivation of the pro-apoptotic protein Bad [57] and inhibiting Jak-Stat pathway [58].

Erk signaling also contributes towards tumor invasion and metastasis by regulating the expression of integrin and matrix metalloproteinases (MMPs). Activated Ras-Mek-Erk pathway drives the production of MMP1 [59,60,61].

8. The PI3K/Akt pathway

The PI3K/Akt pathway is activated in various cancers, mostly on accont of mutations in tumor suppressor PTEN (phosphatase and tensin homolog) [62]. In melanoma, los of PTEN on chromosome 10q 23-24 was first reported by Parmiter et al [63]. The PTEN gene encodes a phosphatase that degrades products of PI3K by dephosphorylating phosphatidylinositol 3,4,5-triphosphate and phosphatidylinositol 3,4-biphosphate at 3 positions [64]. Loss of PTEN increases AKT phosphorylation and activity leading to increased mitogenic signaling and decreased apoptosis [65]. Various studies suggest that 30-40% of melanoma cell lines and 5-15% of uncultured melanoma specimens carry inactivating mutations or homozygous deletions of Pten [63,66,67].

Pten encodes a negative regulator of extracellular growth signals that are transcended via PI3K-Akt pathway. Akt/protein kinase B (PKB), a serine-threonine kinase, is a core component of the PI3K signaling cascade and is activated through the phosphorylation of Ser 473/474 and Thr 308/309 [68,69]. Activated Akt regulates a network of factors that control cell proliferation and survival and this pathway is hyperactive in most metastatic melanomas [70,71,72]. Akt activates the transcription of a wide variety of genes involved in a wide range of cellular activities – those involved in immune activation, cell proliferation, apoptosis and cell survival [69]. Several studies have documented Akt activation in melanoma. Dai et al undertook a 292 sample study of pAkt levels using tissue microarray & immunohistochemistry strategies and identified strong pAkt expression in 17%, 43%, 49% and 77% of the biopsies in normal nevi, dysplastic nevi, primary melanoma and melanoma metastasis respectively. An important cell adhesion protein MelCAM that plays critical roles in melanoma development was increased upon active Akt expression [73,74]. PI3K and Akt is known to increase the expression of MMP2 and MMP9 by a mechanism involving Akt activation of NF-kappaB binding to the MMP promoter [75,76]. Akt overexpression led to upregulation of VEGF, increased production of superoxide ROS. Akt can suppress apoptosis by phosphorylating and inactivating many proapoptotic proteins like caspase 9 and Bad [77,78]. PI3K pathway emerges as the central axis that is deregulated in melanoma and along with constitutively active MAPK pathway makes an important role in melanoma development progression. Thus targeting PI3K is expected to be an important therapeutic target modality for melanoma treatment.

9. Wnt/β-catenin pathway

Beta-catenin (β-catenin) is a key component of the Wnt signaling pathway. Signaling through this pathway controls a wide range of cellular functions and aberrant Wnt/β-catenin signaling can lead to cancer development and progression [79]. Wnts are glycoproteins that act as ligands to stimulate receptor-mediated signal transduction pathways involved in cell survival, proliferation, behavior and fate. Wnt proteins are known to activate 3 different extracellular pathways – Wnt/β-catenin, Wnt/planar-polarity and Wnt/Ca^{2+} pathways [80]. The Wnt/β-catenin also known as the canonical Wnt pathway plays an important role in melanoma development. In the absence of Wnt ligands, free β-catenin binds to the destructive complex of Axin, adenomatous polyposis coli (APC) and glycogen synthase kinase-3β (GSK-3β). GSK-3β mediates the phosphorylation of β-catenin at specific regulatory sites on the N-terminal side marking β-catenin for ubiquitination and subsequent proteosomal degradation. Upon the binding of Wnt ligand, GSK--catenin for ubiquitination and subsequent proteosomal degradation. Upon the binding of Wnt ligand, GSK-3β activity is inhibited resulting in accumulation of β-catenin in the cytoplasm and shuttles into the nucleus where it serves as an essential co-activator of the Tcf/Lef (T-cell factor / lymphoid enhancer factor) family [81]. Numerous genes implicated in the tumorigenic process like c-myc and cyclinD1 have been identified as targets of the canonical Wnt signaling.

Increased nuclear localization of β-catenin – an important indication of activated Wnt signaling pathway is observed in over a third of melanoma specimens [82,83,84]. Mutations in β-catenin have been observed in about 23% of melanoma cancer cell lines and these mutations affect phosphorylation sites at Ser33, Ser37, Thr41 and Ser45 [85] at the N-terminal domain. These mutations render β-catenin resistant to phosphorylation and subsequent degradation. Low rates of β-catenin mutation have been observed in primary melanomas and metastasis indicating that activating mutations is a rare event in melanoma tumorigenesis [82,83,84,86,87,88]. Mutations in APC were observed sporadically in primary melanomas [82, 85,88]. While APC promoter 1A hypermethylation was observed in 17% of melanoma biopsies and 13% of melanoma cell lines. Wnt signaling pathways is activated in tumors through aberration in other genes. ICAT (inhibition of β-catenin & T-cell factor), a gene that negatively regulates the association of β-catenin with TCF4 thus repressing the transactivation of β-catenin-Tcf4 target genes [89]. A study by Reifenberger J et al suggests that loss of ICAT expression may contribute to the progression of melanoma [86]. ICAT mRNA expression analysis in two-third melanoma specimens revealed a 20% or less decrease in ICAT transcription [86]. However the mechanism behind the reduced ICAT mRNA level in melanoma is unclear.

Identification of Wnt target genes is also important towards the study of melanoma progression. Brn1, the POU domain transcription factor is directly controlled by Wnt signaling in transgenic mouse models and melanoma cell lines [90]. Studies indicate that overexpression of Brn2 is associated with increased melanoma progression and tumorigenicity [90,91].MITF (microphthalmia-associated transcription factor), a Wnt target gene, is essential for the development of the melanocyte lineage and has an important role in the control of cell proliferation, survival and differentiation [54,92,93]. The regulation of MITF expression by β-catenin significantly influences the growth and survival behavior of treatment resistant melanoma [94]. A study by Schepsky A et al demonstrated that MITF can directly interact with β-catenin and redirect transcriptional activity away from canonical Wnt signaling-regulated target gene specific for MITF [95]. Induction of Wnt signaling can be blocked by 5 different proteins – Dkk, Wise, sFrp (secreted Frizzled related protein), Wif (wnt inhibitory factor), and Cerebrus that compete for the Wnt ligand or the Lrz-Frp receptor [96]. Interestingly, Dkk1 (Dickkopf 1) expression is negligible in melanomas [97]. Studies by Kuphal et al have demonstrated a downregulated or loss of Dkk-1, -2 and-3 in all melanoma cell lines and most of the melanoma tumor samples that were analyzed [98]. In xenograft mouse model, overexpression of Dkk-1 and Wif-1inhibited melanoma tissue growth [99,100].

10. The JNK/c-Jun pathway

Activation of Jnks is usually in response to diverse stresses. These kinases play an important role in the regulation of cell proliferation, cell survival, cell death, DNA repair and metabolism. A variety of extracellular stimuli by cytokines, growth factors, hormones, UV radiation and tumor promoters are known to activate Jnks [101]. Sequential protein phorphorylation through a MAP-kinase module (MAP3K-MAP2K-MAPK) is responsible for Jnk activation [102]. Depending upon the cellular context, Jnk has been shown to elicit both positive and negative effects on tumor development [103]. Activation of Jnk is required for Ras-mediated transformation and mediate proliferation and tumor growth [104,105]. These observations are consistent with the findings of constitutively active Jnk in tumor samples and cell lines [103,106]. Jnk mediated the phosphorylation at serine 63 & 73 residues enhancing the ability of transcription factor c-Jun, a component of the AP-1 transcription complex [107]. The activation of Jnk leas to the induction of AP-1 dependent target genes that play important roles in cell proliferation, cell death and inflammation. Other members of the AP-1 transcription complex include c-Jun, Jun B, Jun D, c-Fos, Fra1 and Fra 2. The role of Jnk in oncogenesis is emerging; however c-Jun is a well defined oncogene in cancer. c-Jun is amplified and overexpressed in undifferentiated and aggressive sarcomas [108], breast and lung cancer [109,110]. Since the 1990s, the role of Jnk pathway in melanomas was recognized [111,112]. c-Jun, Jun B, c-fos genes play a role in the transformation of melanocytes into malignant melanomas [111].

The possible role Jnk pathway has led research teams to study the clinical relevance of interfering with this pathway. siRNA or chemical inhibitors of Jnk signaling inhibited proliferation in breast and non-small cell lung cancer (NSCLC) [106,113] and also induced apoptosis in prostate cancer cells [114]. A study by Gurzov E et al demonstrated that knock-down of c-Jun and Jun B in B16F10 melanoma cells by siRNA resulted in increased cell cycle arrest and apoptosis also resulting in extended survival of mice inoculated with these modified melanoma cells[115], suggesting that inactivation of c-Jun and Jun B could provide a valuable strategy for antitumor intervention [115].

11. The NFκB (NF-kappaB) pathway

The NFκB family in mammals contains 5 members – p105/p50 (NFκB1), p100/p52 (NFκB2), RelA (p65), RelB and c-Rel (J-206, 207). The canonical activation of NFκB pathway involves TNFα stimulation resulting in the subsequent phosphorylation/activation of IKK (IκB kinase). In turn, IKK-mediated phosphorylation of IκB leading to ubiquitination of IκB and its proteosomal degradation, releasing the NFκB complex which activates a host of target genes [116,117]. The type of genes that get trans-activated depends on the composition of activated NFκB complex. For instance, complexes containing c-Rel activates pro-apoptotic genes (Dr4/Dr5, Bcl-x) and inhibits anti-apoptotic genes (cellular inhibitor of apoptosis (cIAP1, cIAP2), survivin). Complexes containing RelA inhibits the expression of DR4/DR5 and upregulates caspase 8, cIAP1 and cIAP2 [118].

NFκB is activated in various tumors including melanomas and distinct mechanisms have been proposed for the elevated levels of NFκB activity in melanomas. Activation of NFκB in melanomas is also linked to the loss of E-cadherin, a frequent event in melanoma transformation [119]. NIK (NFκB interacting kinase), an activator of IKK is overexpressed in melanoma cells while compared to normal cells. The major contribution of NFκB in melanoma development and progression relates to its function as an important regulator of survival and apoptosis. A study by Meyskens at al demonstrated that in metastatic melanoma cells, an increase in DNA binding activity of NFκB is associated with an increased expression of p50 and RelA resulting in increased expression of anti-apoptotic regulators. Also the expression of c-Rel, the transcriptional activator of pro-apoptotic genes is markedly in melanoma cells compared with normal melanocytes [120]. Strong p50 nuclear staining also correlated with poor prognosis in melanoma patients [121]. Besides eliciting anti-apoptotic activities NFκB mediates the transcription of MMP2 and MMP9 [121,122]. Overexpression of MMPs is associated with tumor invasion, metastasis and angiogenesis.

12. Melanoma stem cells

Stem cells are cells that can self-renew and the ability to differentiate into various cell lineages. These cells are located in the restrictive niche (environment). The interaction between stem cells and their microenvironment is important for the self renewal process. These cells are highly clonogenic and slow cycling (quiescent) in response to proliferation and survival stimuli. Stem cells divide asymmetrically giving rise to a daughter cell that remains a stem cell (capable of self renewal) and another daughter cell that can rapidly divide and differentiate. Melanocytes that are found in the skin and in the choroid layer of the eye is derived from the neural crest (NC). Neural crest cells undergo EMT to migrate along the definite pathways in the embryo. NC cells give rise to a large array of differentiated cells – melanocytes, peripheral neurons & glia, endocrine and cartilage cells [123]. Melanoblasts which are melanocytic precursors – unpigmented cells with the potential to produce melanin, invade the skin areas and differentiate into melanocytes.

The cancer stem theory suggests that cancer originates from a small subpopulation of neoplastic stem cells that have the potential to self renew and are primarily responsible for sustaining the tumor and giving rise to progressively differentiating cells that proliferate rapidly and contribute to the cellular heterogeneity of the tumor (F-194). Cancer stem cells arise either from undifferentiated stem cells or from cells that possess stem cell like characteristics. Evidence suggests that aggressive melanoma cells acquire characteristics of embryonic stem cells having a multipotent plastic phenotype [124]. Studies by Bittner MP et al demonstrated that melanoma cells express genes associated with different cell types like endothelial, epithelial, fibroblastic, neuronal, hematopoietic and progenitor cells [125]. Strangely genes specific for melanocytes are downregulated in metastatic melanomas. Tyrosinase & MLANA (melan A), genes associated with pigmentation are greatly downregulated in aggressive melanomas [124]. Aggressive melanoma cells express endothelial-associated genes and form extravascular fluid-conducting networks which allow melanomas to greatly adapt to the hypoxic microenvironment of rapidly proliferating tumors, a phenomenon called as "vascular mimicry" [124,126]. From different melanoma cell lines, cells with stem cell-like features which have the ability to grow as non-adherent cell aggregates known as spheroids/spheres have been isolated (F-196). These cells have the ability to differentiate into various lineages – adipogenic, osteogenic, chondrogenic and melanogenic. A study by Bittner M et al demonstrated a subset of these spheroid cells express the cell surface marker CD20, a unique molecular signature of aggressive melanomas [125]. For the treatment of non-Hodkin's lymphoma, CD20 is a standard therapeutic target which raises the possibility that CD20 could be used as a potential target for melanoma treatment [127].

Several studies have demonstrated that aggressive melanoma cells share characteristics with embryonic progenitors. Evidence suggests a major role for stromal components in all stages of tumorigenesis (initiation, progression and metastasis) [128]. Noted scientist Stephen Paget had coined the term "seed & soil" hypothesis predicting that metastatic cells only colonize soils (organs) that are permissive to their growth[129,130]. Studies show embryonic microenvironment has the capacity to reverse the metastatic phenotype of cancer cells. The microenvironment of human embryonic stem cells reprograms aggressive melanoma cells towards a less aggressive phenotype [124]. Nodal, an embryonic morphogen of the TGFβ family is important for sustaining melanoma aggressiveness and plasticity. Nodal is regained in highly aggressive melanoma cell lines, invasive VGP (vertical growth phase)-stage melanoma and metastatic melanoma [131], implicating Nodal as a novel diagnostic marker in melanoma progression and could be a therapeutic target for metastatic melanoma treatment [124].

13. Conclusion

Our understanding of melanoma development and progression has evolved tremendously over the past three decades. Unfortunately our understanding of the molecular biology of melanoma is still far from complete despite extensive research and knowledge gained in chromosomal alterations, mutations in important melanoma-associated genes, epigenetic modifications and melanoma microenvironment. Even to this day, the best prognostic significance of primary melanoma is the thickness of the tumor (i.e. RGP → VGP transition) and the presence/absence of ulcerations. Melanoma still remains as a tumor that is refractory to current chemotherapeutic treatments. A further study of the interaction between various signaling pathways will help researchers decipher the complexity of the genetic and epigenetic changes which eventually would lead to better therapeutic modalities for the treatment of primary and metastatic melanomas.

Glossary

AK - actinic keratosis

BCC - basal cell carcinoma

Cdks - cyclin-dependent kinases

CREB - cyclic adenosine monophosphate responsive element-binding

FAMS - familial atypical mole-melanoma syndrome

GSK3β - glycogen synthase kinase-3beta

IKK - Inhibitor of IκB kinase

MAPK - mitogen activated protein kinase

MITF - microphthalmia-associated transcription factor

MMP - matrix metalloproteinase

NF-κB - nuclear factor kappa-B

NIK - NFκB-interacting kinase

Pten - phosphatase and tensin homolog

Rb - retinoblastoma

RGP - radial growth phase

http://dx.doi.org/10.5772/55257

SCC - Squamous cell carcinoma

Tcf4 - T-cell factor-4

UVR - ultraviolet radiation

VGP - vertical growth phase

WIF1 - Wnt-inhibitory factor 1

Author details

Rohinton S. Tarapore

University of Pennsylvania School of Medicine, Philadelphia, PA, USA

References

[1] Jemal, A, Bray, F, Center, M. M, Ferlay, J, Ward, E, et al. (2011). Global cancer statistics. CA Cancer J Clin , 61, 69-90.

[2] Marghoob, A. A. (2011). Skin cancers and their etiologies. Semin Cutan Med Surg 30: S, 1-5.

[3] Eichberger, T, Regl, G, Ikram, M. S, Neill, G. W, Philpott, M. P, et al. (2004). FOXE1, a new transcriptional target of GLI2 is expressed in human epidermis and basal cell carcinoma. J Invest Dermatol , 122, 1180-1187.

[4] Iwasaki, J. K, Srivastava, D, Moy, R. L, Lin, H. J, & Kouba, D. J. (2012). The molecular genetics underlying basal cell carcinoma pathogenesis and links to targeted therapeutics. J Am Acad Dermatol 66: e, 167-178.

[5] Narayanan, D. L, Saladi, R. N, & Fox, J. L. (2010). Ultraviolet radiation and skin cancer. Int J Dermatol , 49, 978-986.

[6] Foster, P. J, Dunn, E. A, Karl, K. E, Snir, J. A, Nycz, C. M, et al. (2008). Cellular magnetic resonance imaging: in vivo imaging of melanoma cells in lymph nodes of mice. Neoplasia , 10, 207-216.

[7] Marugame, T, & Zhang, M. J. (2010). Comparison of time trends in melanoma of skin cancer mortality (1990-2006) between countries based on the WHO mortality database. Jpn J Clin Oncol 40: 710.

[8] Ko, J. M, Velez, N. F, & Tsao, H. (2010). Pathways to melanoma. Semin Cutan Med Surg , 29, 210-217.

[9] Jemal, A, Thun, M. J, Ries, L. A, Howe, H. L, Weir, H. K, et al. (2008). Annual report to the nation on the status of cancer, 1975-2005, featuring trends in lung cancer, tobacco use, and tobacco control. J Natl Cancer Inst , 100, 1672-1694.

[10] Linos, E, Swetter, S. M, Cockburn, M. G, Colditz, G. A, & Clarke, C. A. (2009). Increasing burden of melanoma in the United States. J Invest Dermatol , 129, 1666-1674.

[11] Wargo, J. A, & Tanabe, K. (2009). Surgical management of melanoma. Hematol Oncol Clin North Am x., 23, 565-581.

[12] Glanz, K, Buller, D. B, & Saraiya, M. (2007). Reducing ultraviolet radiation exposure among outdoor workers: state of the evidence and recommendations. Environ Health 6: 22.

[13] Meeran, S. M, Punathil, T, & Katiyar, S. K. (2008). IL-12 deficiency exacerbates inflammatory responses in UV-irradiated skin and skin tumors. J Invest Dermatol , 128, 2716-2727.

[14] Benjamin, C. L, & Ananthaswamy, H. N. (2007). and the pathogenesis of skin cancer. Toxicol Appl Pharmacol 224: 241-248., 53.

[15] Garbe, C, & Leiter, U. (2009). Melanoma epidemiology and trends. Clin Dermatol , 27, 3-9.

[16] Gandini, S, Autier, P, & Boniol, M. (2011). Reviews on sun exposure and artificial light and melanoma. Prog Biophys Mol Biol , 107, 362-366.

[17] Preston, D. S, & Stern, R. S. (1992). Nonmelanoma cancers of the skin. N Engl J Med , 327, 1649-1662.

[18] Gilchrest, B. A, Eller, M. S, Geller, A. C, & Yaar, M. (1999). The pathogenesis of melanoma induced by ultraviolet radiation. N Engl J Med , 340, 1341-1348.

[19] Gloster, H. M. Jr., Neal K ((2006). Skin cancer in skin of color. J Am Acad Dermatol quiz 761-744., 55, 741-760.

[20] Ma, F, Collado-mesa, F, Hu, S, & Kirsner, R. S. (2007). Skin cancer awareness and sun protection behaviors in white Hispanic and white non-Hispanic high school students in Miami, Florida. Arch Dermatol , 143, 983-988.

[21] Schroeder, P, Haendeler, J, & Krutmann, J. (2008). The role of near infrared radiation in photoaging of the skin. Exp Gerontol , 43, 629-632.

[22] Bennett, D. C. (1993). Genetics, development, and malignancy of melanocytes. Int Rev Cytol , 146, 191-260.

[23] Tsao, H, Atkins, M. B, & Sober, A. J. (2004). Management of cutaneous melanoma. N Engl J Med , 351, 998-1012.

[24] Lomas, J, Martin-duque, P, Pons, M, & Quintanilla, M. (2008). The genetics of malignant melanoma. Front Biosci , 13, 5071-5093.

[25] Hussussian, C. J, Struewing, J. P, Goldstein, A. M, Higgins, P. A, Ally, D. S, et al. (1994). Germline mutations in familial melanoma. Nat Genet 8: 15-21., 16.

[26] Kamb, A, Shattuck-eidens, D, Eeles, R, Liu, Q, Gruis, N. A, et al. (1994). Analysis of the gene (CDKN2) as a candidate for the chromosome 9p melanoma susceptibility locus. Nat Genet 8: 23-26., 16.

[27] Pomerantz, J, Schreiber-agus, N, Liegeois, N. J, Silverman, A, Alland, L, et al. (1998). The Ink4a tumor suppressor gene product, interacts with MDM2 and neutralizes MDM2's inhibition of p53. Cell 92: 713-723., 19Arf.

[28] Zhang, Y, Xiong, Y, & Yarbrough, W. G. (1998). ARF promotes MDM2 degradation and stabilizes ARF-INK4a locus deletion impairs both the Rb and p53 tumor suppression pathways. Cell 92: 725-734., 53.

[29] Kamijo, T, Weber, J. D, Zambetti, G, Zindy, F, Roussel, M. F, et al. (1998). Functional and physical interactions of the ARF tumor suppressor with and Mdm2. Proc Natl Acad Sci U S A 95: 8292-8297., 53.

[30] Stott, F. J, Bates, S, James, M. C, Mcconnell, B. B, Starborg, M, et al. (1998). The alternative product from the human CDKN2A locus, ARF), participates in a regulatory feedback loop with p53 and MDM2. EMBO J 17: 5001-5014., 14.

[31] Chin, L, Garraway, L. A, & Fisher, D. E. (2006). Malignant melanoma: genetics and therapeutics in the genomic era. Genes Dev , 20, 2149-2182.

[32] Gandini, S, Sera, F, Cattaruzza, M. S, Pasquini, P, Abeni, D, et al. (2005). Meta-analysis of risk factors for cutaneous melanoma: I. Common and atypical naevi. Eur J Cancer , 41, 28-44.

[33] Gandini, S, Sera, F, Cattaruzza, M. S, Pasquini, P, Picconi, O, et al. (2005). Meta-analysis of risk factors for cutaneous melanoma: II. Sun exposure. Eur J Cancer , 41, 45-60.

[34] Zuo, L, Weger, J, Yang, Q, Goldstein, A. M, Tucker, M. A, et al. (1996). Germline mutations in the binding domain of CDK4 in familial melanoma. Nat Genet 12: 97-99., 16INK4a.

[35] Soufir, N, Avril, M. F, Chompret, A, Demenais, F, Bombled, J, et al. (1998). Prevalence of and CDK4 germline mutations in 48 melanoma-prone families in France. The French Familial Melanoma Study Group. Hum Mol Genet 7: 209-216., 16.

[36] Wolfel, T, Hauer, M, Schneider, J, Serrano, M, Wolfel, C, et al. (1995). A CDK4 mutant targeted by cytolytic T lymphocytes in a human melanoma. Science 269: 1281-1284., 16INK4a.

[37] Eng, C, Li, F. P, Abramson, D. H, Ellsworth, R. M, Wong, F. L, et al. (1993). Mortality from second tumors among long-term survivors of retinoblastoma. J Natl Cancer Inst , 85, 1121-1128.

[38] Fletcher, O, Easton, D, Anderson, K, Gilham, C, Jay, M, et al. (2004). Lifetime risks of common cancers among retinoblastoma survivors. J Natl Cancer Inst , 96, 357-363.

[39] Druker, B. J, Talpaz, M, Resta, D. J, Peng, B, Buchdunger, E, et al. (2001). Efficacy and safety of a specific inhibitor of the BCR-ABL tyrosine kinase in chronic myeloid leukemia. N Engl J Med , 344, 1031-1037.

[40] Demetri, G. D, Von Mehren, M, & Blanke, C. D. Van den Abbeele AD, Eisenberg B, et al. ((2002). Efficacy and safety of imatinib mesylate in advanced gastrointestinal stromal tumors. N Engl J Med , 347, 472-480.

[41] Lynch, T. J, Bell, D. W, Sordella, R, Gurubhagavatula, S, Okimoto, R. A, et al. (2004). Activating mutations in the epidermal growth factor receptor underlying responsiveness of non-small-cell lung cancer to gefitinib. N Engl J Med , 350, 2129-2139.

[42] Curtin, J. A, Busam, K, Pinkel, D, & Bastian, B. C. (2006). Somatic activation of KIT in distinct subtypes of melanoma. J Clin Oncol , 24, 4340-4346.

[43] Albino, A. P. Le Strange R, Oliff AI, Furth ME, Old LJ ((1984). Transforming ras genes from human melanoma: a manifestation of tumour heterogeneity? Nature , 308, 69-72.

[44] Davies, H, Bignell, G. R, Cox, C, Stephens, P, Edkins, S, et al. (2002). Mutations of the BRAF gene in human cancer. Nature , 417, 949-954.

[45] Lopez-bergami, P, Fitchman, B, & Ronai, Z. (2008). Understanding signaling cascades in melanoma. Photochem Photobiol , 84, 289-306.

[46] Pollock, P. M, Harper, U. L, Hansen, K. S, Yudt, L. M, Stark, M, et al. (2003). High frequency of BRAF mutations in nevi. Nat Genet , 33, 19-20.

[47] Gorden, A, Osman, I, Gai, W, He, D, Huang, W, et al. (2003). Analysis of BRAF and N-RAS mutations in metastatic melanoma tissues. Cancer Res , 63, 3955-3957.

[48] Kumar, R, Angelini, S, Czene, K, Sauroja, I, Hahka-kemppinen, M, et al. (2003). BRAF mutations in metastatic melanoma: a possible association with clinical outcome. Clin Cancer Res , 9, 3362-3368.

[49] Carr, J, & Mackie, R. M. (1994). Point mutations in the N-ras oncogene in malignant melanoma and congenital naevi. Br J Dermatol , 131, 72-77.

[50] Van Elsas, A, Zerp, S, Van Der Flier, S, Kruse-wolters, M, Vacca, A, et al. (1995). Analysis of N-ras mutations in human cutaneous melanoma: tumor heterogeneity detected by polymerase chain reaction/single-stranded conformation polymorphism analysis. Recent Results Cancer Res , 139, 57-67.

[51] Kortylewski, M, Heinrich, P. C, Kauffmann, M. E, & Bohm, M. MacKiewicz A, et al. ((2001). Mitogen-activated protein kinases control Kip1 expression and growth of human melanoma cells. Biochem J 357: 297-303., 27.

[52] Lefevre, G, Calipel, A, Mouriaux, F, Hecquet, C, Malecaze, F, et al. (2003). Opposite long-term regulation of c-Myc and through overactivation of Raf-1 and the MEK/ERK module in proliferating human choroidal melanoma cells. Oncogene 22: 8813-8822., 27Kip1.

[53] Lopez-bergami, P, Huang, C, Goydos, J. S, Yip, D, Bar-eli, M, et al. (2007). Rewired ERK-JNK signaling pathways in melanoma. Cancer Cell , 11, 447-460.

[54] Goding, C. R. (2000). Mitf from neural crest to melanoma: signal transduction and transcription in the melanocyte lineage. Genes Dev , 14, 1712-1728.

[55] Wu, M, Hemesath, T. J, Takemoto, C. M, Horstmann, M. A, Wells, A. G, et al. (2000). c-Kit triggers dual phosphorylations, which couple activation and degradation of the essential melanocyte factor Mi. Genes Dev , 14, 301-312.

[56] Kim, D. S, Hwang, E. S, Lee, J. E, Kim, S. Y, Kwon, S. B, et al. (2003). Sphingosine-1-phosphate decreases melanin synthesis via sustained ERK activation and subsequent MITF degradation. J Cell Sci , 116, 1699-1706.

[57] Eisenmann, K. M, Vanbrocklin, M. W, Staffend, N. A, Kitchen, S. M, & Koo, H. M. (2003). Mitogen-activated protein kinase pathway-dependent tumor-specific survival signaling in melanoma cells through inactivation of the proapoptotic protein bad. Cancer Res , 63, 8330-8337.

[58] Krasilnikov, M, Ivanov, V. N, Dong, J, & Ronai, Z. (2003). Erkand P. I K negatively regulate STAT-transcriptional activities in human melanoma cells: implications towards sensitization to apoptosis. Oncogene , 22, 4092-4101.

[59] Tower, G. B, Coon, C. C, Benbow, U, Vincenti, M. P, & Brinckerhoff, C. E. (2002). Erk 1/2 differentially regulates the expression from the 1G/2G single nucleotide polymorphism in the MMP-1 promoter in melanoma cells. Biochim Biophys Acta , 1586, 265-274.

[60] Ishii, Y, Ogura, T, Tatemichi, M, Fujisawa, H, Otsuka, F, et al. (2003). Induction of matrix metalloproteinase gene transcription by nitric oxide and mechanisms of MMP-1 gene induction in human melanoma cell lines. Int J Cancer , 103, 161-168.

[61] Ramos, M. C, Steinbrenner, H, Stuhlmann, D, Sies, H, & Brenneisen, P. (2004). Induction of MMP-10 and MMP-1 in a squamous cell carcinoma cell line by ultraviolet radiation. Biol Chem , 385, 75-86.

[62] Steelman, L. S, Bertrand, F. E, & Mccubrey, J. A. (2004). The complexity of PTEN: mutation, marker and potential target for therapeutic intervention. Expert Opin Ther Targets , 8, 537-550.

[63] Parmiter, A. H, Balaban, G, & Clark, W. H. Jr., Nowell PC ((1988). Possible involvement of the chromosome region 10q24----q26 in early stages of melanocytic neoplasia. Cancer Genet Cytogenet , 30, 313-317.

[64] Simpson, L, & Parsons, R. (2001). PTEN: life as a tumor suppressor. Exp Cell Res , 264, 29-41.

[65] Wu, H, Goel, V, & Haluska, F. G. (2003). PTEN signaling pathways in melanoma. Oncogene , 22, 3113-3122.

[66] Herbst, R. A, Weiss, J, Ehnis, A, Cavenee, W. K, & Arden, K. C. (1994). Loss of heterozygosity for 10q22-10qter in malignant melanoma progression. Cancer Res , 54, 3111-3114.

[67] Healy, E, Rehman, I, Angus, B, & Rees, J. L. (1995). Loss of heterozygosity in sporadic primary cutaneous melanoma. Genes Chromosomes Cancer , 12, 152-156.

[68] Harlan, J. E, Yoon, H. S, Hajduk, P. J, & Fesik, S. W. (1995). Structural characterization of the interaction between a pleckstrin homology domain and phosphatidylinositol 4,5-bisphosphate. Biochemistry , 34, 9859-9864.

[69] Nicholson, K. M, & Anderson, N. G. (2002). The protein kinase B/Akt signalling pathway in human malignancy. Cell Signal , 14, 381-395.

[70] Stahl, J. M, Sharma, A, Cheung, M, Zimmerman, M, Cheng, J. Q, et al. (2004). Deregulated Akt3 activity promotes development of malignant melanoma. Cancer Res , 64, 7002-7010.

[71] Robertson, G. P. (2005). Functional and therapeutic significance of Akt deregulation in malignant melanoma. Cancer Metastasis Rev , 24, 273-285.

[72] Dhawan, P, Singh, A. B, Ellis, D. L, & Richmond, A. (2002). Constitutive activation of Akt/protein kinase B in melanoma leads to up-regulation of nuclear factor-kappaB and tumor progression. Cancer Res , 62, 7335-7342.

[73] Li, G, Kalabis, J, Xu, X, Meier, F, Oka, M, et al. (2003). Reciprocal regulation of Mel-CAM and AKT in human melanoma. Oncogene , 22, 6891-6899.

[74] Johnson, J. P. (1999). Cell adhesion molecules in the development and progression of malignant melanoma. Cancer Metastasis Rev , 18, 345-357.

[75] Kim, D, Kim, S, Koh, H, Yoon, S. O, Chung, A. S, et al. (2001). Akt/PKB promotes cancer cell invasion via increased motility and metalloproteinase production. FASEB J , 15, 1953-1962.

[76] Park, B. K, Zeng, X, & Glazer, R. I. (2001). Akt1 induces extracellular matrix invasion and matrix metalloproteinase-2 activity in mouse mammary epithelial cells. Cancer Res , 61, 7647-7653.

[77] Cardone, M. H, Roy, N, Stennicke, H. R, Salvesen, G. S, Franke, T. F, et al. (1998). Regulation of cell death protease caspase-9 by phosphorylation. Science , 282, 1318-1321.

[78] Datta, S. R, Dudek, H, Tao, X, Masters, S, Fu, H, et al. (1997). Akt phosphorylation of BAD couples survival signals to the cell-intrinsic death machinery. Cell , 91, 231-241.

[79] Giles, R. H, Van Es, J. H, & Clevers, H. (2003). Caught up in a Wnt storm: Wnt signaling in cancer. Biochim Biophys Acta , 1653, 1-24.

[80] Veeman, M. T, Axelrod, J. D, & Moon, R. T. (2003). A second canon. Functions and mechanisms of beta-catenin-independent Wnt signaling. Dev Cell , 5, 367-377.

[81] Elcheva, I, Tarapore, R. S, Bhatia, N, & Spiegelman, V. S. (2008). Overexpression of mRNA-binding protein CRD-BP in malignant melanomas. Oncogene , 27, 5069-5074.

[82] Rimm, D. L, Caca, K, Hu, G, Harrison, F. B, & Fearon, E. R. (1999). Frequent nuclear/cytoplasmic localization of beta-catenin without exon 3 mutations in malignant melanoma. Am J Pathol , 154, 325-329.

[83] Demunter, A, Libbrecht, L, Degreef, H, & De Wolf-peeters, C. van den Oord JJ ((2002). Loss of membranous expression of beta-catenin is associated with tumor progression in cutaneous melanoma and rarely caused by exon 3 mutations. Mod Pathol , 15, 454-461.

[84] Omholt, K, Platz, A, Ringborg, U, & Hansson, J. (2001). Cytoplasmic and nuclear accumulation of beta-catenin is rarely caused by CTNNB1 exon 3 mutations in cutaneous malignant melanoma. Int J Cancer , 92, 839-842.

[85] Rubinfeld, B, Robbins, P, Gamil, M, Albert, I, Porfiri, E, et al. (1997). Stabilization of beta-catenin by genetic defects in melanoma cell lines. Science , 275, 1790-1792.

[86] Reifenberger, J, Knobbe, C. B, Wolter, M, Blaschke, B, Schulte, K. W, et al. (2002). Molecular genetic analysis of malignant melanomas for aberrations of the WNT signaling pathway genes CTNNB1, APC, ICAT and BTRC. Int J Cancer , 100, 549-556.

[87] Pollock, P. M, & Hayward, N. (2002). Mutations in exon 3 of the beta-catenin gene are rare in melanoma cell lines. Melanoma Res , 12, 183-186.

[88] Worm, J, Christensen, C, Gronbaek, K, Tulchinsky, E, & Guldberg, P. (2004). Genetic and epigenetic alterations of the APC gene in malignant melanoma. Oncogene , 23, 5215-5226.

[89] Tago, K, Nakamura, T, Nishita, M, Hyodo, J, Nagai, S, et al. (2000). Inhibition of Wnt signaling by ICAT, a novel beta-catenin-interacting protein. Genes Dev , 14, 1741-1749.

[90] Goodall, J, Martinozzi, S, Dexter, T. J, Champeval, D, Carreira, S, et al. (2004). Brn-2 expression controls melanoma proliferation and is directly regulated by beta-catenin. Mol Cell Biol , 24, 2915-2922.

[91] Thomson, J. A, Murphy, K, Baker, E, Sutherland, G. R, Parsons, P. G, et al. (1995). The brn-2 gene regulates the melanocytic phenotype and tumorigenic potential of human melanoma cells. Oncogene , 11, 691-700.

[92] Hodgkinson, C. A, Moore, K. J, Nakayama, A, Steingrimsson, E, Copeland, N. G, et al. (1993). Mutations at the mouse microphthalmia locus are associated with defects in a gene encoding a novel basic-helix-loop-helix-zipper protein. Cell , 74, 395-404.

[93] Hughes, M. J, Lingrel, J. B, Krakowsky, J. M, & Anderson, K. P. (1993). A Helix-loop helix transcription factor-like gene is located at the mi locus. J Biol Chem , 268, 20687-20690.

[94] Widlund, H. R, Horstmann, M. A, Price, E. R, Cui, J, Lessnick, S. L, et al. (2002). Beta-catenin-induced melanoma growth requires the downstream target Microphthalmia-associated transcription factor. J Cell Biol , 158, 1079-1087.

[95] Schepsky, A, Bruser, K, Gunnarsson, G. J, Goodall, J, Hallsson, J. H, et al. (2006). The microphthalmia-associated transcription factor Mitf interacts with beta-catenin to determine target gene expression. Mol Cell Biol , 26, 8914-8927.

[96] Kawano, Y, & Kypta, R. (2003). Secreted antagonists of the Wnt signalling pathway. J Cell Sci , 116, 2627-2634.

[97] Forget, M. A, Turcotte, S, Beauseigle, D, Godin-ethier, J, Pelletier, S, et al. (2007). The Wnt pathway regulator DKK1 is preferentially expressed in hormone-resistant breast tumours and in some common cancer types. Br J Cancer , 96, 646-653.

[98] Kuphal, S, Lodermeyer, S, Bataille, F, Schuierer, M, Hoang, B. H, et al. (2006). Expression of Dickkopf genes is strongly reduced in malignant melanoma. Oncogene , 25, 5027-5036.

[99] Mikheev, A. M, Mikheeva, S. A, Rostomily, R, & Zarbl, H. (2007). Dickkopf-1 activates cell death in MDA-MB435 melanoma cells. Biochem Biophys Res Commun , 352, 675-680.

[100] Lin, Y. C, You, L, Xu, Z, He, B, Yang, C. T, et al. (2007). Wnt inhibitory factor-1 gene transfer inhibits melanoma cell growth. Hum Gene Ther , 18, 379-386.

[101] Weston, C. R, & Davis, R. J. (2007). The JNK signal transduction pathway. Curr Opin Cell Biol , 19, 142-149.

[102] Karin, M. (1995). The regulation of AP-1 activity by mitogen-activated protein kinases. J Biol Chem , 270, 16483-16486.

[103] Kennedy, N. J, & Davis, R. J. (2003). Role of JNK in tumor development. Cell Cycle , 2, 199-201.

[104] Yang, Y. M, Bost, F, Charbono, W, Dean, N, Mckay, R, et al. (2003). C-Jun NH(2)-terminal kinase mediates proliferation and tumor growth of human prostate carcinoma. Clin Cancer Res , 9, 391-401.

[105] Cui, J, Han, S. Y, Wang, C, Su, W, Harshyne, L, et al. (2006). c-Jun NH(2)-terminal kinase 2alpha2 promotes the tumorigenicity of human glioblastoma cells. Cancer Res , 66, 10024-10031.

[106] Khatlani, T. S, Wislez, M, Sun, M, Srinivas, H, Iwanaga, K, et al. (2007). c-Jun N-terminal kinase is activated in non-small-cell lung cancer and promotes neoplastic transformation in human bronchial epithelial cells. Oncogene , 26, 2658-2666.

[107] Adler, V, Schaffer, A, Kim, J, Dolan, L, & Ronai, Z. (1995). UV Irradiation and heat shock mediate JNK activation via alternate pathways. J Biol Chem , 270, 26071-26077.

[108] Mariani, O, Brennetot, C, Coindre, J. M, Gruel, N, Ganem, C, et al. (2007). JUN oncogene amplification and overexpression block adipocytic differentiation in highly aggressive sarcomas. Cancer Cell , 11, 361-374.

[109] Vleugel, M. M, Greijer, A. E, Bos, R, Van Der Wall, E, & Van Diest, P. J. (2006). c-Jun activation is associated with proliferation and angiogenesis in invasive breast cancer. Hum Pathol , 37, 668-674.

[110] Maeno, K, Masuda, A, Yanagisawa, K, Konishi, H, Osada, H, et al. (2006). Altered regulation of c-jun and its involvement in anchorage-independent growth of human lung cancers. Oncogene , 25, 271-277.

[111] Yamanishi, D. T, Buckmeier, J. A, & Meyskens, F. L. Jr. ((1991). Expression of c-jun, jun-B, and c-fos proto-oncogenes in human primary melanocytes and metastatic melanomas. J Invest Dermatol , 97, 349-353.

[112] Rutberg, S. E, Goldstein, I. M, Yang, Y. M, Stackpole, C. W, & Ronai, Z. (1994). Expression and transcriptional activity of AP-1, CRE, and URE binding proteins in B16 mouse melanoma subclones. Mol Carcinog , 10, 82-87.

[113] Mingo-sion, A. M, Marietta, P. M, Koller, E, & Wolf, D. M. Van Den Berg CL ((2004). Inhibition of JNK reduces G2/M transit independent of leading to endoreduplication, decreased proliferation, and apoptosis in breast cancer cells. Oncogene 23: 596-604., 53.

[114] Uzgare, A. R, & Isaacs, J. T. (2004). Enhanced redundancy in Akt and mitogen-activated protein kinase-induced survival of malignant versus normal prostate epithelial cells. Cancer Res , 64, 6190-6199.

[115] Gurzov, E. N, Bakiri, L, Alfaro, J. M, Wagner, E. F, & Izquierdo, M. (2008). Targeting c-Jun and JunB proteins as potential anticancer cell therapy. Oncogene , 27, 641-652.

[116] Dixit, V, & Mak, T. W. (2002). NF-kappaB Signaling Many roads lead to madrid. Cell , 111, 615-619.

[117] Ghosh, S, & Karin, M. (2002). Missing pieces in the NF-kappaB puzzle. Cell 109 Suppl: S, 81-96.

[118] Chen, X, Kandasamy, K, & Srivastava, R. K. (2003). Differential roles of RelA (and c-Rel subunits of nuclear factor kappa B in tumor necrosis factor-related apoptosis-inducing ligand signaling. Cancer Res 63: 1059-1066., 65.

[119] Poser, I, Dominguez, D, De Herreros, A. G, Varnai, A, Buettner, R, et al. (2001). Loss of E-cadherin expression in melanoma cells involves up-regulation of the transcriptional repressor Snail. J Biol Chem ,. 276, 24661-24666.

[120] Meyskens, F. L. Jr., Buckmeier JA, McNulty SE, Tohidian NB ((1999). Activation of nuclear factor-kappa B in human metastatic melanomacells and the effect of oxidative stress. Clin Cancer Res , 5, 1197-1202.

[121] Boukerche, H, Su, Z. Z, Emdad, L, Sarkar, D, & Fisher, P. B. (2007). mda-9/Syntenin regulates the metastatic phenotype in human melanoma cells by activating nuclear factor-kappaB. Cancer Res , 67, 1812-1822.

[122] Philip, S, & Kundu, G. C. (2003). Osteopontin induces nuclear factor kappa B-mediated promatrix metalloproteinase-2 activation through I kappa B alpha /IKK signaling pathways, and curcumin (diferulolylmethane) down-regulates these pathways. J Biol Chem , 278, 14487-14497.

[123] Dupin, E. Le Douarin NM ((2003). Development of melanocyte precursors from the vertebrate neural crest. Oncogene , 22, 3016-3023.

[124] Hendrix, M. J, Seftor, E. A, Seftor, R. E, Kasemeier-kulesa, J, Kulesa, P. M, et al. (2007). Reprogramming metastatic tumour cells with embryonic microenvironments. Nat Rev Cancer , 7, 246-255.

[125] Bittner, M, Meltzer, P, Chen, Y, Jiang, Y, Seftor, E, et al. (2000). Molecular classification of cutaneous malignant melanoma by gene expression profiling. Nature , 406, 536-540.

[126] Hendrix, M. J, Seftor, E. A, Hess, A. R, & Seftor, R. E. (2003). Molecular plasticity of human melanoma cells. Oncogene , 22, 3070-3075.

[127] Coiffier, B, Lepage, E, Briere, J, Herbrecht, R, Tilly, H, et al. (2002). CHOP chemotherapy plus rituximab compared with CHOP alone in elderly patients with diffuse large-B-cell lymphoma. N Engl J Med , 346, 235-242.

[128] Lee, J. T, & Herlyn, M. (2007). Microenvironmental influences in melanoma progression. J Cell Biochem , 101, 862-872.

[129] Paget, S. (1989). The distribution of secondary growths in cancer of the breast. 1889. Cancer Metastasis Rev , 8, 98-101.

[130] Fidler, I. J. (2003). The pathogenesis of cancer metastasis: the'seed and soil' hypothesis revisited. Nat Rev Cancer , 3, 453-458.

[131] Topczewska, J. M, Postovit, L. M, Margaryan, N. V, Sam, A, Hess, A. R, et al. (2006). Embryonic and tumorigenic pathways converge via Nodal signaling: role in melanoma aggressiveness. Nat Med , 12, 925-932.

[132] Miller, S. A, Hamilton, S. L, Wester, U. G, & Cyr, W. H. (1998). An analysis of UVA emissions from sunlamps and the potential importance for melanoma. Photochem Photobiol , 68, 63-70.

[133] Lautenschlager, S, Wulf, H. C, & Pittelkow, M. R. (2007). Photoprotection. Lancet , 370, 528-537.

[134] Brenner, M, & Hearing, V. J. (2008). The protective role of melanin against UV damage in human skin. Photochem Photobiol , 84, 539-549.

[135] Bastian, B. C. LeBoit PE, Hamm H, Brocker EB, Pinkel D ((1998). Chromosomal gains and losses in primary cutaneous melanomas detected by comparative genomic hybridization. Cancer Res , 58, 2170-2175.

[136] Curtin, J. A, Fridlyand, J, Kageshita, T, Patel, H. N, Busam, K. J, et al. (2005). Distinct sets of genetic alterations in melanoma. N Engl J Med , 353, 2135-2147.

[137] Balazs, M, Adam, Z, Treszl, A, Begany, A, Hunyadi, J, et al. (2001). Chromosomal imbalances in primary and metastatic melanomas revealed by comparative genomic hybridization. Cytometry , 46, 222-232.

[138] Hausler, T, Stang, A, Anastassiou, G, Jockel, K. H, Mrzyk, S, et al. (2005). Loss of heterozygosity of 1p in uveal melanomas with monosomy 3. Int J Cancer , 116, 909-913.

[139] White, J. S, Mclean, I. W, Becker, R. L, Director-myska, A. E, & Nath, J. (2006). Correlation of comparative genomic hybridization results of 100 archival uveal melanomas with patient survival. Cancer Genet Cytogenet , 170, 29-39.

[140] Speicher, M. R, & Prescher, G. du Manoir S, Jauch A, Horsthemke B, et al. ((1994). Chromosomal gains and losses in uveal melanomas detected by comparative genomic hybridization. Cancer Res , 54, 3817-3823.

[141] Vajdic, C. M, Hutchins, A. M, Kricker, A, Aitken, J. F, Armstrong, B. K, et al. (2003). Chromosomal gains and losses in ocular melanoma detected by comparative genomic hybridization in an Australian population-based study. Cancer Genet Cytogenet , 144, 12-17.

[142] Garraway, L. A, Widlund, H. R, Rubin, M. A, Getz, G, Berger, A. J, et al. (2005). Integrative genomic analyses identify MITF as a lineage survival oncogene amplified in malignant melanoma. Nature , 436, 117-122.

[143] Jonsson, G, Dahl, C, Staaf, J, Sandberg, T, Bendahl, P. O, et al. (2007). Genomic profiling of malignant melanoma using tiling-resolution arrayCGH. Oncogene , 26, 4738-4748.

[144] Alonso, S. R, Tracey, L, Ortiz, P, Perez-gomez, B, Palacios, J, et al. (2007). A high-throughput study in melanoma identifies epithelial-mesenchymal transition as a major determinant of metastasis. Cancer Res , 67, 3450-3460.

[145] Hoek, K, Rimm, D. L, Williams, K. R, Zhao, H, Ariyan, S, et al. (2004). Expression profiling reveals novel pathways in the transformation of melanocytes to melanomas. Cancer Res , 64, 5270-5282.

[146] Seftor, R. E, Seftor, E. A, Koshikawa, N, Meltzer, P. S, Gardner, L. M, et al. (2001). Cooperative interactions of laminin 5 gamma2 chain, matrix metalloproteinase-2, and membrane type-1-matrix/metalloproteinase are required for mimicry of embryonic vasculogenesis by aggressive melanoma. Cancer Res , 61, 6322-6327.

[147] Jaeger, J, Koczan, D, Thiesen, H. J, Ibrahim, S. M, Gross, G, et al. (2007). Gene expression signatures for tumor progression, tumor subtype, and tumor thickness in laser-microdissected melanoma tissues. Clin Cancer Res , 13, 806-815.

[148] Weeraratna, A. T, Jiang, Y, Hostetter, G, Rosenblatt, K, Duray, P, et al. (2002). Wnt5a signaling directly affects cell motility and invasion of metastatic melanoma. Cancer Cell , 1, 279-288.

[149] Becker, B, Roesch, A, Hafner, C, Stolz, W, Dugas, M, et al. (2004). Discrimination of melanocytic tumors by cDNA array hybridization of tissues prepared by laser pressure catapulting. J Invest Dermatol , 122, 361-368.

[150] Winnepenninckx, V, Lazar, V, Michiels, S, Dessen, P, Stas, M, et al. (2006). Gene expression profiling of primary cutaneous melanoma and clinical outcome. J Natl Cancer Inst , 98, 472-482.

[151] Haqq, C, Nosrati, M, Sudilovsky, D, Crothers, J, Khodabakhsh, D, et al. (2005). The gene expression signatures of melanoma progression. Proc Natl Acad Sci U S A , 102, 6092-6097.

Chapter 4

Current Management of Malignant Melanoma: State of the Art

Zekayi Kutlubay, Burhan Engin,
Server Serdaroğlu and Yalçın Tüzün

Additional information is available at the end of the chapter

http://dx.doi.org/10.5772/55304

1. Introduction

The word "melanoma" was first used by *Rene Laennec,* inventor of the stethoscope, in his manuscript reporting a case of disseminated melanoma in 1812 [1]. Cutaneous malignant melanoma (CMM) arises from the malignant transformation of the pigment producing melanocytes, which are located and evenly distributed in the basal epidermal layer of human skin. These pigment-producing cells (melanocytes) are located predominantly in the skin, but also found in the eyes, ears, GI tract, leptomeninges, and oral and genital mucous membranes [2].

The incidence of cutaneous malignant melanoma has increased significantly among all Caucasian populations over the last several decades. The rate of incidence of cutaneous melanoma continues to rise almost inexorably in populations of European origin worldwide. Diagnosis of melanoma at an early stage is almost curable but there is currently no effective treatment for advanced melanoma. Probably a large proportion of melanomas can be ascribed to a single (modifiable) risk factor-sun exposure. It has not been established whether medical intervention of any kind influences the outcome in the case of melanoma. Major initiatives in recent years have concentrated on education about sun avoidance, the importance of skin awareness and skin examination, and the screening of populations at high risk for melanoma. However, it is unclear whether any of the latter measures have had any significant influence on mortality from melanoma. The annual increase in incidence rate varies between populations, but in general has been in the order of 3–7% per year for fair-skinned Caucasian populations. CMM represents a significant and growing public health burden because of the increase in incidence and the consequent mortality [3].

The cancer statistic in the United States was reported to be 6 cases per 100.000 inhabitants at the beginning of the 1970s and 18 cases per 100.000 and year at the beginning of 2000, thus demonstrating a threefold increase in incidence rates. Incidence rates in central Europe increased in the same time period, from 3 to 4 cases to 10 to 15 cases per 100.000 inhabitants and year, which is very similar to the increase in the United States. The highest incidence rates were reported in Australia and New Zealand, with 30 to 60 cases per 100.000 inhabitants and year [4]. Cutaneous melanoma ranks as the sixth most common cancer in American men and women, the second most common cancer in patients between the ages of 20 and 35, and the leading cause of cancer death in women ages 25 to 30 years [5]. Although melanoma accounts for 5% of all skin cancers in the United States, it is responsible for the most common skin cancer-related deaths (it accounts for 79 percent of all skin cancer deaths) because of its high mortality when identified at an advanced stage [6, 7]. The number of deaths due to CMM has also increased in most fair-skinned populations throughout the world in the past few decades. However, melanoma mortality rates have been rising at a rate of increase lower than that for melanoma incidence. Between 1955 and 1984, mortality from CMM had been rising both in young adults (20–44 years) and in middle-aged populations (45–64 years) in most European countries, North America, Australia and New Zealand, with a rate of increase of 2–4% annually. In Australia in 1985–1999 the mean age-standardized mortality rates were 4.8 and 2.5 per 100.000 in men and women, respectively. In 1990–1994 the rate rose by 3.7% in men to 5.0 per 100.000 and in women it fell by 5.2% to 2.4 per 100.000 [3]. Although mortality rates have increased, 5-year survival has steadily improved over recent decades, and is now greater than 85%, but melanoma causes disproportionate mortality in those of young and middle age, such that an average of 18.6 years of potential life are lost for each melanoma death in the USA, one of the highest rates for adult-onset cancers [8]. Predicted 1-year survival for stage IV disease ranges between 41% and 59% [5].

The etiology of melanoma is multifactorial that environmental, host, and genetic factors contribute to its development. The most important environmental risk factor is ultraviolet radiation (UVR) exposure [6]. Most melanomas are thought to be caused by periodic, intense sun exposure (particularly during the critical time period of childhood and adolescence), termed the *intermittent exposure* hypothesis, though exposure in adulthood certainly also plays a part. In older people, melanomas appear to be more related to chronic exposure. This is suggested by the body site distribution of melanomas in the elderly, with more melanomas on chronically exposed body sites [7, 9]. The most important host risk factor for CMM in fair-skinned people is the presence of both common acquired and atypical (dysplastic) melanocytic naevi. Patients with a family history of melanoma are at increased risk. Around 5–12% of patients with melanoma have a family history of CMM in one or more first-degree relatives. Some of these patients have an inherited mutation in highly penetrant susceptibility genes which are associated with a significantly increased risk of melanoma [3].

Cutaneous malignant melanoma is currently classified into four major clinical subtypes: Superficial spreading, nodular, acral lentiginous, and lentigo maligna, of which superficial spreading melanoma is by far the most common form (approximately 70%) of CMM [10]. CMM that is less invasive and locally defined at diagnosis has a five-year survival rate of more than

http://dx.doi.org/10.5772/55304

95% after treatment by surgical excision alone. Fortunately, the vast majority of CMM (approximately 80%) are diagnosed at this early stage. If the cancer is more advanced, however, survival rates drop substantially to 30% to 60% after five years, depending on the tumor thickness in millimeters (*Breslow*'s depth). Metastatic disease has poor patient outcomes as treatment options are limited [10].

The prognosis for a patient with a newly diagnosed cutaneous melanoma depends mainly on two factors— the thickness of the primary tumour and the presence or absence of metastasis to regional lymph nodes. However, other prognostic factors are very important, including tumour ulceration, mitotic rate, and presence of regression, as well as sex and age of the patient, and tumour site [8].

For the primary prevention, physical protection from exposure to sunlight is generally accepted as the most important element of melanoma risk reduction. It seems particularly meaningful to prevent multiple erythemas during childhood, convincing parents and care takers not to let children stay too long under the sun. Sun-protective clothing and hats should be worn and peak hours of sun intensity should be avoided. For these purposes, mass media campaigns and widespread public education programmes would be most effective to make changes in attitude and behaviour towards sun protection [8,11]. The wavelength of light that is causal for melanoma is still not known and therefore sunscreens should be broad-spectrum types, providing protection across both UVB and UVA ranges. Advice should be to use sunscreens that are water proof, and sunscreens must be applied regularly and in sufficient quantities [12]. Regular screening of the total population for CMM does not seem useful and is not propagated in any country in the world. However, it seems likely that people with a familial risk of developing melanomas (those with familial or sporadic dysplastic naevus syndrome, xeroderma pigmentosum and large congenital naevi, representing approximately 10% of all melanoma patients) can benefit from regular check-ups. Screening in these populations, and regular checks (every 6–12 months) lead to earlier detection [11].

2. Etiopathogenesis

2.1. Risk factors

The etiology of melanoma is multifactorial, with environmental, host, and genetic factors contributing to its development. Ultraviolet radiation exposure is the most important environmental risk factor [6]. The precise type of sun exposure that is causal has been controversial but the data are now strong that the dominant cause is intermittent sun exposure [12]. Periodic and intense sun exposure rather than long, heavy sun exposure especially during childhood and adolescence is the feature of intermittent sun exposure. Also, sunburn history particularly blistering and peeling burns are important indicators for intermittent sun exposure [7].

In a meta-analysis by *Dennis* et al., an increased risk of melanoma was seen with an increasing number of sunburns for all time-periods, including childhood, adolescence, adulthood, and lifetime [13]. The relationship between melanoma and exposure to ultraviolet light is complex that lower incidence of melanoma among people who work outdoors is seen compared with those working indoors. The possible explanation for this is that chronically tanned skin is less melanoma-prone than untanned skin exposed to bursts of high intensity sun, in particular sunburns [14].

The geographic distribution of melanoma supports the importance of UVR exposure in its pathogenesis. Living closer to the equator, where there is the greatest ambient solar radiation, is consistently associated with increased melanoma risk [6]. When the incidence and mortality rates of melanoma compared between Europe and Australia it was reported 5 to 10 times higher incidence rates in Australia [4]. Melanoma incidence and mortality among Caucasians correlate inversely with latitude of residence and dose of UV radiation, termed *latitude gradient*. In the United States, SEER (Surveillance Epidemiology and End Results) data from 1992 to 2001 demonstrate that the latitude gradient applies only to non-Hispanic whites; melanoma incidence was not associated with latitude and UV index in Afro-Americans, Hispanics, Asians and Native Americans [7]. Migration studies also provide evidence for the effect of ambient UVR exposure levels on melanoma risk [6]. Younger migrants to sunny areas have an increased risk for melanoma as compared with adult immigrants [7].

The anatomic distribution of melanoma also offers insight into the pathogenesis of the disease and the role of UVR. The most common sites for melanoma are the trunk in men and the lower legs in women which are areas of high levels of acute, intermittent sun exposure. In older people, there is a greater incidence of melanomas located on chronically sun exposed areas with maximal cumulative sun exposure that the face is the most common location [6,7].

Cust et al. reported that UV radiation exposure from sunbeds is a risk factor for early-onset melanoma, particularly melanoma diagnosed between ages 18 and 29 years [15]. Artificial lights (psoralen and ultraviolet A light (PUVA), UVB and tanning booths) have been associated with the development melanoma [7].

Weaker phenotypic risk factors are related to; the presence of skin that burns easily in the sun such as: skin phototype I-II, high density of freckles, fair complexion/sun sensitivity, an increased number of common or atypical/dysplastic nevi (moles), blue eye colour and red hair colour [12]. *Loria* et al. reported that the crude relative risk increased significantly for individuals with red hair, but hair color was no longer significant in multivariate analysis and light-colored eyes were an independent risk factor even after controlling for the number of nevi, skin type, and other relevant factors [16].

The strongest phenotypic risk factor for melanoma is the presence of increased numbers of melanocytic naevi [12]. With growing numbers of melanocytic nevi, the melanoma risk increases nearly linearly. In addition, the presence of atypical melanocytic nevi was found to be an independent risk factor [4]. Adults with more than 100 clinically typical-appearing nevi, children with more than 50 typical-appearing, and any patient with atypical nevi are at risk. Large congenital nevi are recognized potential precursors of melanoma, although the degree of risk varies depending on the size of the lesion [7]. Twin studies have provided strong evidence that naevus number is predominantly genetically determined with a smaller effect of environmental factors, particularly sun exposure. It is theorized, therefore, that the genes

http://dx.doi.org/10.5772/55304

that determine naevus number are also common melanoma susceptibility genes [12]. Many of the oncogenic mutations initially identified in melanomas have also been detected in benign melanocytic proliferations [5].

Any family history increases the risk of melanoma. Familial melanoma comprises 10-15% of all patients with melanoma [7,12]. The presence of more than one case of melanoma in a family may occur by chance alone, or may be due to low penetrance alleles and/or sun exposure habits common to affected relatives. However, an estimated 25% of familial melanoma is associated with germline mutations of the CDKN2A gene on chromosome 9 (which codes for the cell cycle inhibitor protein, p16) and often presents with an autosomal dominant pattern of transmission [17].

2.2. Genetics

Melanoma develops as a result of accumulated abnormalities in genetic pathways within the melanocyte. These abnormalities promote cell proliferation and prevent normal pathways of apoptosis in response to DNA damage [8]. The driving force behind the initiation and progression of melanoma development is the acquisition of somatic mutations in key regulatory genes. The first gene found to be specifically altered in melanoma was *NRAS*, which harbors mutations in 15–25% of melanoma cell lines and primary tumors [14]. *NRAS* mutations tend to occur in melanomas arising from intermittently sun-exposed skin [5]. *NRAS* mutations are more common in patients with nodular melanomas and melanomas arising on chronically sun-damaged skin. Recent data have shown that *NRAS* mutations may be associated with thicker tumors (>1 mm) and higher mitotic rate (>1/mm2) compared with mutations in *BRAF*. In response to a variety of cellular stimuli, including ligand-mediated activation of receptor tyrosine kinases (RTKs), RAS assumes an activated, GTP-bound state, leading to recruitment of RAF to the plasma membrane and phosphorylation-driven activation of the RAF-MEK-ERK cascade [14]. RAS genes acquire their transforming activity following the acquisition of a single-point mutation that impairs their GTPase activity and leads to constitutive signaling through the mitogen-activated protein kinase (MAPK), PI3K/AKT, and Ral-GDS pathways [18]. *Omholt* et al. demonstrated that *NRAS* mutations are present in the radial growth phase (RGP) of primary melanoma lesions as well as in tumor-associated nevi and that they are preserved in corresponding vertical growth phase (VGP) and metastatic lesions [19].

BRAF is a serine/threonine kinase, which is a major player in the Ras-Raf-Mek-Erk mitogen-activated protein kinase (MAPK) signaling transduction pathway that regulates cell growth, proliferation, and differentiation in response to various stimuli [7]. Mutations in *BRAF* have been found in about 60% of melanoma samples and cell lines. *BRAF* mutations are common in benign and dysplastic nevi pointing to a potential initiating role of *BRAF* in melanocyte transformation [20]. *BRAF* mutations are more common in intermittently UV-exposed skin compared with chronically sun exposed skin or relatively unexposed skin (eg, acral sites, mucosal sites), which more frequently demonstrate *KIT* mutations. Acral and mucosal melanomas have infrequent *BRAF* mutations, and show greater numbers of chromosomal aberrations. There can also be frequent gains in *CCND1* and regions of chromosome 22, and losses from chromosome 4q. *Curtin* et al. demonstrated that melanomas arising on skin without chronic sun-induced damage had frequent mutations in *BRAF* and frequent losses of chromosome 10, whereas melanomas on skin with chronic sun-induced damage had infrequent mutations in *BRAF* and frequent increases in the number of copies of the *CCND1* gene [21]. *Omholt* et al. demonstrated that *BRAF* mutations occur at an early stage during melanoma pathogenesis rather than being associated with metastasis initiation. Although the *BRAF* mutations do not seem to be important for metastasis initiation, the finding that they are preserved throughout tumor progression suggests that they may still influence tumor maintenance [19]. Although *BRAF* mutations are highly prevalent (59%) in melanomas occurring on skin without chronic sun damage, *BRAF* mutations are significantly less frequent in acral and mucosal melanomas. *BRAF* mutations are more commonly detected in superficial spreading melanomas and melanomas that arise on nonchronically sun-damaged skin [5].

The two recognized major melanoma susceptibility genes, *CDKN2A,* located on chromosome 9p21.3, and *CDK4* both, are involved in controlling cell division. *CDKN2A* mutations are found in approximately 20% of tested melanoma families, while *CDK4* mutations have been found to date in only a few families. *CDKN2A* encodes for two gene products, p^{14ARF} (alternative reading frame) and p16 (also known as INK4A, inhibitor of kinase 4a), which regulate cell cycle entry at the G1 checkpoint and stabilize p53 expression [18, 22, 23]. When defective, p16 is unable to inactivate CDK4 and CDK6, which phosphorylate Rb, releasing the transcription factor E2F and leading to cell cycle progression [8].

The *PTEN* gene, located on chromosome 10, encodes a tumor suppressor protein and has also gained considerable attention as the understanding of melanoma pathogenesis has increased [24]. The negative regulation of cell interactions with the extracellular matrix could be the way PTEN phosphatase acts as a tumor suppressor. PTEN gene plays an essential role in human development. Mutations in *PTEN* are found in 10%-20% of primary melanomas and have also been associated with thyroid, breast, and prostate cancer [5,25]. *PTEN* encodes a negative regulator of extracellular growth signals that are transmitted via the phosphatidylinositol-3-kinase (PI3K)-AKT pathway [14]. Inactivation of *PTEN* allows signaling through the AKT pathway, which contributes to aberrant cell growth and escape from apoptosis [5].

3. Epidemiology

Generally, an individual's risk for developing melanoma depends on two groups of factors; intrinsic and extrinsic that is environmental. "Intrinsic" factors are generally an individual's family history and inherited genotype, while the most relevant environmental factor is sun exposure. Epidemiologic studies suggest that exposure to ultraviolet radiation (UVA and UVB) is one of the major contributors to the development of melanoma. UV radiation causes damage to the DNA of cells, typically thymine dimerization, which when unrepaired can create mutations in the cell's genes. When the cell divides, these mutations are propagated to new generations of cells. If the mutations occur in protooncogenes or tumor suppressor genes, the rate of mitosis in the mutation-bearing cells can become uncontrolled, leading to the formation of a tumor [26].

Cutaneous malignant melanoma is the most serious form of skin cancer. In general cutaneous melanoma most commonly affects adult Caucasians and is rarely observed before puberty. Melanoma may occur at any age, although children younger than age 10 years rarely develop a de novo melanoma. It was reported that in 2002 there were 53.600 new cases, and 7.400 deaths from cutaneous malignant melanoma in the United States. The incidence rate of MM has increased 4% per year since 1973 [27]. This epidemic of MM is also evident in other parts of the industrialized world, including Australia and southern Europe. It is predicted that the incidence of MM will continue to increase as a result of the continuing decrease in the concentration of stratospheric ozone and increasing leisure time for sunlight-related recreation, including sunbathing, which increases exposure to solar UV radiation [28].

3.1. Environmental factors

Sunlight and most particularly the ultraviolet spectrum of sunlight is the only environmental factor that has been compellingly implicated as a cause of melanoma [29].

Possible significant elements in determining risk include the intensity and duration of sun exposure, the age at which sun exposure occurs, and the degree of skin pigmentation. Exposure during childhood is a more important risk factor than exposure in adulthood [30, 31].

Individuals with blistering or peeling sunburns (especially in the first twenty years of life) have a significantly greater risk for melanoma. This does not mean that sunburn is the cause of melanoma. Instead it is merely statistically correlated [32].

Fair and red-headed people, individuals with multiple atypical nevi or dysplastic nevi and people born with giant congenital melanocytic nevi are at increased risk [33]. Melanoma incidence is 10–20-fold higher among the fair-skinned than the dark-skinned people. Among fair-skinned people, melanoma incidence generally increases with proximity to the equator (some exceptions occur, particularly in continental Europe, where the association is confounded by pigmentation). Fair-skinned migrants from high- (e.g. the UK) to low-latitude countries (e.g. Australia) have lower melanoma rates than native-born residents, and vice versa [29].

History of melanoma in melanoma-prone families due to mutations in some genes were found to greatly increase the risk of a person. (e.g. CDKN2A and CDK4). Patients with a history of melanoma are at risk of developing a second primary tumor [34, 35].

Looking at the geographical distribution of the incidence of malignant melanoma in Europe has increased in Northern Europe, especially Scandinavian countries (20.7 per 100.000 person-year). Incidence rates were lowest in Southern and Eastern Europe for both males and females, with rates between 5-10 per 100.000 person-year. mortality rates in studies conducted in Europe (5.1 per 100 000 person-years ranging from 2.5) was found to be different in a lot less. Death rates lower in women than men had been established. In the 1990s compared the incidence and mortality rates in southern and eastern Europe, northern and western Europes have been identified as the highest and lowest [36].

Between the years 1970-2009, a study conducted among young adults in the United States the incidence of cutaneous melanoma is increasing rapidly, especially among women. This high-risk population should be closely monitored constantly [37]. The incidence may be higher due to melanoma underreporting to cancer registries, particularly for tumors that are diagnosed and managed in the outpatient setting [38].

While melanoma accounts for roughly 4% of all skin cancers, it causes more than 75% of skin cancer deaths. Treatment of melanoma in its early stages provides the best opportunity for cure. In the United States, an estimated approximately 9.000 deaths will occur in 2012. Melanoma incidence has continued to increase worldwide, with the highest incidence in Australia and New Zealand. The most recent analysis of global cancer statistics for melanoma, from 2002, demonstrated a prevalence of 37.7 cases per 100.000 men and 29.4 cases per 100.000 women in Australia and New Zealand, compared with 6.4 cases per 100,000 men and 11.7 cases per 100.000 women in North America [39].

Differing melanoma incidence between males and females, and the tendency for females to develop excess melanin pigmentation during periods of hormonal stimulation such as pregnancy, has led to a number of studies investigating the role of pregnancy, oral contraceptives and hormone replacement therapy both as risk factors for melanoma and also as events that may affect prognosis. Cumulative data from publications on these topics provide no evidence that prior pregnancy is a risk factor for melanoma. Similarly, there is no evidence to indicate that oral contraceptive or hormone replacement use contributes to melanoma risk, nor that either factor alters the prognosis for those in whom melanoma has already been diagnosed [40, 41].

3.2. Occupation and melanoma

Airline crews, particularly pilots, have been recorded in a number of studies as having a higher-than-expected incidence of melanoma. It is suggested that this may be due to greater opportunities for recreational sun exposure during regulation breaks between flights in areas of the world with a high solar exposure [42].

A number of publications show conflicting results concerning the risk of melanoma developing after renal transplantation and the necessary immunosuppression. Studies from Sweden and the Netherlands show no increase in melanoma incidence over that expected in these countries [43], while studies from the USA and UK show a significantly increased risk, 3.6- and 8-fold higher for USA and UK patients, respectively. While some of these differences may relate to time frames of studies and changes in immunosuppressive regimes over time, further large long-term contemporary studies are required to determine the degree of increased cutaneous surveillance required for transplant patients [44].

3.3. Pesticide exposure

A case–control study comparing melanoma on the palms and soles in both the UK and Australia observed that melanoma patients reported greater exposure to pesticides than that reported by controls, and recently, an Italian case–control study has confirmed higher use of pesticides in a residential setting in melanoma patients compared with that in controls. Interpretation of these data is complex, as over the past decade there have been many regulatory changes in *Europe* regarding the range of pesticides available for domestic use. However, data from these studies indicate that questions regarding the type and frequency of pesticide use should be added to future case–control studies [43, 44].

3.4. Genetic factors

Xeroderma pigmentosum (XPD) is a genetic disorder with a mutation of the XPD gene leading to nucleotide excision repair defects. Patients experience 1000-fold greater risk of melanoma as they are unable to repair UV-induced DNA damage. The relative ability to repair DNA modifies the risk in the presence of other host factors such as age, poor tanning ability and dysplastic naevi. Two polymorphisms of the XPD gene are associated with a decreased risk of melanoma among women with five or more severe sunburns or high cumulative sun exposure.

Mutations of the melanocortin-1 receptor gene variants are more common among fair-skinned and red-haired people. Polymorphism of this gene is associated with melanoma. The risky factors are the phenotype of pigmentation of the individual, the presence of atypical naevi, >50 melanocytic naevi, high recreational and occupational sun exposures [45]. People with a past history of other types of skin cancer (basal cell carcinomas and squamous cell carcinomas) caused by high doses of solar UV radiation have threefold higher risks of melanoma than the average population [46].

3.5. Artificial light

Several forms of artificial light have been associated with the development of melanoma in some studies: fluorescent lighting and suntan beds and parlors. Although exposure to fluorescent lighting was hypothesized to increase risk for developing melanoma there have been no studies to support this idea. On the other hand, the use of tanning lamps and tanning parlors may increase risk for melanoma [47, 48].

3.6. Female sex hormones and melanoma

Differing melanoma incidence between males and females, and the tendency for females to develop excess melanin pigmentation during periods of hormonal stimulation like pregnancy, have led to a number of studies investigating the role of pregnancy, oral contraceptives and hormone replacement therapy both as risk factors for melanoma and also as events that may affect prognosis. Cumulative data from publications on these topics provide no evidence that prior pregnancy is a risk factor for melanoma. Similarly, there is no evidence to indicate that oral contraceptive or hormone replacement use contributes to melanoma risk, nor that either factor alters the prognosis for those in whom melanoma has already been diagnosed [41, 49, 50].

4. Clinical presentation

The most common sites that melanomas are found include the trunk (back) followed by the upper extremities, and head and neck for men; and the lower extremities followed by the back, upper extremities, and head and neck for women. Amelanotic melanoma and those resembling keratoses are particularly difficult to diagnose without a high index of suspicion. Acral melanoma is the most frequent form of melanoma among Asians, Africans, and other ethnic groups of color. Subungual melanoma (SM) is a distinctive variant of acral melanoma that most often involves the nail bed of the great toe or thumb. Clinical types include;

4.1. Lentigo malign melanoma

Lentigo maligna melanoma is one of the 4 main subtypes of invasive melanoma and constitutes 10 to 15% of cutaneous melanomas. Generally, patients with lentigo maligna are older than 40 years, with a mean age of 65 years. The peak incidence occurs in the seventh to eighth decades of life [51]. The incidence of lentigo maligna subtypes (in situ and invasive) appears to be rising in the United States [52].

Sir *John Hutchinson* first described lentigo maligna in 1890; the disease continues to be called *Hutchinson* melanotic freckle on occasion. The lesion has subsequently been characterized as malignant lentigo of elderly people, junctional nevus, and melanoma in situ. Most authors currently refer to it as lentigo maligna when it is confined to the epidermis and lentigo maligna melanoma when it violates the dermis [39].

Lentigo maligna melanoma has evolved from a lentigo maligna.They are usually found on chronically sun damaged skin such as the face and the forearms of the elderly people. The risk increases as the number of years spent in sunny districts increases, as well as with increased hours of exposure to sunlight. The incidence of melanoma is highest in Australia, where lentigo maligna accounts for 10-15% of all melanomas. Approximately 10-30% of all cutaneous melanoma arise in head and neck regions. The other risk factors for lentigo malign melanoma are large or giant congenital naevi, fair skin and history of severe sunburn [53].

Many authors consider lentigo maligna to be a preinvasive lesion induced by long-term cumulative ultraviolet injury. Conceptually, the term melanoma is used when atypical melanocytes invade the rich vascular and lymphatic networks of the dermis, thereby establishing metastatic potential [12, 51, 53].

Most malignant melanomas arise as superficial tumors confined to the epidermis, which is often known as horizontal growth. At some point, a stepwise accumulation of genetic abnormalities leads to proliferation and progression to the vertical growth phase, which leads to dermal and deeper involvement and subsequently nodal metastases [54].

Initially the lentigo maligna is a flat, brown or black, irregularly shaped lesion. These lesions will grow very slowly, over months or years, and there may be central regression while the peripheral margin continues to extend. In time, a raised central nodule will develop, indicating transition to the vertical growth phase [12, 51, 53, 54].

Differantial diagnosis of lentigo malign melanom are solar lentigo, pigmented actinic keratosis, seborrheic keratosis, common acquired nevi and dysplastic nevi [12].

Lentigo maligna is basically in situ melanoma and is characterized by epidermal atrophy, extensive solar, lentiginous, and back-to-back proliferation of melanoma cells. Only 5% of

http://dx.doi.org/10.5772/55304

patients with lentigo maligna progress to lentigo maligna melanoma, and it usually takes several years. Several methods of therapy can be used to treat lentigo maligna including cryotherapy, superficial radiation therapy, and surgical excision with mapping and modified *Mohs* surgery [55, 56].

Some imaging methods before proceeding to the treatment of lentigo maligna melanoma can be made. Especially, in patients with suspected metastatic disease, PET scan, CT scan and MR can be made to detect lymph node and internal organ metastases [57].

The treatment of the melanoma is as for other sites in that the margin of excision for tumours thinner than 2 mm is 1 cm minimum and for thicker tumours should be 2 to 3 cm. It is recognized, however, that on the face these margins may not be attainable without unacceptable cosmetic deficit. The surgery is also subject to the same constraints as described above for lentigo maligna, in that there is a high local recurrence rate of the in situ component [12, 58].

4.2. Superficial spreading melanoma

Superficial spreading melanoma is the most common type of cutaneous melanoma. It accounts for nearly 70% of cutaneous melanoma. The mean age at diagnosis is in the fifth decade. The commonest sites are the female leg and the male back (Figure 1), but every site may be affected [12].

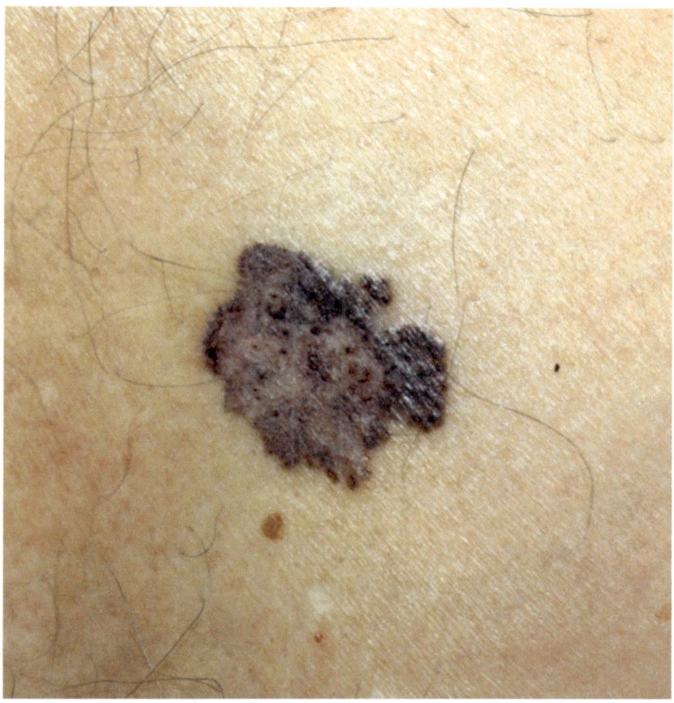

Figure 1. Superficial spreading melanoma with characteristic asymmetry, irregular borders.

Superficial spreading melanoma occurs in two phases: At first, superficial spreading melanoma grows horizontally on the skin surface (radial growth phase). The lesion constitutes as a slowly-enlarging flat area of discoloured skin. At second, superficial spreading melanoma becomes invasive, the melanoma cells cross the basal membrane of the epidermis. A rapidly-growing nodular melanoma can start to proliferate more deeply within the skin [59].

The main risk factors for superficial spreading melanoma are: age, previous invasive melanoma or melanoma in situ, nonmelanoma skin cancer, many melanocytic moles, multiple atypical naevi, family history of melanoma, fair skin and sun damage. Other risk factors include blue or green eyes and red or blond hair [60, 61].

Superficial spreading melanoma presents as a slowly growing or changing flat patch of discoloured skin. At first, it often resembles a mole or freckle. It becomes more distinctive in time, often growing over months to years or even decades before it is detected. Like other flat forms of cutaneous melanoma, it can be detected by the ABCDE rule: Asymmetry, border irregularity, colour variation, large diameter and evolving [51].

The characteristics of superficial spreading melanoma are larger size, irregular shape, variable pigmentation (colours may include light brown, dark brown, black, blue, grey) and irregular surface. It is generally greater than 6 mm in diameter. Irregular asymmetric borders are characteristic [12, 51, 59, 60].

Dermoscopy can be very helpful in distinguishing superficial spreading melanoma from other skin lesions, such as melanocytic naevi, solar lentigines, seborrhoeic keratoses and pigmented basal cell carcinoma (Figure 2) [62].

The initial treatment of a primary melanoma is to cut it out; the lesion should be completely excised with a 2-3 cm margin of normal tissue. Further treatment depends mainly on the *Breslow* thickness of the lesion. After initial excisional biopsy; the radial excision margins are measured clinically from the edge of the melanoma. Occasionally, the pathologist will report incomplete excision of the melanoma, despite wide margins. This means further surgery or radiotherapy will be recommended to ensure the tumour has been completely removed [12].

4.3. Acral lentiginous melanoma

Acral lentiginous melanoma (ALM) is a rare variant occuring exclusively on the sole, with the palm and subungual locations [7, 63]. Subungual melanomas often are mistaken for subungual hematomas (splinter hemorrhages). Subungual melanoma may show itself as a longitudinal pigmented band (melanonychia striata) within the nail plate. This variant of melanoma may also affect the oral and nasal mucosa and involve the anogenital area [64]. This is the least common subtype of melanoma in white people (2-8% of melanoma cases). It is the most common subtype of melanoma in dark skinned patients (ie, Afro-American, Asian, and Hispanic people), representing 29-72% of melanoma cases [65, 66]. Not all palmo-plantar melanomas are ALMs; a minority are superficial spreading or nodular melanomas [7]. ALM shows typically as an asymmetric, brown to black macule with variegations in colour and irregular borders [67]. They usually arise from the nail matrix or, less often, from the nail bed

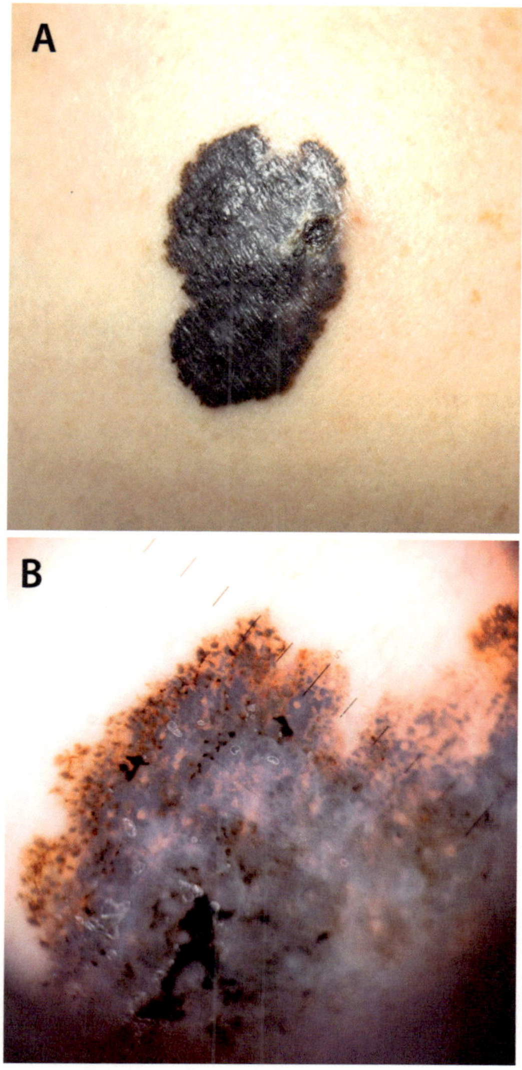

Figure 2. Macroscopic view of a superficial spreading melanoma (A), dermoscopic view characterized by blue-white veil (B).

or nail fold. ALM is similar to lentigo maligna melanoma in that an irregular pigmented macule is present for a long time [68].

Although the pathogenesis of ALM remains unknown, it has been theorized that the more intense and chronic trauma experienced in acral locations may be a predisposing factor [69].

ALM has key demographic and life-style differences to differentiate ALM from other melanoma subtypes: it occurs in an older patient population, and is associated with a lower number of common and atypical nevi, a lower incidence of familial melanoma, and a lower incidence of sunburn but a higher personal and family history of noncutaneous cancers [69].

There is often a delay in the diagnosis of ALM.The presence of invasion can be deceptive and may be present in entirely flat lesions [63]. The clinical differential diagnosis of ALM include a planter wart, which is common reason of delayed diagnosis, black heel (talon noir), lentigines, melanocytic nevi, tinea nigra, traumatic haemorrhage and tattoos such as by silver nitrate. Any growing, tender nodule, or an "ulcer" won't heal, on the sole of the foot, should give rise to concern that the lesion is a melanoma and biopsy should be considered [12, 70].

4.4. Subungual melanoma

Subungual melanoma, considered a variant of ALM, generally arises from the nail matrix. They are the most common on the thumb or great toe. It may manifest as diffuse nail discoloration, a longitidunal pigmented band (melanonychia striata) within the nail plate or growth in the nail bed. Furthermore, 20% of subungual malignant melanomas may present with amelanocytic lesions rather than melanonychia [7, 71].

Pigment spread to the proximal or lateral nail folds is termed the *Hutchinson* sign, which is a hallmark for subungual melanoma. Benign lesions that can mimic subungual melanoma include longitidunal melanonychia (Figure 3), subungual hematoma, pyogenic granuloma or even onychomycosis with pigmentation or hemorrhage [7]. Nonresponsiveness to antifungal drugs should prompt more thorough evaluation, including potential biopsy. Subungual melanomas are most commonly confused with traumatic hemorrhage. This process is persistent, often lasting for more than 1 year, but in contrast to melanoma the dark area moves forward with the nail plate, leaving a normal appearing proximal component. Moreover, melanoma usually shows distal tapering, with the proximal portion being wider. The possibility of melanoma should be considered for all pigmented nail bands in fair-skinned patients, especially if they are darkly pigmented and/or have a width >3mm [67]. If any pigmented lesion of the nail unit that is strongly suspected of being melanoma, an excisional or incisional biopsy of the affected area that includes nail matrix should be performed [70].

Overall 5 year survival is disproportionately poor (25-51%) compared to other histological subtypes [71].

4.5. Nodular melanoma

Nodular melanoma (NM) is the second most common subtype after superficial spreading melanoma and accounts for approximately 15% to 30% of all melanomas. It is diagnosed most frequently in patients in their sixth decade of life [63, 67]. NM tends to affect men more than women. The most common locations are head, neck, the trunk in men (Figure 4) and legs in women [70].

NM clinically lacks an apparent radial growth phase. It is more common for NM to begin de novo than to arise in a pre-existing nevus. Typically, it presents as a black or blue-black nodule, but 5 percent are amelanotic and often misdiagnosed clinically. Thus, any rapidly growing flesh-colored lesion that persists after 1 month or ulcerates or bleeds should prompt medical evaluation [7].

http://dx.doi.org/10.5772/55304

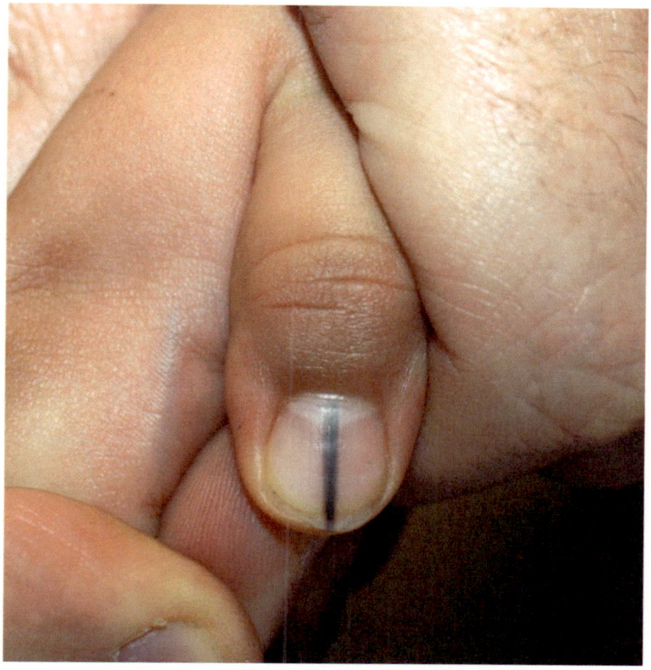

Figure 3. Longitidunal melanonychia: longitudinal pigmented band within the nail plate.

It tends to lack the typical ABCDE melanoma warning signs and thus, may elude early detection. Histologically, it is believed to lack a preceding radial or in situ growth phase. The prognosis of NM is generally worse than other forms of melanoma because there is involvement of the dermis and the lesion is in the "vertical growth phase" at the time of diagnosis.

The clinical differential diagnosis includes hemangioma, pyogenic granuloma, blue nevi, dermatofibroma, pigmented basal cell carcinoma, as well as other cutaneous neoplasms (Figure 5). As a general rule, a firm papule or nodule should never be subjected to any form of monitoring-biopsy if the diagnosis is in doubt [63, 70].

4.6. Mucosal melanoma

Mucosal melanoma is a rare cancer that is clearly distinct from its cutaneous counterpart in biology, clinical course, and prognosis. It accounts for 1.3%-1.4% of all melanomas; that they tend to occur near the mucocutaneous junctions of squamous and columnar epithelia. The most common sites are the head and neck region (conjuctival, intranasal, sinus and oral cavities), vulva, anorectal, or even urethral melanoma. Activating mutations in the c-KIT gene are detected in a significant number of patients with mucosal melanoma [72].

Sun exposure does not play a role in the pathogenesis of these lesions. Irritants and carcinogenic compounds in the air, such as tobacco smoke and formaldehyde, have been implicated in the devolepment of head and neck melanoma, the potential role of these compounds is not clear. The most common presenting trait of mucosal melanoma is the presence of extensive,

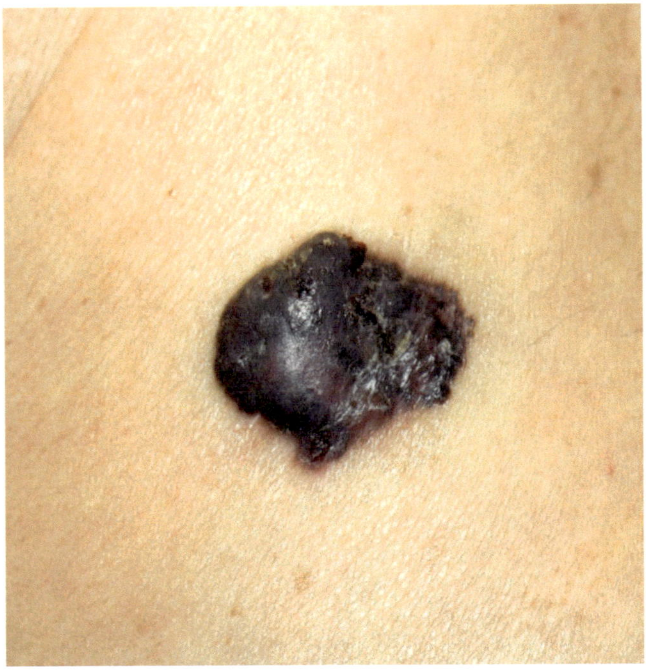

Figure 4. Nodular melanoma manifests as a dark brown-to-black dome-shaped nodule.

irreguler macular pigmentation. Most mucosal melanomas are lentiginous (mucosal lentiginous melanoma), followed in incidence by superficial spreading and nodular types.

Because of its hidden location and rich vascularization, mucosal melanoma usually presents at a more advanced stage and is therefore associated with a higher mortality rate than cutaneous melanoma [7, 12, 73].

4.7. Childhood melanomas

Childhood melanoma is very rare, particularly before puberty. Approximately 1% to 4% occur in patients younger than 20 years of age, and only 0.3 to 0.4% occur in pubertal children. After puberty the incidence of melanoma starts to rise slowly.

As in adults, childhood melanomas mainly affect the white population. Previous surveys have shown slight female predominance of melanoma in children. The most common primary tumor sites are the extremities, followed by trunk. Location in head and neck and trunk has been related to poor prognosis. The risk factors for melanoma in children are parallel those in adults. There are three known predispositions in childhood melanoma: congenital naevi, the atypical mole syndrome, familial melanoma and other family cancer syndromes such as xeroderma pigmentosum and retinoblastoma. Increasing age, UV exposure, and *Caucasian* background were also found to be important in pediatric melanoma.

http://dx.doi.org/10.5772/55304

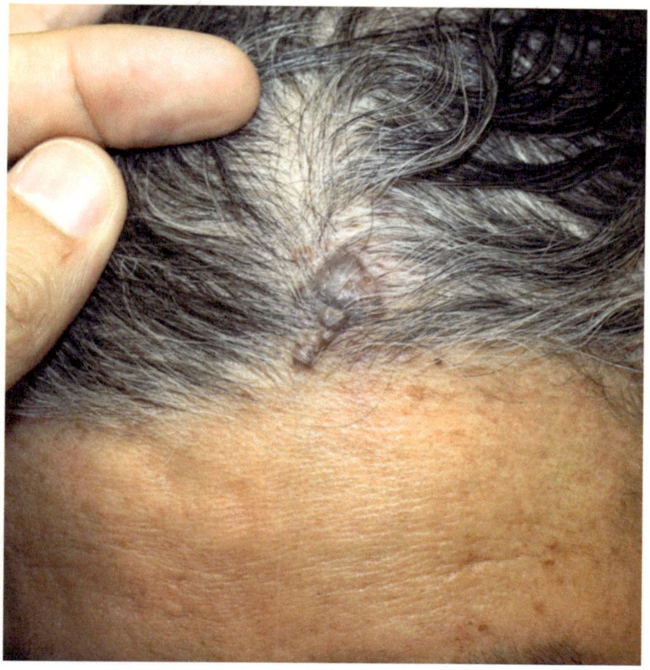

Figure 5. Nodular melanoma must be differentiated from pyogenic granuloma, blue nevi, and pigmented basal cell carcinoma.

Histologically, childhood melanomas may resemble those of adults, but small cell melanomas and melanomas with features of *Spitz* nevus are reported to be more common in this age group. The differentiation of melanoma from Spitz nevi with atypical features remains a major challenge for physicians.

Congenital melanoma is extremely rare; most melanomas in children are acquired after birth. In addition, a mother with visceral metastases can transfer tumor cells transplacentally, giving birth to a newborn with disseminated metastases.

Although, it seems that pediatric patients with melanoma may have a better prognosis than adults showing the same type of lesions, a number of children will still develop metastasis and die of their disease, especially when melanoma is diagnosed after puberty. Treatment follows the same rationale as in adults, with the aim of early detection and appropriate resection of the primary melanoma [12, 67, 68, 74, 75].

4.8. Unusual variants of melanoma

4.8.1. Desmoplastic-neurotropic melanoma

Desmoplastic melanoma (DM) is a rare sub-type melanoma that provokes a scar-like tissue reaction and is frequently associated with neurotropism. It makes up <1% of all melanomas. It is most commonly develops in older persons and has a male predominance 2:1. The head and neck are the most frequently involved sites, although lesions may develop on the trunk and extremities, palate, gingiva, lip, vulva, anus, and conjunctiva. DMs usually arise on the skin that has been severely damaged by long-standing sun exposure, although they have been reported to develop on skin damaged by ionizing radiation and in burn scars [63, 70, 76-78].

Its clinical features are similar to nonmelanoma (keratinocytic) skin cancer. It may occur in association with macular, lentigo maligna-type pigmentation, or it may present de novo as a firm, amelanotic nodule or scar. Fifty percent of the time it is amelanotic and may be mistaken for something as innocent as a scar. In the other 50% of cases it is associated with an overlying lentigo maligna or superficial spreading melanoma [64, 78]. Lack of pigmentation and clinical features more suggestive of keratinocytic skin cancer may result in delay in detection and thicker tumors at diagnosis [39].

Histologically, the tumor is composed of collections of spindle cells diffusely infiltrating the dermis and often the subcutis, associated with abundant stromal collagen. Many DMs are deeply invasive at diagnosis and have a tendency to infiltrate perineurally, otherwise called neurotropic melanoma. Neurotropism is related to increase the frequency of local recurrences. Also, it seems that neurotropism is associated with a signifiant decrease in survival in patients with DM. Occasionally, there are some lesions with prominent perineural invasion and no evidence of an intraepidermal component. These lesions are designated neurotropic melanoma. This seen particularly in lesions on the head and neck area, and may cause severe, relentless pain. In the recent studies, the percentage of desmoplastic melanomas with neurotropism ranged from 16.7 to 77.8% [7, 79].

The clinical differential diagnosis is broad, because these lesions often do not have features that suggest melanoma. Some of the clinical diagnoses that may be rendered include, scar, basal cell carcinoma, squamous cell carcinoma, fibroma, recurrent nevus, and metastatic carcinoma. Deep tissue samples are necessary to establish the diagnosis. The use of immunochemistry (testing for S100 antigen) is suggested as a useful tool in establishing the diagnosis. This sub-type of melanoma usually lacks any valuable dermoscopic features [12, 76-78].

Local recurrence is common, in 22% to 70% of cases, largely because of the tendency of DM to exhibit neurotropism. Although deeply invasive, DM is associated with lower metastatic rates than other sub-types of melanoma when matched for depth of invasion. When they metastasize, these tumors, unlike most melanomas may by-pass regional lymph nodes and spread hematogenously [7, 64, 70].

4.8.2. Angiotropic melanoma

Angiotropic melanoma is defined by cuffing of (close apposition to) the external surfaces of either blood microvessels or lymphatic channels by melanoma cells in a pericytic location without evidence of intravasation in at least two or more foci. Angiotropic metastasis is not synonymous with vascular invasion. The mechanism of angiotropism of melanoma is not clear. There may be a special affinity between the tumor cells and the vascular wall. Angiotropism is seen with greater frequency in melanomas also showing desmoplasia and neurotropism.

http://dx.doi.org/10.5772/55304

Angiotropism has been suggested to be a prognostic factor strongly predicting risk for metastasis of melanoma [77, 80].

4.8.3. Nevoid melanoma

Nevoid melanoma describes a heterogeneous grup of rare lesions that they may resemble a *Spitz* nevus or an acquired or congenital melanocytic nevus. Nevoid melanoma equally affects women and men and the mean age of diagnosis is 47 years. It occurs anywhere, but lower extremities and trunk are preferential sites. Clinically, this may correspond to a tan nodule typically greater than 1 cm in size, located on the trunk or proximal limbs of a young adult.

Histologically, the architectural pattern appears very similar to that of a compound or intradermal nevus with an overall symmetry, well-defined lateral margins, minimal or no intraepidermal pagetoid spread. Histological features mentioning melanoma include the absence of maturation of dermal tumor cells, slight cytological atypia with some mitoses in the dermal component [77, 78].

The differential diagnosis includes *Spitz* nevus, congenital melanocytic nevus, minimal-deviation melanoma, nodular melanoma and melanoma arising in a dermal nevus. Although only one study has reported a better biological behavior for this lesion, there is no evidence that nevoid melanoma has a better prognosis than ordinary melanoma [77, 78, 81].

4.8.4. Verrucous melanoma

Clinically, verrucous melanomas are usually small hyperkeratotic papules without areas of regression and mimic either a verruca, seborrheic keratosis, or a compound or congenital naevus. Some studies reported a greater frequency on the extremities of women, but this has not been confirmed. The back of men also frequently is involved. Histologically, the verrucous component is represented by marked epithelial hyperplasia. It has the same prognosis as conventional melanoma [68, 77, 82].

4.8.5. Small cell melanoma

Small cell melanoma describes a heterogeneous group of melanomas arising in different settings whose common denominator is a population of small cells. A first type, developing particularly in adults, is comprised of small cells with roundish, hyperchromatic nuclei, slight cytoplasm, and numerous mitoses resembling *Merkel*'s cells. A second variant of small cell melanoma has been described arising de novo in children and adolescent on the scalp or developing in a congenital nevus. A third type of small cell melanoma has been described in sun-damaged skin of old patients in the setting of solar melanocytic neoplasia or atypical lentiginous nevi.

A recent report suggested that a small-cell morphology in melanomas is significantly associated with positive sentinel lymph node involvement. Melanomas manifesting this morphology are invariably in vertical growth phase and have an aggressive course [77, 78, 83].

4.8.6. Spitzoid melanoma

Spitzoid melanoma is a rare sub-type of melanoma that resembles clinically and histologically a *Spitz* nevus. But it tends to be larger and have asymmetry and irregular coloration. It can occur in children but are more common in adults. Clinically, spitzoid melanomas are changing nodular lesions, often reaching 1 cm or more in diameter. The nodules are usually amelanotic. They can mimic hemangiomas, pyogenic granulomas, xanthogranulomas, or basal cell carcinomas. Less often, the lesions are pigmented and variegated in color. Nodular lesions can be crusted and ulcerated. The head and extremities are common sites.

Some spitzoid melanomas can evolve from a preexisting *Spitz* nevus, whereas other spitzoid melanomas can develop *de novo*. Differentiation between two of them is sometimes very difficult, especially in younger patients. The presence of mitoses, the nuclear and nucleolar pleomorphism of the cells, the asymmetric distribution of the pigment, and an inflammatory infiltrate with irregular disposition should prompt us to spitzoid melanoma.

The prognosis of spitzoid melanoma in adults is the same as that for other variants of melanoma of equal *Breslow* thickness [7, 77, 84].

4.8.7. Balloon cell melanoma

Balloon cell malignant melanoma (BCMM) is the rarest histological type of primary cutaneous melanoma and is composed of large, polyhedral, foamy cells with abundant cytoplasmic vacuoles. Clinically, lesions appear as soft, rubbery, or firm nodules with a polypoid or papillomatous contour whose cut surfaces are grayish white or brown. The differential diagnosis includes balloon cell change in benign nevi including blue nevi and common acquired nevi, with which balloon cell melanoma may coexist, as well as other malignant clear cell neoplasms. The presence of cytological atypia, nuclear pleomorphism, and mitoses are important for its distinction from the more common balloon-cell nevus. The expression of the usual immunohistochemical markers such as S-100 protein and HMB-54 helps to distinguish this lesion from other clear cell tumors of the skin. The prognosis is similar to that of other types of melanoma matched for depth of invasion [70, 77, 78, 85].

4.8.8. Clear cell sarcoma: Melanoma of soft parts

Clear-cell sarcoma (CCS) is a perplexing tumor considered by some authors as a soft tissue sarcoma derived from the neural crest and by others as an unusual variant or subtype of melanoma. CCS shows a predilection for the deep soft tissues of the lower extremities close to the tendon, fascia, or aponeuroses. The tumor presents as a slowly growing deep-seated mass in close relation with tendons and aponeuroses associated with tenderness and pain. It generally appears in young adults between the ages of 20 and 40 years.

Histologically, the tumor has a multilobulated apperance made by nests and fascicles of uniform plump spindle cells seperated by fine to coarse fibrous septa. CCS is an aggressive neoplasm with a poor prognosis similar to that of sarcomas, with a high rate of local recurrences and metastases to lymph nodes and lungs. Both survival and distant metastases seem to correlate with the tumor size more than the histological parameters [12, 67, 77, 86].

5. Differential diagnosis

Melanoma must be distinguished from a variety of several cutaneous and mucosal lesions. The differential diagnosis change according to the subtype of melanoma.

5.1. Superficial spreading melanoma

This is the most common type of melanoma. It is usually seen on sun-exposed areas, mostly on the lower extremities of women, and the upper back of men. Superficial spreading melanoma can present as an irregular macule with variation in color and texture. A papule or nodule may arise from the macule as the tumor progresses from radial to vertical growth. Superficial spreading melanoma can present de novo or within a preexisting nevus. Atypical nevus, melanocytic nevus, lentigo, seborrheic keratosis, *Spitz* nevus and superficial basal cell carcinoma must be distinguished from superficial spreading melanoma [87-89].

There are several features that can aid in distinguishing the common melanocytic nevus from melanoma. The "ABCD" rule, which has been expanded to the "ABCDE" rule, provides a helpful aid in the diagnosis of pigmented lesions:

A = Asymmetry

B = Border irregularity

C = Color variegation

D = Diameter greater than 6 mm/Difference

E = Elevation/Evolving

Atypical nevus may be misdiagnosed as melanoma because of focal or minimal pagetoid spread, confluence of cellular aggregates along the dermal-epidermal junction, prominent variation in nesting pattern, significant cytologic atypia, entrapment of nests of dermal nevus cells in the papillary dermis, and dense mononuclear cell infiltrates. On occasion, the distinction of atypical nevus from melanoma is exceedingly difficult. The discrimination of melanoma from atypical nevus is usually possible because of the larger size, greater asymmetry, disorder, cellularity, and cytologic atypia encountered in melanoma. Usually atypical nevus will maintain an overall symmetry, a nevic appearance as exemplified by fairly organized junctional nesting, a basilar proliferation of melanocytes that is still concentrated along the epidermal rete and with greater density toward the lower poles of the rete [89-91]. Melanoma may mimic seborrheic keratoses but also may arise within the seborrheic keratosis. *Spitz* nevus is usually domeshaped but may be soft or hard, sessile or pedunculated. It is usually pink to red but may be brown. In contrast to melanoma, the patient can usually pinpoint the onset of the tumor. The nevus may persist but more commonly evolves into an intradermal melanocytic nevus. Histologically, the spindle and epithelioid nevi are characterized by a cellular uniformity, as opposed to the pleomorphism that characterizes malignancy. The development of an apparent spindle and epithelioid nevi after puberty should be regarded with concern. [7, 92, 93].

5.2. Nodular melanoma

Nodular melanoma is the second common subtype of melanoma. It is mostly seen on trunk. This type grows rapidly and enlarge. Instead of arising from the nevus, nodular melanoma begins de novo. Pigmented nodules may be mistaken with blue nevus, pigmented *Spitz* nevus, pigmented basal cell carcinoma, squamous cell carcinoma, metastatic melanoma, *Kaposi* sarcoma and angiosarcoma. Amelanotic nodules can be mistaken with basal cell carcinoma, hemangioma, pyogenic granuloma and *Merkel* cell carcinoma.

Metastatic melanoma is often fairly monomorphous with little stromal response while nodular melanoma are often polymorphous and exhibits greater stromal response.

The blue nevus is a dark blue or black, hairless, dome-shaped nodule, ranging in diameter from a few millimeters to several centimeters, but usually measuring about 5 mm. Its color results from the *Tyndall* light-scattering effect of light reflected from deeply placed dermal pigment through the colloidal medium of the dermis. It most commonly occurs on the head and neck, dorsum of the hands and feet, and buttocks [87, 94, 95].

The keratoacanthoma, in common with the spindle and epithelioid nevus of *Spitz*, may produce the sudden onset of a rapidly growing pigmented nodule, a presentation similar to that of nodular melanoma. Several vascular lesions, including pyogenic granuloma, thrombosed hemangioma, and capillary aneurysm may also produce similar findings.

Kaposi's sarcoma usually appears as multiple violaceous plaques or nodules on the lower extremity. Older tumors tend to assume a reddish brown hue, a pigmentation produced by extravasated red blood cells, and may regress as new ones appear. Ulceration and hemorrhage are frequently seen [96-98].

When there is a doubt in clinically; dermoscopic images and histopathological examination must be done and the exact decision must be made by that.

5.3. Lentigo maligna and lentigo maligna melanoma

Lentigo maligna (LM) has a long radial growth phase that may progress to invasive lentigo malign melanoma. Some authors consider LM as in situ melanoma. Both subtypes are seen in older population. The most common locations are cheeks, nose, neck and scalp. It is related to cumulative sun exposure. Most cases presenting as LM remain in situ lesions; these lesions commonly occur in cosmetically sensitive areas on the head and neck and can abut critical anatomic sites, such as the eyelids, ears, nose, and lips [7, 87, 88]. In dermoscopic examination; hyperpigmented follicular opening, annular-granular pattern, pigmented rhomboidal structures, obliterated hair follicles are seen. Classical dermoscopic features of extrafacial melanoma (atypical pigment network, irregularly distributed globules, dots, streaks and pseudopods) and vertical growth phase-associated dermoscopic criteria (ulceration, blue papular areas and black structureless areas) can also be seen. [99-101].

Lentigo malign melanoma is confused with solar lentigo, ephelids, pigmented actinic keratosis, solar melanocytic hyperplasia, flat seborrheic keratosis and superficial pigmented basal cell carcinoma. Solar lentigines and its amount in excess are predisposed to LMM [7, 99]. Ephelids appear early in childhood. They darken in the summer in response to UV irradiation and lighten in the winter. LM develops irregularities of color, margins, and surface characteristics and enlarges progressively, unlike a common ephelid. Benign lentigines are usually tan to brown, flat, and oval, measuring 5 to 10 mm in diameter. Lentigines, whether benign or lentigo maligna, do not fade when shielded from light. Histologically, they are characterized by an increased number of normal dendritic melanocytes along the dermo-epidermal junction. The solar lentigo appears on sun-exposed surfaces during middle to late life, in common with lentigo maligna, and may closely resemble lentigo maligna [87, 94, 102].

5.4. Acral lentiginous melanoma

The frequency of this subtype in various ethnic groups is different from each other. ALM represents the most common type in darker-pigmented individuals (in blacks 60-72 %, in Asians 29-46 %). ALM is diagnosed in fifth or sixth decades. The most common sites for ALM are the soles, palms and subungual locations. Subungual melanoma may be first evident as a split nail, a swelling of part of the nail bed, an ulceration with a bloody crust, or a longitudinal black or brown streak in the nail bed. The great toe and thumb are most often affected. ALM may be confused with plantar wart, hematoma, palmoplantar nevus and pyogenic granuloma. Subungual melanoma must be differentiated from glomus tumor, hemorrhage, infection, onychomycosis, *Kaposi*'s sarcoma, *Bowen*'s disease, tinea nigra, melanosis and keratoacanthoma [103-106].

Acral lentiginous melanoma, the most common clinicohistologic type of acral melanoma, shares some histologic features with LMM but differs from LMM in its younger age at onset, its anatomic site, the absence of chronic sun exposure, and the greater depth of penetration at diagnosis [71].

The differential diagnosis for acral melanoma primarily includes lentigines and lentiginous melanocytic nevi of acral skin. Lentigines of acral skin usually do not exhibit the frequency of melanocytic proliferation or cytologic atypia that is typical of acral melanoma [7, 97].

5.5. Mucosal melanoma

Mucosal melanomas can arise on the head, neck, vulva, anorectal region and even urethra. With the exception of conjunctiva, patients present with delayed diagnosis. Because of a radial growth phase manifesting as a macular pigmentation any suspicious area in these locations must be biopsied. It can be mistaken with melanotic macules, amalgam tattoo, venous lake, *Kaposi*'s sarcoma, genital lentiginosis and atypical intraepidermal melanocytic proliferation [107-109].

Melanoma of the vulva is really mistaken with vulvar melanosis. Lesions of vulvar melanosis manifest irregular pigmentation with skip areas up to several centimeters in size, but the borders are regular and sharp. Histologically, vulvar melanosis manifests prominent basal layer keratinocytic pigmentation with either a normal or slightly increased density of cytologically basal melanocytes having prominent elongated dendrites. Pigmented *Bowen*'s disease manifests hyperkeratosis and comprises nested neoplastic keratinocytes containing melanin granules. Oral mucosal melanoma usually presents as an irregular brown patch or mass on the oral mucosa extending to the gingival margins. Esophageal and nasal mucosal melanomas are occult and present with obstruction or bleeding [108].

5.6. Desmoplastic melanoma

This subtype is rare and locally aggressive. Commonly it arise in the sixth or seventh decades. The sun-exposed head and neck regions are most effected parts. The lesions have typically have a firm, sclerotic, or indurated. One half of these melanomas are amelanotic. Desmoplastic melanoma is usually diagnosed at an advanced stage, because of the difficulty of its diagnosis.

Sclerosing blue nevus, desmoplastic *Spitz* nevus, dermatofibroma, leiomyosarcoma, malignant fibrous histiocytoma, atypical fibroxanthoma, spindle cell squamous cell carcinoma and, neurothekeoma should be thought in differential diagnosis. The desmoplastic *Spitz* nevus has an inverted wedge-shaped pattern, manifesting an admixture of spindle cells with delicate elongated nuclei and ganglion like cells. Early desmoplastic melanoma shows a infiltrative pattern of growth in which large atypical hyperchromatic spindle cells deform the dermal architecture and invade the dermis of hair follicles. The neurotropism and foci of chronic inflamation that exist in desmoplastic melanoma usually are absent in *Spitz* nevus [110-112].

5.7. Nevoid melanoma

Nevoid melanoma describes a heterogeneous group of rare lesions that histologically resembles benign nevus by their symmetry and apparent maturation with descent in the dermis. Histopathologic features include marked hyperchromasia of the nuclei of tumor cells, the presence of mitoses, and an expansile growth of the dermal cells with effacement of the adventitia in affected area. It may be seen as a papule or nodule that is more than 1 cm in diameter. Minimal deviation melanoma, nodular melanoma, and melanoma arising in dermal nevus must be considered in the differential diagnosis [51, 87].

5.8. Dermoscopy

Dermoscopy, dermatoscopy, epiluminescence microscopy, diascopy, surface microscopy and incident light microscopy are all synonym. Dermoscopy is a noninvasive technique in which a handheld device is used to examine a lesion through a film of liquid, mainly immersion oil, using nonpolarized light, or the lesion is examined under polarized light without a contact medium. Digital dermoscopy permits computerized digital dermoscopic images to be retrieved and examined at a later date so that comparisons could be made and changes detected over time. Confocal scanning laser microscopy and multispectral digital dermatoscopy are new imaging instruments used for early detection of cutaneous melanomas. Dermoscopy improves sensitivity up to 30% and specificity of melanoma diagnosis compared with clinical diagnosis. Morphologic features which are invisible to the naked eye, could be seen with the help of this technique.

Various diagnostic dermoscopic algorithms such as the ABCD rule, the seven-point checklist, pattern analysis, *Menzies* method, and CASH (color, architechture, symmetry, and homogeneity) have been developed for cutaneous melanoma.

Melanomas are multicolored in brown colors and other colors such as black, blue, and pink.

Usually a multicomponent pattern of three or more distinctive features can be seen. Atypical pigment network (Figure 6), irregular dots and globules, irregular streaks (pseudopods, radial streaming), irregular blotches, blue-white veil, abrupt cut-off of the trabeculae (Figure 7), regression structures (peppering), and atypical vascular architecture are common in invasive melanomas.

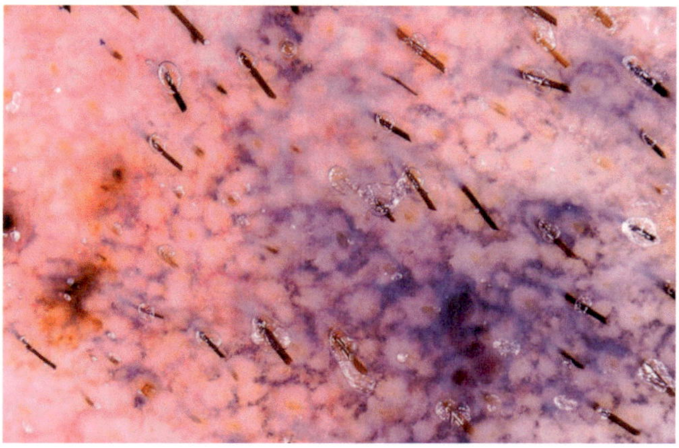

Figure 6. Irregular pigment network is seen (By the courtesy of Prof. Dr. Oya Oğuz).

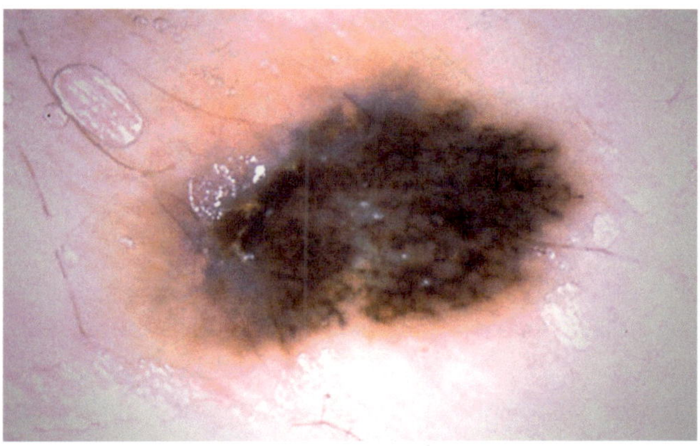

Figure 7. Notice the abrupt cut-off of the trabeculae (By the courtesy of Prof. Dr. Oya Oğuz).

Highly specific surface microscopic features of cutaneous malignant melanoma metastases are as follows: saccular pattern (red-blue, red-light brown, reddish-brownish-gray, blue-gray, dark brown to black); gray streaks surrounding the lesion (melanoma cell infarcts); red-brown globules irregular in size and color; polymorphic angiectatic base pattern and/or aneurysms; areas of polymorphic ectatic vessels running parallel to the skin surface; peripheral erythema (red corona); microscopic ovoid blood lakes; and homogeneous pattern (brown or blue to black) [12, 51, 87].

6. Histopathological examination

Essentially all melanomas begin as a proliferation of melanocytes initially confined to the epidermis. Increasing cytologic atypia of melanocytes accompanies the aberrant architectural appearance of melanomas. After the period of intraepidermal proliferation, there is often invasion of the papillary dermis, primarily as single cells and small aggregates of cells. *Breslow* thickness (in mm) of melanoma is one of the most important factors determining prognosis and theraphy. Melanomas with prominent invasive components may display polypoid morphologies.

6.1. Lentigomaligna/ Lentigomaligna Melanoma (LM/LMM)

Lentigomaligna (known as *Hutchinson*'s melanotic freckle) which is the precursor lesion of LMM is characterized by reproduction of atypical melanocytes mainly present in the basal layer of the epidermis. Tumor cells contain polygonal-shaped, pleomorphic irregularly hyperchromatic, angulated nuclei (Figure 8). In approximately 85% of cases of LM, multi-nucleated melanocytes are seen in the basal layer. These cells are named as "starburst giant cell". The presence of atypical melanocytes in the hair follicles and sweat duct epithelium is a characteristic feature but sometimes it may lead to difficulties in evaluation of tumor thickness [109, 113, 114]. Also there is effacement of rete ridges [115]. Due to chronically actinic damage, epidermis is usually atrophic and solar elastosis is seen in the dermal layer [116]. The upper part of the dermis usually contains melanophages and lymphocytes to a lesser extent [114]. If the lesion progresses, pagetoid spread may be observed within the epidermis [109]. When invasion occurs into the dermis, spindled cells and tumor cell pigmentation can be seen [117].

6.2. Superficial spreading melanoma

Superficial spreading melanoma is also known as pagetoid melanoma which characterized by a proliferation of atypical melanocytes singly and in nests in all layers of the epidermis [114]. Atypical melanocytes sometimes show "buckshot scatter" within the epidermis (Figure 9) [113]. The large tumor cells contain dark, atypical nuclei and abundant, pale cytoplasm [118]. The epidermis may have normal or hyperplastic appearance [119]. There is a continuous spread of tumor growth from one rete ridge to another [114]. If the tumor progresses to vertical growth phase, microinvasive tumor which contains nested and dispersed cells is seen within the dermis [109].

http://dx.doi.org/10.5772/55304

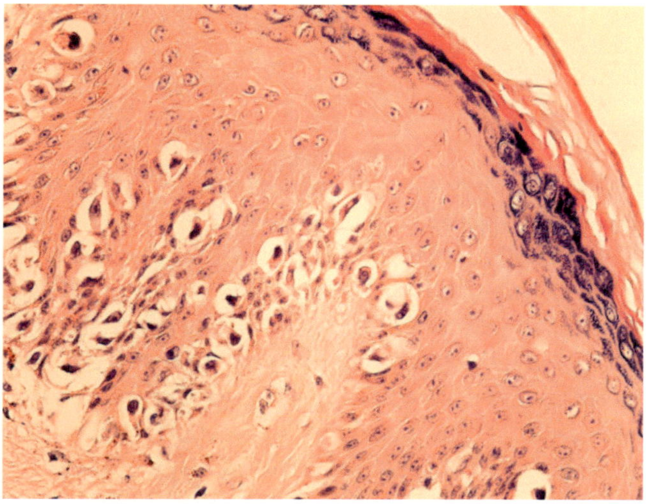

Figure 8. Lentigo maligna: in this in situ lesion, tumor cells are hyperchromatic and distributed in a lentiginous pattern (By the courtesy of Dr. Ahmet Cemil Kaur).

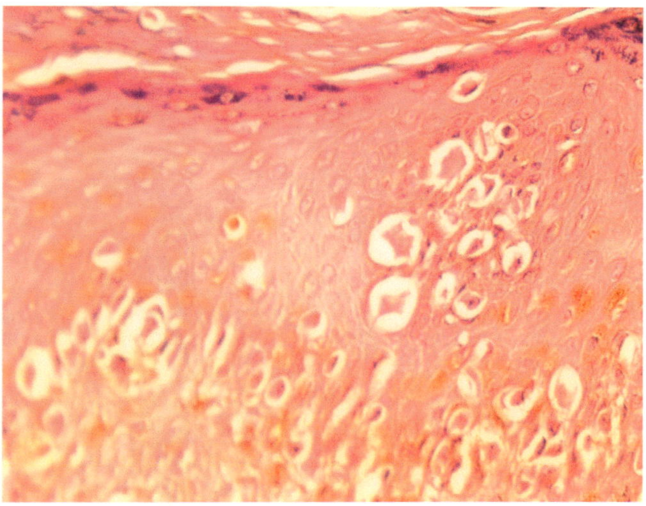

Figure 9. Superficial spreading melanoma: atypical melanocytes are scattered throughout the epidermis. Tumor cells compose cell groups at basal layer, The melanocytes have abundant eosinophilic cytoplasm and pleomorphic vesicular nuclei. Nucleoli are prominent (By the courtesy of Dr. Ahmet Cemil Kaur).

6.3. Nodular melanoma

Nodular melanoma has no concomitant or preexisting radial growth phase [109]. It grows vertically from the beginning and thus may invade the epidermis [113, 114]. Cellular features include a large nucleoli and frequent mitosis [118]. Epidermal melanocytic proliferation is so minimal which typically extending less than three epidermal ridges on both sides of tumor

[120]. The tumor mass contains small nests and aggregates of atypical melanocytes (Figure 10, 11, 12) [117].

6.4. Acral lentiginous melanoma

Histological changes are not fully clear in the early stages which may be seen irregular epidermal hyperplasia and dispersed, localized to the basal layer, atypical melanocytes [114]. Atypical cells proliferate as diffuse along to dermoepidermal junction in the radial growth phase. These cells create a lentiginous pattern by scattered severally [121]. Atypical melanocytes have marked nuclear atypia and also seen around the adnexal structures [109]. In contrast to acral nevi, pigment is seen throughout the stratum corneum [105]. Other changes in the epidermis include acanthosis and elongation of the rete ridges.Tumor infiltration of lymphocytes and tumor regression are common findings in ALM. Kim et al. observed that the frequencies of these findings are 75% and 25% of ALM cases, respectively [122]. The dermal invasive component is predominantly spindle cell type, but epitheloid or nevoid cells may be seen. The presence of small nevus cells may indicate a worse prognosis. Additionally lack of elastosis in dermis is prominent [105, 113, 123].

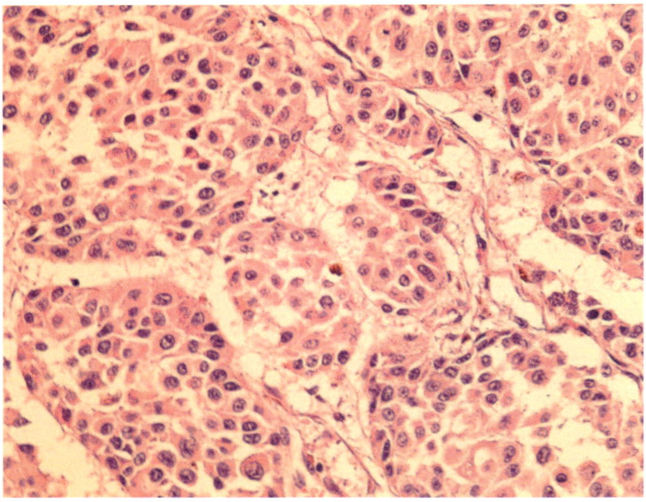

Figure 10. Nodular melanoma: characteristic melanoma morphology, the tumor is composed of cell groups (By the courtesy of Dr. Ahmet Cemil Kaur).

6.5. Desmoplastic melanoma

Desmoplastic melanoma is characterized by intensive atypical spindle-shape melanocytes within dense collagen bundles [124]. Tumor cells have hyperchromatic, elongated nuclei but usually no contain pigment in their cytoplasm [125, 126]. There are often nodular lymphocytic aggregates that are helpful in diagnosis [114, 127]. Perineural invasion has been reported in some studies. In a study by Lens et al., the percentage of desmoplastic melanoma with

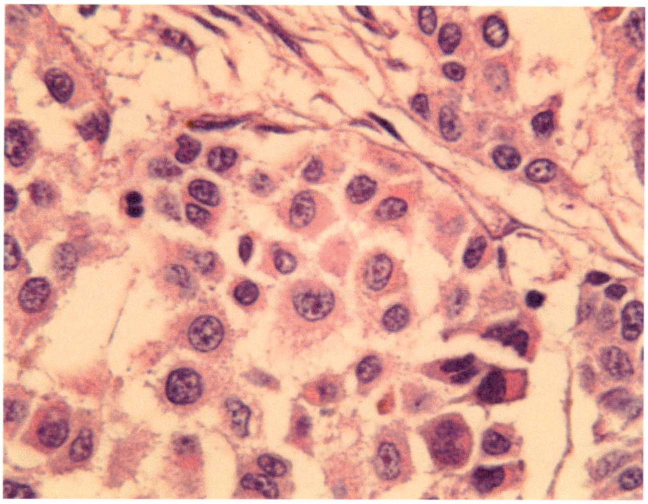

Figure 11. Nodular melanoma: close view, the tumor cells are pleomorphic with abundant cytoplasm, large vesicular nuclei and prominent nucleoli (By the courtesy of Dr. Ahmet Cemil Kaur).

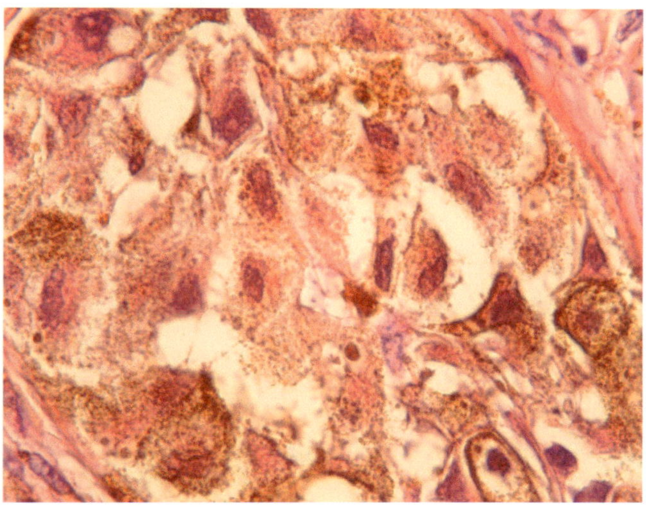

Figure 12. Nodular melanoma: in this example there is heavy melanin pigmentation (By the courtesy of Dr. Ahmet Cemil Kaur).

nuerotropism ranged from 16.7% to 77.8% [76]. *Kay* et al. reported that perineural invasion was 82% [128]. There are two subtypes of desmoplastic melanoma histologically; i) pure desmoplastic melanoma that characterized by desmoplasia through out the tumor, ii) and mixed desmoplastic melanoma that characterized by desmoplasia associated with non-desmoplastic invasive melanoma [129].

6.6. Minimal deviation melanoma

Minimal deviation melanoma is a variant of invasive melanoma that characterized by a nodule with minimal histologic deviation compared to ordinary nevus. It may be confined into the papillary dermis or may invade into the reticular dermis or beyond. This melanoma variant is divided into 6 subtypes according to cytological features (Spitz, halo-nevus like, pigmented spindle cell, desmoplastic, small cell and dermal variant). The average thickness is 3, 40 mm. The infiltration into the subcutaneous fat tissue is not often seen. Necrosis is absent while perineural invasion, mitoses and inflammation with desmoplasia can be seen. Mitotic activity is usually quite low [78, 114, 130, 131].

6.7. Special variants

6.7.1. Follicular melanoma

This rare variant is characterized by a deep-seated follicular structure in which atypical melanocytic cells extend downward along the follicular epithelium and mainly involves follicular unit as well as adjacent dermal layer [113, 132, 133].

6.7.2. Myxoid melanoma

Myxoid variant is characterized by spindle and stellate-shaped cells embedded within myxoid stroma. There is no cytoplasmic mucin in tumor cells. The stroma stains with *Alcian* blue. HMB-45 is showed less often while tumor cells strongly express S-100 protein [109, 113].

6.7.3. Balloon cell melanoma

The tumor is composed of large cells that exhibit an abundant quantity of clear or finely vacuolated cytoplasm. The other histopathological features include nuclear pleomorphism, mitotic activity, cytological atypia and necrosis [78, 113].

6.8. Histopathologic prognostic factors in melanoma

6.8.1. Tumor thickness

Primary tumor thickness is the most powerful predictor of melanoma survival. The *Breslow* thickness that is measured from the most superficial aspect of the granular cell layer to the deepest point of invasion of the tumor is the better prognostic indicator. If the tumor is ulcerated, the measurement should be from the base of the ulcer to the deepest dermal melanoma cell. In AJCC staging system (2001), the thickness thresholds have been revised as ≤1.0 mm, >1.0-2.0 mm, 2.1-4.0 mm and >4 mm. The *Breslow* thickness increases with increasing rate of sentinel lymph node involvement: 4% in melanoma smaller than 1.00 mm, 12% in melanoma 1.01 to 2.00 mm, 28% in melanoma 2.01 to 4.00 mm, and 44% in melanoma exceeding 4.00 mm.

Clark's level which is other tumor thickness indicator is described by *Clark* as anatomic levels in melanoma invasion (Table 1):

Level I	Melanomas confined to the
Level II	Penetration by melanomas into the papillary dermis
Level III	Tumor cells fill and expand the papillary dermis
Level IV	Spreading into the reticular dermis
Level V	Penetration into the subcutaneous fat

Table 1. *Clark* level of invasion

If Clark's level increases, the mean life span is decreased [119, 134-137].

6.8.2. Ulceration

Ulceration is defined as disappearance of the all layers of epidermis (including basement membrane), evidence of host response, and thinning, effacement or reactive hyperplasia of adjacent epidermis. The presence of ulceration shows that the lesion has aggressive feature. Ulceration due to trauma should be excluded. The presence of ulceration is associated with a higher risk of metastases. According to the presence or absence of ulceration, each T category is divided into two as "a" and "b" in the AJCC cutaneous melanoma classification 2009 (Table 2). This system classifies melanomas on the basis of their local, regional, and distant characteristics, as follows: [39, 51, 135, 138]

- Stage I and II - Localized primary melanoma
- Stage III - Metastasis to single regional lymph node basin (with or without in-transit metastases)
- Stage IV – Distant metastatic disease.

6.8.3. Mitotic rate

The mitotic rate is important prognostic indicator that is determined by the number of mitotic figures/1 mm^2 of tumor in the most mitotically active area. The increased mitotic activity is associated with poor prognosis [51, 114].

6.8.4. Satellite deposites

Microsatellites are defined as discrete tumor aggregates separated from the main body of the tumor mass. These deposites settled to 0,05 mm or more away from the main tumor mass are associated with an increased risk of local recurrence, regional lymph node metastases and diminished survival [114, 134].

Stage	T	N	M	Clinical-Histopathological Features
0	Tis	N0	M0	In situ melanoma (ıntraepithelial)
IA	T1a	N0	M0	≤1 mm without ulceration
IB	T1b	N0	M0	≤1 mm with ulceration
	T2a	N0	M0	1.01-2 mm without ulceration
IIA	T2b	N0	M0	1.01-2 mm with ulceration
	T3a	N0	M0	2.01-4 mm without ulceration
IIB	T3b	N0	M0	2.01-4 mm with ulceration
	T4a	N0	M0	4 mm without ulceration
IIC	T4b	N0	M0	"/>4 mm with ulceration
IIIA	T1-4a	N1a	M0	Single regional nodal micrometastasis, without ulceration
	T1-4a	N2a	M0	2-3 microscopic positive regional nodes, without ulceration
IIIB	T1-4b	N1a	M0	Single regional nodal micrometastasis, with ulceration
	T1-4b	N2a	M0	2-3 microscopic positive regional nodes, with ulceration
	T1-4a	N1b	M0	Single regional nodal macrometastasis, without ulceration
	T1-4a	N2b	M0	2-3 macroscopic regional nodes, without ulceration
	T1-4a/b	N2c	M0	In-transit met(s)/ satellite lesion(s) without metastatic lymph nodes
IIIC	T1-4b	N1b	M0	Single regional nodal macrometastasis, with ulceration
	T1-4b	N2b	M0	2-3 macroscopic regional nodes, with ulceration
	Any T	N3	M0	4 or more metastatic nodes, matted nodes, or in-transit met(s)/satellite lesion(s) with metastatic nodes
IV	Any T	Any N	Any M1	M1a: Distant skin, subcutaneous, or nodal mets with normal LDH levels M1b: Lung metastases with normal LDH M1c: All other visceral metastases with normal LDH or any distant metastasis with elevated LDH

T=tumor size; N=node status; M=metastasis; Ta=without ulceration; Tb=with ulceration;

Table 2. Cutaneous Melanoma Staging

6.8.5. Lymphocytic infiltration

Tumor-infiltrating lymphocytes are an important indicator of host immune response against melanoma. This response is divided into 3 categories and should be reported as brisk, non-brisk and absent. Although the presence of host inflammatory response is generally associated with a better prognosis in melanoma, there are also studies reporting that no significant correlation between lymphocytic infiltration and prognosis [119].

6.8.6. Histological subtype

There is no survival difference among three histological subtypes (superficial spreading, nodular and acral lentiginous) when these are corrected for thickness. But lentigo malign melanoma, particularly in woman, has been reported to have a better prognosis, independent of thickness [51].

6.8.7. Regression

Regression is caused by the interaction between melanoma cells and host immune system. Tumor tissue replaced with degenerative melanoma cells, melanophages, lymphocytic proliferation, haphazard fibrosis and telangiectasias. Complete regression is characterized by total absence of malignant melanoma cells in both dermis and epidermis. The correlation between regression and prognosis is still controversial [119, 134].

6.8.8. Vascular invasion

Tumor cells may invade the vessel lumen. It correlates with the development of in-transit metastases, when the presence of blood vessel and lymphatic invasion should be reported. Vascular invasion is associated with poor prognosis and decreased survival in thick cutaneous malignant melanomas [109, 119]. Angiogenesis is a distinct histological prognostic indicator that is defined as the increasing development of new blood vessels at the base of the tumor mass. Increasing angiogenesis is associated with thick tumors, surface ulceration, relapse and tumor related death [114].

6.9. Immunohistochemistry of melanoma

Immunohistochemical staining is often used for differentiate melanomas from tumors that they mimic in conventionally stained sections [139].

S-100 is a commonly used sensitive marker for melanoma. But its positivity appears some tumors such as nerve sheath and granular cell tumors and myoepitheliomas. Although its sensitivity is 97-100%, its specificity for melanocytic lesions is limited. The specificity of S-100 is ranged from 75% to 87%. S-100 A6 is one of the subtypes of S-100 protein, expressed in both benign and malignant melanocytic lesions. S-100 A6 has been reported that it is expressed in approximately 62-100% of metastatic and primary melanomas [140, 141].

HMB-45 is an antibody formed against the cytoplasmic premelanosomal glycoprotein gp100 while its sensitivity is lower than S-100, its specificity is greater. HMB-45 expression is maximal (77-100%) in primary melanomas. This rate is lower (58-83%) in patients with metastatic lesions [139].

Melan-A, also known as melanoma antigen recognized by T cells-1 (MART-1), is an important melanocytic marker. Sensitivity and specificity of Melan-A are similar to HMB-45 that ranged from 75-92% and 95-100%, respectively. It is less positive in lesions with metastatic melanomas than primary melanoma [139].

MIB-1, also known as Ki-67, is a proliferation marker that is expressed by proliferating cells. It provides guidance about presence or absence of "maturation". MIB-1 has an important role in distinguishing between melanocytic nevi and melanoma. While less than 5% of nuclei is positive in melanocytic nevi, this ratio is greater (25% or more) in melanoma [114, 141].

Tyrosinase is an enzyme that plays a role in hydroxylation of tyrosine in the synthesis of melanin. Its sensitivity for melanoma is slightly better than HMB-45 at 84-94%. The sensitivity is reduced in advanced diseases and metastatic lesions (79-93%). The specificity is very high for melanoma (97-100%) [139].

Microphthalmic transcription factor (MITF) is expressed in most benign melanocytic nevi and melanomas. Nuclear staining occurs with MITF unlike cytoplasmic markers. MITF expression has been reported in 81-100% of melanomas [51, 113].

There are also numerous immunohistochemical markers such as epithelial markers (keratin, EMA, CEA), histiocytic markers (eg. CD68, Mac 378, alpha-1 antitrypsin), Bcl-2, Cyclin D1, p16, CD40, CD44, melanoma cell adhesion molecule (Mel-CAM) [114].

7. Treatment

7.1. Staging workup

Any lesion that is clinically suspicious for melanoma should ideally undergo an complete elliptical excisional biopsy with narrow margins (such as 2 mm) [12]. Wide excisions should be avoided for obtaining an accurate result of the subsequent sentinel lymph node biopsy, if necessary. Examination of the entire pigmented lesion allows for the greatest chance of accurate diagnosis and also for the measurement of *Breslow* thickness and the assessment of other prognostic factors [142]. Although there is evidence that an incisional biopsy does not adversely affect survival, this approach should be an exception and reserved for cases in which the tumor is too large to be excised, or when it is not practical to perform an excision. If the lesion is large or located on certain anatomical sites such as palm/sole, digit, face or ear, a full-thickness incisional biopsy can be performed, reaching to the adipose tissue. This biopsy should be obtained from the most elevated or darkest area of the lesion, although there is not always a correlation between clinical appearance and the thickest part of the lesion. If initial biospy confirms melanoma with subtotal excision and if there is significant amount of residual lesion, a narrow margined re-excision should be immediately made, to evaluate if the patient is a candidate for sentinel lymph node biopsy.

Although cutaneous melanoma is rare in children and young adults, the incidence is rising annually in this population. Staging work up is almost similar, in children and adults [143].

7.2. Evaluation for regional metastasis

7.2.1. *Macroscopic metastases*

First step should always be history taking and physical examination. A careful lymph node examination of the whole body should be made, particulary the regions close to the site of the primary lesion. Also because of the aberrant lymphatic drainage pathways to unexpected nodal basins and to interval nodes between the primary site and expected regional nodal basin, a search for clinically detectable nodal disease in unexpected locations is crucial. If there is a palpable lymph node during physical examination, first a fine needle aspiration biopsy should be performed to make a histological confirmation. If the result of the fine needle aspiration is inconclusive, an excisional biospy can be made. For the detection small nodal metastases, best noninvasive methods seem to be ultrasound imaging and positron emission tomography, with sensitivity and specificity being lower than tissue diagnosis [144].

7.2.2. *Microscopic metastases*

Sentinel lymph node biopsy (SLNB) as elective lymph node dissection (ELND) does not offer a survival advantage to melanoma patients, a new approach, SLNB has become the choice of biopsy type. *Morton* developed sentinel node biopsy as a means of ensuring that the node biopsied was the one most likely to be the first draining lymph node. This technique was widely adopted although the first randomized clinical trial to evaluate it was only published in 2006. In SLNB, lymphoscintigraphy is used to identify the lymphatic drainage pattern from the site of the primary melanoma, by injecting radiolabelled colloid and/or blue dye at the site of the primary melanoma [145]. The tracer/dye is concentrated in the sentinel node and is detected using a hand-held gamma probe (neoprobe) and examination by naked eye for the blue stained node. Sometimes there is more than one sentinel node and sometimes these sentinel nodes are in different lymph node basins. The node is removed and subjected to pathological examination using immunohistochemistry (S100 and HMB-45) The surgical technique must be learnt and false-negative results are more common in trainees, so an experienced medical team is vital. The pathological examination of the nodes is also a skilled procedure; naevus cells may be seen, for example, in the subcapsular area of the node and must be distinguished from melanoma cells. The likelihood of a positive SLNB result is correlated with *Breslow* thickness. Use of SLNB to stage patients for trials of adjuvant therapies would appear reasonable but the patient should be aware that the risk of positivity is low. In patients with melanoma of *Breslow* thickness from 1.5 to 4.0 mm, the risk of positive SLNBs is significantly higher at 23% [146]. The value of SLNB in patients with tumours of *Breslow* thickness 4 mm or thicker is questionable (if the intent is therapeutic as well as being a staging tool) because the risk of haematogenous spread is so high. At present SLNB is of proven staging value but of no established therapeutic value. Its use in identifying patients for adjuvant therapies means that it will continue to be used, but its role must be evaluated in the long term.

7.3. Evaluation for distant metastasis

For the evaluation of distant metastases, a thorough examination of the neurologic, psychiatric, musculoskeletal, skin, lymphatic, endocrine, cardiovascular, and respiratory systems is necessary. Patients with newly diagnosed melanoma require a complete cutaneous and physical examination with particular attention to lymphadenopathy and hepatomegaly, and a baseline chest radiograph. If the latter examinations fail to detect any evidence of metastatic disease and the patient has no other symptoms or signs, no further laboratory evaluation is indicated. Current imaging technics like computed tomography, magnetic resonance imaging, PET, chest X-ray and laboratory tests like LDH are not routinely indicated as their sensitivity ans specificity are low. According to current guidelines, no additional work up is necessary in stage 0 and 1A, optional chest X-ray may be performed in stage 1B and 2, optional chest X-ray and LDH for stage 3 and chest X-ray and/or chest CT and LDH for stage 4 can be done [146].

7.4. Treatment of primary melanoma

The Standard treatment for primary cutaneous melanoma is wide local excision. The aim of wide excision is to reach histopathologically confirmed tumor-free margins, as well as preventing local recurrence. Recommended clinical margins around the residual lesion or biopsy scar for melanoma in situ, non lentigo maligna pattern, is 0.5 to 1 cm; for melanoma <1 mm *Breslow* depth a 1-cm margin; for melanoma 1 to 2 mm a 1- to 2-cm margin as anatomically possible; for melanoma ≥ 2 mm a 2-cm margin. lesion excision at special sites, such as the digits, soles, ears, vagina or anus, also requires individual surgical and functional consideration. For subungal melanoma, partial or complete amputation of the digit is the choice of treatment.

Lentigo maligna and lentigo maligna melanoma have high potential for sub-clinical peripheral extension, as their clinical margins are usually poorly defined and obscured by background photo-damage. For lentigo maligna melanoma, the probability of a macular invasive desmoplastic component is increased. Thus, standard surgical safety margins recommended, are often insufficient for these two subtypes [12, 51].

7.5. Treatment of regional metastasis

7.5.1. Macrometastatic nodal disease

One of the main causes of melanoma-related morbidity with an important negative effect on quality of life is the poor control of the nodal disease. Therefore, current standard of therapy for microscopic or macroscopic melanoma in lymph nodes is complete dissection of the node in the involved regional basin. According to the current guidelines, adequate lymphadenectomy is described as at least 10 nodes in the groin region, 15 lymph nodes in the axillary region and 15 lymph nodes in the neck area. There are also some complications, leading to significant morbidity, of the lymph node dissection, like wound infection, delayed wound healing, seroma, lymphedema and nerve damage. In the case of regional metastatic melanoma, complete lymph node dissection is associated with long-term survival rates [87].

7.5.2. Micrometastatic nodal disease

For micrometastatic disease, elective lymph node dissection was the procedure of choice, historically. It is the dissection of regional lypmh nodes draining the site of a primary cutaneous melanoma, with no clinically palpable lymph nodes or overt metastatic disease. With today's knowledge, according to multiple prospective randomized-controlled trials, survival rates of the patients undergoing elective lymph node dissection were found to be no higher than other patients. Thus there is no role for elective lypmh node dissection today, especially considering its significant morbidity and the availability of sentinel lypmh node biopsy [144]. For the identification of micrometastatic nodal disease, sentinel node biopsy is the tool of choice. The only handicap of sentinel node biopsy is that, it can not be classified as therapeutic yet. If the result of the sentinel lymph node biopsy returns as positive, always a complete lymph node dissection should be performed. According to current trials of investigations, immediate complete lymph node dissection has a higher survival rate than delayed dissection.

7.5.3. Adjuvant therapy

Adjuvant therapy is usually given after surgical resection of the primary lesion. It is preferred in patients with increased relapse risk. When thickness of the primary lesion is higher than 4 mm or when there is nodal involvement, adjuvant therapy is necessary. Up to now, interferon-α2b (IFN- α2b) is the only form of adjuvant therapy, which is approved by U.S. Food and Drug Administration. It has been shown that interferon-α2b improves disease-free survival for stage 2B and 3 melanoma, and it also improves overall survival. Interferon-α2b is used in high doses. There are two phases of treatment with interferon, first phase is induction phase. During induction, 20 million units per square meter of body surface area per day, are given intravenously, 5 days a week, for 4 weeks. After this high dose period, during the maintenance period, 10 million units per square meter per day, given subcutaneously three times a week for 48 weeks. During or after interferon treatment, autoantibodies like antithyroid, anti-nuclear, anti-DNA, anticardiolipin autoantibodies may appear in blood tests of the patients and some autoimmune diseases may develop. Both autoantibody positivity and development of autoimmune diseases are associated with increased survival in those patients. High dose interferon treatment may cause flu-like symptoms, fatigue, malaise, fever, nausea and headache, depression, elevated levels of transaminases and myelosupression [147].

Melanoma vaccines: Vaccines stimulate specific immune response against melanoma-associated antigens. They can be of autologous, allogenic or peptide type and also immunologic adjuvants like bacille Calmette-Guérin or DETOX are added. Target of the vacines can be autologous tumor cells, allogenic melanoma cells, or more specifically heat shock proteins and T cell defined antigens glycoprotein 100, tyrosinase, MART-1. Up to now, none of the trials showed increased survival for the patients using these vaccines but more research on this area should be done.

7.5.4. Satellite metastases

For localized disease, limited to one extremity only, first choice of treatment should ideally be surgical excision with clear margins if possible. But in case of multiple lesions, chance of performing an ideal excision may be low, so in that case, isolated limb perfusion can be considered. It is a simple and less invasive, yet more effective treatment. Main idea about isolated limb perfusion is giving high doses of chemotherapeutic agents locally, to avoid systemic toxicity, and obtain more therapeutic effect. The technique of this method involves perfusing an isolated arm or leg, in a hyperthermic environment, with cytotoxic agents. Conventinally chemotherapeutic agent used in this procedure is melphalan. Approximately in half of the patients, complete disappearance of the lesion is observed. Although systemic side effects of this method is fairly less, when compared to conventinal chemotherapy, local side effects can be serious. Significant tissue damage due to high concentrations of cytotoxic agent can be seen. Compartment syndrome is one of the most severe morbidities. Advanced age and patients with serious co-morbidities are usually not preferred for this type of treatment. A new approach is isolated limb infusion, which is a less invasive method, for appliance on patients with older age or worse general health conditions. Isolated limb infusion can be done with melphalan and actinomycin D [51, 67].

7.6. Treatment of distant or disseminated metastasis

In case of stage 4 melanoma, with distant metastasis, mean survival is 6 to 8 months and there is currently no effective systemic treatment, to increase survival rate. For this reason, main treatment goal is the palliation of symptoms. For the patients with increased age and serious comorbidities, observation and conservative treatment may also be the option of choice [146]. If there are symptomatic visceral metastasis, surgical excision to perform metastasectomy can be tried. Also excision of skin metastasis or lymph node metastasis may improve the locoregional control of the disease and may help to decrease morbidity.

In one case report [148], a 44-year-old *Caucasian* woman who underwent extensive surgical resection of a melanoma on the right side of her scalp, came with a new metastasis, a large nodule in her right cheek. The patient underwent two sessions of electrochemotherapy with intravenous injections of bleomycin, as neoadjuvant treatment permitting conservative surgery three months later. In this case, electrochemotherapy offers the option of more conservative surgery and an improved cosmetic effect with complete local tumor control.

Although melanoma is known to be radiotherapy resistant, for brain metastasis, spinal cord compression and painful bone metastasis, local radiation can be used.

7.7. Radiation therapy

Radiation therapy plays a role in the management of primary cutaneous melanoma in definitive, adjuvant, and palliative settings. The role for radiation therapy in early stage primary melanom is limited as the treatment is adequate excision. However desmoplastic melanoma and those with neurotropism invasion are exceptions, due to frequent local recurrence [149]. The greatest controversy regarding radiotherapy lies with its use in stage III disease, particularly as postoperative treatment after lymph node dissection. A recently completed randomized trial confirmed the benefit of adjuvant radiotherapy in improvement in nodal field control after nodal dissection for patients who are at moderate to high risk for regional relapse [150].

For primary melanoma, adequate surgery is usually the best option for local control and cure. Factors often considered indicative of the need for adjuvant radiation therapy include primary site in the head and neck region, close or positive margins not amenable to further excision, lymphatic space invasion, multiple recurrences, and desmoplastic neurotropic growth [149]. Apart from its use in an adjuvant setting, radiation therapy has been used as the definitive treatment of primary melanomas, locally advanced acral lentiginous melanoma, and as a substitute for wide excision after limited excision.

Radiation therapy has a well-established role in patients with metastatic melanoma Symptoms of pressure, mass effect, and bleeding from metastases in a variety of locations may benefit from palliative radiation. The development of stereotactic techniques has improved the efficacy of radiation for brain metastases. Expansion of this methodology to stereotactic body radiation metastases has the potential to improve further palliation of unresectable metastases.

7.8. Systemic therapies

7.8.1. Chemotherapy

For systemic chemotherapy, first line chemotherapeutic agent is dacarbazine, an alkylating agent. It is an U.S. Food and Drug Administration (FDA) approved chemotherapy drug for metastatic melanoma. It is thought to be the most effective single agent therapy. Approximately 10 to 20% of the patients response to treatment and the mean duration of response is 4 to 6 months. Dose of the treatment does not affect the response rate. Major side effects of dacarbazine are nausea and vomiting. Temozolomide is also an alkylating agent. This chemotherapeutic agent can also be used orally. Another advantage is that, temozolomide can cross the blood-brain barrier. Thus for patients with central nervous system involvement, temozolomide can be preferred. According to a randomized phase 3 study, its efficacy is equal to dacarbazine. For metastatic melanoma to brain, a combination of temozolomide and thalidomide, along with radiation, can be benefical. For dacarbazine, increased response rates are reported, when combined with other cytotoxic agents like cisplatin, vinblastine, carmustine or tamoxifen [144].

7.8.2. Immunotherapy

Among immunotherapeutic agents, interleukin 2 (IL-2) is the only agent, which has an approval form FDA. Overall response rate of this agent is 16%, but a durable response rate is 5 to 8%. Approximately the time for the duration of response is 9 months. Of the 28% of the patients with metastatic melanoma who responded to IL-2 treatment, no progression was observed at a follow-up period of 62 months. Also patients who responded longer than 30 months, did not show any sign of relapse afterwards. On the other hand, there are some important side effects of IL-2 treatment. Most common side effect of IL-2 is hypotension. It can also cause capillary leak syndrome, supraventricular tachycardia, transient renal insufficiency, respiratory distress, increased susceptibility to infections. There are also newer investigations about combining IL-2 with tumor-infiltrating lymphocytes and lymphokine activated killer cells. These immunologically active cells are considered to be helpful in transferring and adoptive immune force, to generate an antitumor effect.

In a case study [151], patient with cutaneous metastasis with significant comorbidities, including advanced age, anticoagulation for a metallic valve, chronic anemia, macular degeneration, and history of hematopoietic malignancy (high-grade lymphoma, *Waldenstrom* macroglobulinemia) was treated with a novel method. 1% gentian violet was applied to the wounds, and the patient was instructed to apply gentian violet and imiquimod to the base of the lesions daily. This was accompanied by a brisk inflammatory response. At the time of reexamination, 4 months after the procedure, no clinical recurrence was noted. This method can be useful when surgery is not an option.

In another case [152], 82-year-old man who presented with rapidly progressing cutaneous melanoma metastases, together with inguinal lymph nodes and bilateral pulmonary involvement, treated with topical immunotherapy with diphencyclopropenone (DPCP) in aqueous cream weekly to elicit moderate contact hypersensitivity. Larger lesions were also treated with intralesional 5-fluorouracil (50 mg/mL). One month later, cutaneous metastases began to regress, and during the following 4 months his inguinal lymphadenopathy and pulmonary lesions disappeared. He remains clinically disease free 18 months after his metastases began to regress. This can show the potential for some patients to overcome even widespread and extensive disease, presumably via immune-mediated regression, and raises the possibility that topical immunotherapy may play a role even in patients with bulky disease.

7.8.3. Biochemotherapy

Biochemotherapy alone has not shown any increase in overall survival rate, but when compared to other systemic chemotherapeutic agents like dacarbazine, or interferon, vaccines, IL-2, it can show better results.

7.8.4. Novel therapies

About the etiopathology of intrinsic resistance of malignant melanoma to chemotherapy, the anti-apoptotic protein B-cell lymphoma 2 (Bcl-2) is found to play an important role. A new antisense Bcl-2 oligonucleotide, Oblimersen, is targeting Bcl-2 messenger RNA selectively and this leads to the degradation of the Bcl-1, thus decreasing the levels of Bcl-2 in the body. Oblimersen can also be used in combination with conventional systemic chemotherapeutic agents, like dacarbazine.

Also in two-thirds of melanomas, there is a mutation in B-raf gene. A RAF inhibitor, Sorafenib, inhibits both B-raf and C-raf, and also used orally. Since the evaluation of sorafenib, a new generation of BRAF inhibitors has been developed. These drugs show higher potency against mutated BRAF and have fewer off-target effects; the list of those currently under preclinical investigation includes SB590885, dabrafenib (GSK2118436), AZ628, XL281, GDC-0879, and vemurafenib (RG704, PLX4032/4720) [153]. PLX4032 (and its analogue PLX4720) are adenosine triphosphate (ATP)-competitive RAF inhibitors (wild-type BRAF 50% inhibitory concentration [IC50]-100 nmol/L, mutated BRAF IC50-31 nmol/L) that selectively inhibit growth in melanoma cell lines harboring the BRAF V600E mutation in both in vitro and in vivo mouse xenograft models [154].

Much of the foundation for the development of these treatments is the realisation that melanoma growth and progression is driven by somatic activating mutations in signalling molecules such as BRAF, KIT, NRAS and GNAQ/GNA11 [147]. Active drugs targeting BRAF and KIT are available and and the anti-CTLA4 antibody ipilimumab has shown an overall survival benefit and the possibility of prolonged disease control in the metastatic setting.

Although there are many phase III trials in progress, about treatment of metastatic melanoma, up to now, no curative adjuvant or systemic therapies have been approved for stage 4 metastatic melanoma. Among these treatments some may have serious side effects. According to one study [7], patients with metastatic melanoma are treated with the selective BRAF inhibitor, dabrafenib. Keratinocyte proliferation is characteristic of BRAF inhibitor induced cutaneous toxicities, and the spectrum of lesions ranges from benign seborrhoeic keratoses, *Grover*'s disease and plantar hyperkeratosis through to verrucal keratoses of undetermined prognosis and malignant well differentiated SCCs.

In the future of metastatic melanoma treatment, molecular profiling of patient tumors will play an important role in the part of therapy selection for medical oncologists. Recent preclinical studies shows that inhibitors of BRAF paradoxically activate MAPK signaling in tumors that lack activating BRAF mutations [153]. Reports from six independent groups have shown that BRAF inhibition activates MAPK in cell lines with NRAS and KRAS mutations, as well as those cell lines where the MAPK pathway is activated through other oncogenes such as HER2. Studies showed that although vemurafenib and other BRAF inhibitors were able to profoundly inhibit the activity of BRAF V600E-containing complexes in melanoma cells, they instead promoted the activity of CRAF-CRAF dimers in cells with RAS mutations, leading in turn to MEK activation. There is also evidence that PLX4032 increases the invasive potential of NRAS-mutated melanoma cells through the activation of ERK and FAK signaling. Additional studies demonstrated that BRAF inhibitors may even contribute to the progression of NRAS-mutated melanomas in part by suppressing apoptosis through the modulation of Mcl-1 expression.

According to one study [155], data of 97 patients with melanoma show substantial clinical activity of trametinib, MEK inhibitor. Differences in response rates during this treatment, according to mutations indicate the importance of mutational analyses.

These studies are extremely important for approaching the development of new cancer therapies as they indicate that simple empiric evaluation of novel cancer therapeutics in patients could be associated with adverse outcomes. Instead they affirm the approach of rationally developing therapies in cancer patients based on strong preclinical data and individual patient molecular profiling.

7.9. Vaccines

Melanoma is considered as a rather "immunogenic" tumor. One can understand it by the spontaneous immune-mediated regression of primary tumors, association between infiltrating T lymphocytes and improved survival, response to nonspecific immunotherapy agents, including interferon-alpha, IL-2, and ipilimumab and identification of tumor-associated melanoma antigens and human leukocyte antigen (HLA)-restricted epitopes within these anti- gens [156].

A variety of strategies, including peptide and protein vaccines, recombinant DNA and viral vectors, and the use of autologous and allogeneic whole cell vaccines, have been tested in patients. Although many studies have not had significant clinical benefit, there are some important data that have emerged from these clinical trials. There also have been at least two randomized phase III vaccine trials that have shown a clinical benefit in melanoma [157].

There has been considerable interest in the identification of patient-specific and tumor-specific biomarkers that may predict therapeutic response and clinical outcomes. These studies would help select patients more likely to respond to a particular vaccine approach and might identify new strategies for improving the potency of individual vaccines so that more patients might benefit from immunotherapy.

8. Prognosis

Malignant melanoma is the most fatal type of the skin cancers. The best survival rates of melanoma arise if it is detected at the early stages, this is generally when the size of the tumours is small and treatable. After detection the prognosis of the melanoma can be determined by assessing a number of histopathological (morphological) factors such as the thickness of lesions, levels of invasion, presence of ulceration and the number of metastatic lymph nodes involved. Clinical prognostic factors such as age, sex, anatomical location of the tumour can also be used to determine the possible progression of the cancer and the likely survival rates of the patient. The thickness of the tumor is the dominant prognostic factor in determining risk of metastasis and prognosis for cutaneous melanoma [158, 159]. The American Joint Committee on Cancer (AJCC) tumor node metastasis committee has approved a new melanoma staging system, which was implemented in 2009 [160]. The prognostic factors included in AJCC staging system are tumor thickness, ulceration, level of invasion (*Clark*'s level) and mitotic rate [160, 161].

In the AJCC staging system, tumor thickness is the most powerful independent prognostic factor for patients with cutaneous melanoma. Melanoma thickness is measured from the granular layer of the epidermis to the greatest depth of tumor invasion, this was originally described by *Breslow* in 1970. Now it is correlated with a thickness of ≤1 mm (T1), 1.01 to 2 mm (T2), 2.01 to 4 mm (T3), or ≥4 mm (T4) [159]. In it, invasive tumor thickness is used to predict

5-year survival. In general, the higher the *Breslow* thickness, the worse the prognosis (Table 3) [161,162].

Breslow thickness	5-year survival
≤1 mm (T1)	95% to 100%
1.01 to 2 mm (T2)	80% to 96%
2.01 to 4 mm (T3)	60% to 75%
>4 mm (T4)	37% to 50%

Table 3. The relation of *Breslow* thickness and prognosis

The depth of the tumor is most accurately measured by evaluating the entire tumor via an excisional biopsy. Determination from specimens obtained using other biopsy techniques, such as a wedge or punch biopsy, is less accurate. Tumor depth cannot be calculated from a shave biopsy that only contains a portion of the tumor because it leads to an underestimation of its thickness. Excisional biopsy should extend down to the subcutaneous fat tissue [163].

Clark level of invasion is a method for determining the prognosis (outlook) with melanoma. This method was devised by the pathologist *Wallace Clark* and measured the depth of penetration of a melanoma into the skin according to anatomic layer. There are five *Clark* levels of invasion (Table 1).

The *Clark* levels provide a system to relate the degree of penetration of melanoma into the skin to the 5-year survival rate after surgical removal of the melanoma [158, 161, 164].

Ulceration is the second most powerful factor for poor prognosis. The presence of ulcerations on the surface of the tumour causes a reduction in the survival rate. Ulcerations appear when an intact epidermis is not present around the tumour and is usually a result of an aggressive tumour. The presence of ulceration in tumours less than 1mm, causes a reduction in survival rate by 4% compared to non-ulcerated tumour. Survival rates can be reduced by up to 22% if the tumour thickness is greater than 4mm.This therefore, indicates that tumour thickness and ulceration have strong relationship with survival rates and so the prognosis of thin non-ulcerated melanoma is excellent [51].

Current studies have shown that tumor mitotic rate is a powerful independent prognostic factor. But the prognostic importance of mitotic rate in melanoma recurrences is not known. A high mitotic rate also correlates with a greater likelihood of having a positive sentinel lymph node biopsy. The mitotic rate is measured by simply examining the excised tumor with a microscope and manually counting the number of cells exhibiting mitosis, an easily identifiable characteristic of dividing cells. Most often, the mitotic rate is reported as one of three categories :

- less than 1 per square millimeter
- 1 to 4 per square millimeter

- greater than 4 per square millimeter

The higher the mitotic count, the more likely the tumor is to have metastasized. The logic is that the more cells are dividing, the more likely they will invade the blood or lymphatic systems and thus spread around the body. Research has shown that the odds of survival for patients with stage I melanoma and a mitotic rate of 0 per square millimeter is twelve times better than that of patients with a mitotic rate of greater than 6 per square millimeter. Also, only 4% of lesions with low mitotic rate recur compared to 24% of those with a high mitotic rate. Mitotic rate can also help to predict that your sentinel lymph node biopsy will be positive or not. Although mitotic rate has no role in the current staging system for melanoma, research has demonstrated that it is a more important prognostic factor than ulceration, which does have an important role in staging. The American Academy of Dermatology argues that mitotic rate should be optional in biopsy reports or not. On the other hand, the National Comprehensive Cancer Center recommends that mitotic rate should be reported for all lesions in stage I to II patients. Still other experts argue that measuring the mitotic rate should only be done in large academic medical centers for future research purposes. Increasing mitotic rate is related with a decreasing survival [165, 166].

Tumor-infiltrating lymphocytes (TILs) describe the patient's immune response to the melanoma. One marker used to determine immune activity in melanoma is the presence in sentinel lymph node biopsy samples, which has been variably associated with a favorable prognosis. Some investigators assessed whether the presence of tumor-infiltrating lymphocytes was an independent predictor of sentinel lymph node biopsy status and survival or not [167, 168].

Microscopic satellites are defined as dermal or subcutaneous nodules. Microscopic satellites in primary melanomas are considered to be localized micrometastases developing in close proximity to the main tumoral portion of melanomas and show bad prognosis. In particular, the presence of angiotropism predicts the detection of microscopic satellites, and microscopic satellites probably develop as a result of extravascular migration. Consequently the linkage between microscopic satellites and angiotropism provides additional support for extravascular migratory metastasis as a mechanism of melanoma metastasis. Finally, ongoing investigations to develop a more specific biomarker for angiotropism and extravascular migratory metastasis are essential for the more precise recognition of extravascular migratory metastases and the explaining of its biological and prognostic significance. This pericytic angiotropism of melanoma cells, without any sign of intravasation, suggests that melanoma cells may migrate along the external surface of vessels, a mechanism we have termed extravascular migratory metastasis (EVMM), as distinct from intravascular dissemination [51, 169].

Common cell types are epithelioid and spindle cells, although mixed cells may also be seen. Generally, spindle cells are associated with better prognosis than other cell types.

The incidence of malignant melanoma appears to be increasing at an alarming rate throughout the world over the past 35-40 years and continues to increase in the USA, Canada, Asia, Australia, and Europe. The behavior of head and neck melanoma is aggressive, and it has an overall poorer prognosis than that of other skin sites. Correlations between different factors were found, e.g. tumour localisation predominating on the back in males and on the legs in female. In one study, 11.734 patients were analyzed, 49.3% were male. Between 1978 and 1992, most of the newly registered melanoma patients were female, but after 1992 there was a higher incidence of male patients. Men exhibited a disadvantaged distribution for almost all prognostic indicators being significantly older at diagnosis, having thicker melanomas, and having more melanomas localized on the trunk or head and neck. In analyses of histological subtypes, females had significantly more lentigo maligna melanomas and acral lentiginous melanomas, but the incidence of superficial spreading melanoma and nodular melanoma did not differ across gender. Males more often presented with lymph node metastases or distant metastases at the time of diagnosis than did females (5.2 vs. 3.0% and 1.7 vs. 1.1%, respectively). Whereas overall disease progression, lymph node metastasis, and distant metastasis occurred significantly more often in males than in females, local recurrence and in-transit/satellite metastases were equally common [170-172].

If we summarize, prognostic factors include tumor thickness (mm), levels of invasion, presence of ulceration, increased mitotic rate. Prognosis is better if there happens to be tumor-infiltrating lymphocytes around the lesion. There is stil controversy going on about regression. Some studies have shown an adverse outcome while others no effect, or a favorable outcome. Presence of microscopic satellites shows bad prognosis and also angiotropism is a bad prognostic marker. Vascular/lymphatic invasion, although seen very rarely, indicates unfavorable prognosis. Tumor cell type also has an effect on prognosis. Better prognosis with spindle cells versus other cell types. Prognosis worsens with increasing age and women have better prognosis than men. Extremity lesions have better prognosis than axial lesions (trunk, head and neck, palms and soles) [12, 173].

9. Patient education

Melanoma is the most dangerous form of skin cancer [174]. The incidence of melanoma is increasing worldwide, more than other cancers. The clinicians has the greatest impact on reducing these cases. They educate patients about early detection, treatment and prevention methods [175]. UV light is the most important risk factor for melanoma development. The risk of developing melanom may be reduced by protecting from UV light exposure. We must educate others as to the importance of sun protection [174]. Patients should be educated to avoid intense intermittent sun exposure and minimize cumulative sun exposure [176]. Avoiding overexposure to direct sunlight during the peak daylight hours, wearing protective clothing, and applying sunscreen are the ways to protect the skin [177].

Clinicians must educate patients as to the importance of using sunscreens that protects against both UVA and UVB light and with an SPF 30 or greater [174, 175]. It is important to emphasize the correct application of the recommended amount of sunscreen and the need for reapplication of sunscreen [176]. Sunscreen should be applied to exposed dry skin 15 to 30 minutes before sun exposure. The standard amount of sunscreen used in SPF testing is 2 mg/cm^2. Sunscreen should be reapplied every 2 hours or after swimming or heavy perspiration; many water-resistant sunscreens lose effectiveness after 40 minutes in the water [177]. Clinicians recommend patients sun protective clothing such as sunglasses, hats or long sleeve clothing. Patients should be avoided direct exposure to the sunlight between 9 AM - 3 PM and tanning beds [174]. There is great concern in regard to the total amount of sun exposure during infancy and early childhood [175]. The importance of sun protection in childhood should be emphasized [176].

Self-examination of skin by informed patients in terms of suspicious nevi is an important contributory factor in the early diagnosis of melanoma [178].

Skin self examination has the potential to significantly reduce melanoma mortality. One retrospective study concluded that skin self examination has the potential to reduce melanoma mortality by 63% [179]. One study found that 44% of diagnosed recurrent melanoma was initially detected by patients based on symptoms that raised suspicion of metastasis [180]. For this reason, patients shoul be educated about the skin self examination. Patient education in skin self examination includes information on the warning signs of melanoma. Also it includes directions on how to perform a thorough whole-body skin examination [176]. Patients at higher risk should carefully examine their own skin monthly and also be frequently examined by dermatologists professionally [174].

Older individuals are both more likely to acquire and to die from cutaneous melanoma; thus, elderly people should be a primary target for secondary melanoma prevention. We must be careful for the early detection and patient routine screening. Also secondary melanoma prevention should be focused on targeted education to older men and their spouses for early detection and reduction of mortality in this extremely high-risk group [181].

Following the diagnosis of cutaneous melanoma, all patients should be educated on the risks of developing a second primary melanoma. In addition, counselling on the common clinical characteristics of cutaneous melanomas and instruction on how to perform a skin self examination should be provided. In the event of the development of new pigmented lesions or changes in preexisting pigmented lesions, patients should be advised to seek medical attention. In addition, appropriate lifelong follow-up surveillance is critical for the detection of thinner, more curable melanomas [182].

Most of the studies suggested that many cancer patients want to get detailed information about their disease, treatment options and prognosis of the disease. The most common complaint of these patients is not to told what is wrong with them, during the treatment. Cancer care professionals are beginning to recognize that patients' information needs and preferences [183].

With growing evidence that well-informed patients are more satisfied with their care and do better clinically. Efforts are needed to improve the information provision to melanoma patients. Exploration of the patients' personal information needs must lead to a more patient-tailored approach of informing melanoma patients. A good opportunity would be the implementation of a survivorship care plan, which aims at providing a cancer survivor with a summary of their course of treatment, management of late effects, and strategies for health promotion [184].

http://dx.doi.org/10.5772/55304

The importance of malignant melanoma as a potentially fatal skin cancer among Caucasian populations worldwide has received critical attention in recent years. As compared to other life-threatening malignancies such as breast or prostate carcinoma, melanoma may be diagnosed by simple inspection of the skin surface with 80 to 90% accuracy. Sun avoidance, regular self-examination are important measures that can easily be applied. Future investigations is needed to establish whether education and modification of behavior such as reduced sun exposure and various methodologies of skin examination have a significant impact in reducing mortality from melanoma.

Author details

Zekayi Kutlubay*, Burhan Engin, Server Serdaroğlu and Yalçın Tüzün

*Address all correspondence to: zekayikutlubay@hotmail.com

İstanbul University, Cerrahpaşa Medical Faculty, Department of Dermatology, İstanbul, Turkey

References

[1] Chin L, Merlino G, DePinho RA. Malignant melanoma: modern black plague and genetic black box. Genes Dev. 1998; 12: 3467-3481.

[2] Jhappan C, Noonan FP, Merlino G. Ultraviolet radiation and cutaneous malignant melanoma. Oncogene 2003; 22: 3099–3112.

[3] Lens MB, Dawes M. Global perspectives of contemporary epidemiological trends of cutaneous malignant melanoma. Br J Dermatol 2004; 150: 179–185.

[4] Garbe C, Leiter U. Melanoma epidemiology and trends. Clin Dermatol 2009; 27: 3–9.

[5] Ko JM, Velez NF, Tsao H. Pathways to Melanoma. Semin Cutan Med Surg 2010; 29: 210-217.

[6] Kanavy HE, Gerstenblith MR. Ultraviolet Radiation and Melanoma. Semin Cutan Med Surg 2011; 30: 222-228.

[7] Paek SC, Sober AJ, Tsao H, Mihm MC, Johnson TM. Cutaneous Melanoma In: Wolff K, Goldsmith LA, Katz SI, Gilchrest B, Paller AS, Leffell DJ. (eds): Fitzpatrick's Dermatology in General Medicine, 7th ed. New York: Mc Graw Hill Companies, 2008; 1134-1157.

[8] Thompson JF, Scolyer RA, Kefford RF. Cutaneous melanoma. Lancet 2005; 365: 687–701.

[9] De Vries E, Bray FI, Coebergh JW, Parkin DM. Changing Epidemiology of Malignant Cutaneous Melanoma in Europe 1953–1997: Rising Trends in Incidence and Mortali-

ty but Recent Stabilizations in Western Europe and Decreases in Scandinavia. Int. J. Cancer 2003; 107; 119–126.

[10] van den Hurk K, Niessen HE, Veeck J, Van den Oord JJ, Van Steensel MA, Hausen AZ, van Engeland M, Winnepenninckx VJ. Genetics and epigenetics of cutaneous malignant melanoma: A concert out of tune. Biochimica et Biophysica Acta 2012; 1826: 89–102.

[11] De Vries E, Coebergh JW. Cutaneous malignant melanoma in Europe. Eur J Cancer 2004; 40: 2355–2366.

[12] Bishop J.A.N. Lentigos, Melanocytic Naevi and Melanoma In: Burns T, Breathnach S, Cox N, Griffiths C (eds): Rook's Textbook of Dermatology, 8th ed. Oxford, Blackwell publishing, 2010; 54.32-54.56.

[13] Dennis LK, Vanbeek MJ, Beane Freeman LE, et al: Sunburns and risk of cutaneous melanoma: Does age matter? A comprehensive meta-analysis. Ann Epidemiol 2008; 18: 614-627.

[14] Dahl C, Guldberg P. The genome and epigenome of malignant melanoma. APMIS 2007; 115: 1161–1176.

[15] Cust AE, Armstrong BK, Goumas C, et al: Sunbed use during adolescence and early adulthood is associated with increased risk of early-onset melanoma. Int. J. Cancer 2011; 128: 2425–2435.

[16] Loria D, Matos E. Risk factors for cutaneous melanoma: a case control study in Argentina. Int J Dermatol 2001; 40: 108-114.

[17] Ashton-Prolla P, Bakos L, Junqueira G, et al: Clinical and Molecular Characterization of Patients at Risk for Hereditary Melanoma in Southern Brazil. J Invest Dermatol 2008; 128: 421–425.

[18] Rebecca VW, Sondak VK, Smalleya KS. A brief history of melanoma: from mummies to mutations. Melanoma Research 2012; 22: 114–122.

[19] Omholt K, Platz A, Kanter L, Ringborg U, Hansson J. *NRAS* and *BRAF* Mutations Arise Early during Melanoma Pathogenesis and Are Preserved throughout Tumor Progression. Clin Cancer Res 2003; 9: 6483-6488.

[20] Pons M, Quintanilla M. Molecular biology of malignant melanoma and other cutaneous tumors. Clin Transl Oncol 2006; 8: 466-74.

[21] Curtin JA, Fridlyand J, Kageshita T. Distinct Sets of Genetic Alterations in Melanoma. N Engl J Med 2005; 353: 2135-47.

[22] Demierre MF, Sondak VK. Cutaneous melanoma: pathogenesis and rationale for chemoprevention. Crit Rev Oncol Hematol 2005; 53: 225–239.

[23] Nikolaou V, Kang X, Stratigos A et al. Comprehensive mutational analysis of CDKN2A and CDK4 in Greek patients with cutaneous melanoma. Br J Dermatol. 2011; 165: 1219-22.

[24] Romano C, Schepis C. PTEN gene: a model for genetic diseases in dermatology. ScientificWorldJournal. 2012; 2012: 252457.

[25] Kim M. Cooperative interactions of PTEN deficiency and RAS activation in melanoma metastasis. Small GTPases. 2010; 1: 161-164.

[26] Wang S, Setlow R, Berwick M, Polsky D, Marghoob A, Kopf A, Bart R. "Ultraviolet A and melanoma: a review". J Am Acad Dermatol 2001; 44 (5): 837–846.

[27] Geller AC, Miller DR, Annas GD, Demierre MF, Gilchrest BA, Koh HK. Melanoma incidence and mortality among US whites, 1969-1999. JAMA. 2002; 288: 1719-20.

[28] Wei Q. Repair of UV-induced DNA damage and Melanoma Risk. From melanocytes to melanoma. Eds. Hearing Vj, Leong Spl. Totowa: Humana Pres Inc. 2006: 441-453.

[29] Whiteman D.C, Whiteman C.A, Green, A.C. Childhood sun exposure as a risk factor for melanoma: a systematic review of epidemiologic studies. Cancer Causes Control 2001; 12: 69–82.

[30] Khlat M, Vail A, Parkin M, Green A. "Mortality from melanoma in migrants to Australia: variation by age at arrival and duration of stay". Am J Epidemiol 1992; 135 (10): 1103–1113.

[31] Hausauer AK, Swetter SM, Cockburn MG, Clarke CA. Increases in melanoma among adolescent girls and young women in California: trends by socioeconomic status and UV radiation exposure. Arch Dermatol. 2011; 147: 783-9.

[32] Wolf P, Donawho C K, Kripke M L. "Effect of Sunscreens on UV radiation-induced enhancements of melanoma in mice". J. Nat. Cancer. Inst. 1994; 86 (2): 99–105.

[33] Bliss J, Ford D, Swerdlow A, Armstrong B, Cristofolini M, Elwood J, Green A, Holly E, Mack T, MacKie R. "Risk of cutaneous melanoma associated with pigmentation characteristics and freckling: systematic overview of 10 case-control studies. The International Melanoma Analysis Group". Int J Cancer 1995; 62 (4): 367–376.

[34] Miller A, Mihm M. "Melanoma". N Engl J Med. 2006; 355 (1): 51–65.

[35] Rhodes A, Weinstock M, Fitzpatrick T, Mihm M, Sober A. "Risk factors for cutaneous melanoma. A practical method of recognizing predisposed individuals". JAMA 1987; 258 (21): 3146–3154.

[36] Esther de Vries, Freddie I Bray, Jan Willem W Coebergh, Donald M Parkin. Changing epidemiology of malignant cutaneous melanoma in Europe 1953-1997: rising trends in incidence and mortality but recent stabilizations in western Europe and decreases in Scandinavia. International Journal of Cancer. 2003; 107(1): 119-126.

[37] Reed KB, Brewer JD, Lohse CM, Bringe KE, Pruitt CN, Gibson LE. Increasing incidence of melanoma among young adults: an epidemiological study in Olmsted County, Minnesota. Mayo Clin Proc. 2012; 87(4): 328-834.

[38] Cockburn M, Swetter SM, Peng D, Keegan TH, Deapen D, Clarke CA. Melanoma underreporting: why does it happen, how big is the problem, and how do we fix it? J Am Acad Dermatol. 2008; 59: 1081-5.

[39] Swetter SM. Cutaneous Melanoma. Elston DM (Eds). http://emedicine.medscape.com/article/1100753-overview#a0199 (accessed 5 September 2012).

[40] Karagas MR, Zens MS, Stukel TA, et al. Pregnancy history and incidence of melanoma in women: a pooled analysis. Cancer Causes Control 2006; 17: 11-19.

[41] MacKie RM, Bray CA. Hormone replacement therapy after surgery for stage 1 or 2 cutaneous melanoma. Br J Cancer 2004; 90: 770-772.

[42] Pukkala E, Aspholm R, Auvinen A, et al Incidence of cancer among Nordic airline pilots over five decades: occupational cohort study. BMJ 2002; 325: 567.

[43] Bastiaannet E, Homan-van der Heide JJ, Ploeg RJ, Hoekstra HJ No increase of melanoma after kidney transplantation in the northern part of The Netherlands. Melanoma Res. 2007; 17: 349-353.

[44] Lindelof B, Sigurgeirsson B, Gabel H, Stern RS Incidence of skin cancer in 5356 patients following organ transplantation. Br J Dermatol 2000; 143: 513-519.

[45] Kitchener S. Epidemiology of Melanoma Color Atlas of Melanocytic Lesions of the Skin. Ed. Soyer HP, Argenziano G, Hofmann-Wellenhof R, Berlin Heideberg: Springer-Veriag; 2007; 185-195.

[46] Green AC, O'Rourke MG. Cutaneous malignant melanoma in association with other skin cancers. J. Natl. Cancer Inst. 1985; 74: 977–980.

[47] Berwick M, Wiggins C, The current epidemiology of cutaneous malignant melanoma. Journal Article Frontiers in Bioscience 2006; 11: 1244-1254.

[48] Purdue MP, Freeman LE, Anderson WF, Tucker MA. Recent trends in incidence of cutaneous melanoma among US Caucasian young adults. J Invest Dermatol. 2008; 128: 2905-8.

[49] Lea CS, Holly EA, Hartge P, et al. Reproductive risk factors for cutaneous melanoma in women: a case-control study. Am J. Epidemiol 2007; 165: 505-513.

[50] Driscoll MS, Grin-Jorgensen CM, Grant-Kels JM. Does pregnancy influence the prognosis of malignant melanoma?. J Am Acad Dermatol. 1993; 29(4): 619-30.

[51] Bailey EC, Sober AJ, Tsao H, Mihm MC, Johnson TM. Cutaneous melanoma. In: Goldsmith LA, Katz SI, Barbara AG, Paller AS, Leffell DJ, Wolff K. (Eds). Fitzpatrick's Dermatology in General Medicine 8th Edition. New York, Mc Graw Hill Medical, 2012; 1416-1444.

[52] Swetter SM, Boldrick JC, Jung SY, Egbert BM, Harvell JD. Increasing incidence of lentigo maligna melanoma subtypes: northern California and national trends 1990-2000. J Invest Dermatol. 2005; 125(4): 685-91.

[53] Holman CD, Armstrong BK. Cutaneous malignant melanoma and indicators of total accumulated exposure to the sun: an analysis separating histogenetic types. J Natl Cancer Inst. Jul 1984; 73: 75-82.

[54] Liu V, Mihm MC. Pathology of malignant melanoma. Surg Clin North Am. 2003; 83(1): 31-60.

[55] Clark GS, Pappas-Politis EC, Cherpelis BS, Messina JL, Möller MG, Cruse CW, Glass LF. Surgical management of melanoma in situ on chronically sun-damaged skin. Cancer Control. 2008; 15(3): 216-24.

[56] Gross EA, Andersen WK, Rogers GS. Mohs micrographic excision of lentigo maligna using Mel-5 for margin control. Arch Dermatol. 1999; 135(1): 15-7.

[57] King DM. Imaging of metastatic melanoma. Cancer Imaging 2006; 6: 204–208.

[58] McKenna JK, Florell SR, Goldman GD, Bowen GM. Lentigo maligna/lentigo maligna melanoma: current state of diagnosis and treatment. Dermatol Surg. 2006; 32(4): 493-504.

[59] Gürer MA, Adışen E. Kutanöz melanoma. In: Dermatoloji. Tüzün Y, Gürer M, Serdaroğlu S, Oğuz O, Aksungur V. (eds). 3rd Edition. İstanbul, Nobel Tıp Kitabevleri, 2008; 1791-1823. (Turkish)

[60] Langholz B, Richardson J, Rappaport E, Waisman J, Cockburn M, Mack T. Skin characteristics and risk of superfcial spreading and nodular melanoma. Cancer Causes and Control, 2000; 11: 741-750.

[61] Elwood JM, Jopson J. Melanoma and sun exposure: an overview of published studies. Int J Cancer. 1997; 73(2): 198-203.

[62] Interactive Medical Media. Dermatology lectures on line. Dermoscopy. http://www.dermlectures.com

[63] Chamberlain A, Ng J. Cutaneous melanoma--atypical variants and presentations. Aust Fam Physician. 2009; 38(7): 476-82.

[64] Lang PG. Current concepts in the management of patients with melanoma. Am J Clin Dermatol. 2002; 3(6): 401-26.

[65] Cress RD, Holly EA. Incidence of cutaneous melanoma among non-Hispanic whites, Hispanics, Asians, and blacks: an analysis of california cancer registry data,1988-93. Cancer Causes Control. 1997; 8(2): 246-52.

[66] Byrd KM, Wilson DC, Hoyler SS, Peck GL. Advanced presentation of melanoma in African Americans. J Am Acad Dermatol. 2004; 50(1) :21-4; discussion 142-3.

[67] Nestle FO, Halpern AC. Melanoma. In: Dermatology. Volume 2. Eds. Bolognia JL, Jorizzo JL, Rapini RP. 2nd Edition. Spain. Mosby, 2008; 1745-1771.

[68] Roesch A, Volkenandt M. Melanoma. In: Braun-Falco's Dermatology. Burgdorf WHC, Plewig G, Wolff HH, Landthaler M. eds. 3rd Edition. Heidelberg, Springer; 2009; 1416-1432.

[69] Piliang MP. Acral lentiginous melanoma. Clin Lab Med. 2011; 31(2): 281-8.

[70] Porras BH, Cockerell CJ. Cutaneous malignant melanoma: classification and clinical diagnosis. Semin Cutan Med Surg. 1997; 16(2): 88-96.

[71] Miranda BH, Haughton DN, Fahmy FS. Subungual melanoma: An important tip. J Plast Reconstr Aesthet Surg. 2012; 23.

[72] Rogers RS 3rd, Gibson LE. Mucosal, genital, and unusual clinical variants of melanoma. Mayo Clin Proc. 1997; 72(4): 362-6.

[73] Seetharamu N, Ott PA, Pavlick AC. Mucosal melanomas: a case-based review of the literature. Oncologist. 2010; 15(7): 772-81.

[74] Paradela S, Fonseca E, Prieto VG. Melanoma in children. Arch Pathol Lab Med. 2011; 135(3): 307-16.

[75] Pustišek N, Situm M, Mataija M, Vurnek Živković M, Bolanča Z. Malignant melanoma in childhood and adolescence. J Eur Acad Dermatol Venereol. 2012; 23.

[76] Lens MB, Newton-Bishop JA, Boon AP. Desmoplastic malignant melanoma: a systematic review. Br J Dermatol. 2005; 152(4): 673-8.

[77] Rongioletti F, Smoller BR. Unusual histological variants of cutaneous malignant melanoma with some clinical and possible prognostic correlations. J Cutan Pathol. 2005; 32(9): 589-603.

[78] Magro CM, Crowson AN, Mihm MC. Unusual variants of malignant melanoma. Mod Pathol. 2006; 19 Suppl 2: 41-70.

[79] Jain S, Allen PW. Desmoplastic malignant melanoma and its variants. A study of 45 cases. Am J Surg Pathol. 1989; 13(5): 358-73.

[80] Saluja A, Money N, Zivony DI, Solomon AR. Angiotropic malignant melanoma: a rare pattern of local metastases. J Am Acad Dermatol. 2001; 44(5): 829-32.

[81] Diwan AH, Lazar AJ. Nevoid melanoma. Clin Lab Med. 2011; 31(2): 243-53.

[82] Steiner A, Konrad K, Pehamberger H, Wolff K.Verrucous malignant melanoma. Arch Dermatol. 1988; 124(10): 1534-7.

[83] Kirkham N.Small cell melanoma. Histopathology. 2002; 40(2): 196-8.

[84] Kamino H.Spitzoid melanoma. Clin Dermatol. 2009; 27(6): 545-55.

[85] Lee L, Zhou F, Simms A, et al. Metastatic balloon cell malignant melanoma: a case report and literature review. Int J Clin Exp Pathol. 2011; 4(3): 315-21

[86] Hocar O, Le Cesne A, Berissi S, et al. Clear cell sarcoma (malignant melanoma) of soft parts: a clinicopathologic study of 52 cases. Dermatol Res Pract. 2012; 2012:984096.

[87] Schwartz RA. Skin Cancer Recognition and Management. 2nd Ed. Massachusetts, Blackwell Publishing, 2008; 152-199.

[88] Nouri K. Skin Cancer. New York, Mc Graw Hill, 2008; 140-167.

[89] Choi JN, Hanlon A, Leffell D. Melanoma and nevi: detection and diagnosis. Curr Probl Cancer 2011; 35: 138-161.

[90] van Kempen LC. 5th Canadian Melanoma Conference: research frontiers. Expert Rev Anticancer Ther 2011; 11: 845-848.

[91] Rolfe HM. Accuracy in skin cancer diagnosis: a retrospective study of an Australian public hospital dermatology department. Australas J Dermatol 2012; 53: 112-117.

[92] BJ Nickoloff. The Many Molecular Mysteries of Melanoma. Melanoma Techniques and Protocols Molecular Diagnosis, Treatment, and Monitoring. Ed. BJ Nickoloff. Totowa, Humana Press; 1-14.

[93] Harris K, Florell SR, Papenfuss J, Kohlmann W, Jahromi M, Schiffman JD, et all. Melanoma mimic: a case of multiple pagetoid Spitz nevi. Arch Dermatol 2012; 148: 370-374.

[94] D'Ath P, Thomson P. Superficial spreading melanoma. BMJ. 2012; 344.

[95] Liebman TN, Rabinovitz HS, Balagula Y, Jaimes-Lopez N, Marghoob AA. White shiny structures in melanoma and BCC. Arch Dermatol 2012; 148: 146.

[96] Yang GB, Barnholtz-Sloan JS, Chen Y, Bordeaux JS. Risk and survival of cutaneous melanoma diagnosed subsequent to a previous cancer. Arch Dermatol 2011; 147: 1395-1402.

[97] Liu Z, Sun J, Smith L, Smith M, Warr R. Distribution quantification on dermoscopy images for computer-assisted diagnosis of cutaneous melanomas. Med Biol Eng Comput 2012; 50: 503-513.

[98] Scolyer RA, Thompson JF, Stretch JR, Sharma R, McCarthy SW. Pathology of melanocytic lesions: new, controversial, and clinically important issues. J Surg Oncol 2004; 86: 200-211.

[99] Bowen GM, Bowen AR, Florell SR. Lentigo maligna: one size does not fit all. Arch Dermatol 2011; 147: 1211-1213.

[100] Kvaskoff M, Siskind V, Green AC. Risk factors for lentigo maligna melanoma compared with superficial spreading melanoma: a case-control study in Australia. Arch Dermatol 2012; 148: 164-170.

[101] Pralong P, Bathelier E, Dalle S, Poulalhon N, Debarbieux S, Thomas L. Dermoscopy of lentigo maligna melanoma: report of 125 cases. Br J Dermatol 2012 doi: 10.1111

[102] Moreno M, Schmitt RL, Lang MG, Gheno V. Epidemiological profile of patients with cutaneous melanoma in a region of southern Brazil. J Skin Cancer 2012; 2012: 917346.

[103] Lee HY, Chay WY, Tang MB, Chio MT, Tan SH. Melanoma: differences between Asian and Caucasian patients. Ann Acad Med Singapore 2012; 41: 17-20.

[104] Chow WT, Bhat W, Magdub S, Orlando A. In situ subungual melanoma: Digit salvaging clearance. J Plast Reconstr Aesthet Surg 2012; 1-3.

[105] Bravo Puccio F, Chian C. Acral junctional nevus versus acral lentiginous melanoma in situ: a differential diagnosis that should be based on clinicopathologic correlation. Arch Pathol Lab Med 2011; 135: 847-852.

[106] Rashid OM, Schaum JC, Wolfe LG, Brinster NK, Neifeld JP. Prognostic variables and surgical management of foot melanoma: review of a 25-year institutional experience. ISRN Dermatol 2011; 2011: 384729.

[107] Ramos JA, Ramos WE, Ramos CV. Melanoma of the female urethra. Indian J Urol 2011; 27: 448-450.

[108] Hajar-Serviansky T, Gutierrez-Mendoza D, Galvan IL, Lammoglia-Ordiales L, Mosqueda-Taylor A, Hernandez-Cázares Mde L, Toussaint-Caire S. A case of oral mucosal melanoma. Clinical and dermoscopic correlation. J Dermatol Case Rep 2012; 6: 1-4.

[109] Crowson AN, Magro CM, Barnhill RL, Mihm MC. Pathology. Cutaneous Melanoma. Ed. Balch CM, Houghton AN, Sober AJ, Soong S. 4th Edition. Missouri, Quality Medical Publishing, 2003; 171-206.

[110] Hung CT, Wu BY. Cutaneous combined desmoplastic melanoma. Indian J Dermatol Venereol Leprol 2012; 78: 230.

[111] Fish LM, Duncan L, Gray KD, Bell JL, Lewis JM. Primary cutaneous melanoma arising in a long-standing irradiated keloid. Case Rep Surg 2012; 2012: 165319.

[112] Koc MK, Sudogan S, Kavala M, Kocaturk E, Büyükbabani N, Altintas S. Desmoplastic spitz naevus can be mistaken for desmoplastic malignant melanoma and dermatofibroma. Acta Derm Venereol 2011; 91: 74-75.

[113] Weedon D. Lentigines, nevi, and melanomas. Weedon's Skin Pathology. 3rdEd. Churchill Livingstone Elsevier. 2010; 709- 756.

[114] Mckee PH, Calonje E, Granter SR. Melanoma. Pathology of the skin with clinical correlation. 3rd Ed. Elsevier Mosby. 2005; 1309-1356.

[115] Smalberger GJ, Siegel DM, Khachemoune A. Lentigo maligna. Dermatol Ther 2008; 21: 439-446.

[116] Reed JA, Shea CR. Lentigo maligna: melanoma in situ on chronically sun-damaged skin.Arch Pathol Lab Med 2011; 135: 838-841.

[117] Duncan LM. The classification of cutaneous melanoma. Hematol Oncol Clin North Am 2009; 23: 501-513.

[118] Su WP. Malignant melanoma: basic approach to clinicopathologic correlation. Mayo Clin Proc 1997; 72: 267-272.

[119] Payette MJ, Katz M 3rd, Grant-Kels JM. Melanoma prognostic factors found in the dermatopathology report. Clin Dermatol 2009; 27: 53-74.

[120] Stoff B, Salisbury C, Parker D, O'Reilly Z, Wald F. Dermatopathologyof skin cancer in solid organ transplant recipients. Transplant Rev 2010; 24: 172-189.

[121] Phan A, Touzet S, Dalle S, Ronger-Savlé S, Balme B, Thomas L. Acral lentiginous melanoma: histopathological prognostic features of 121 cases. Br J Dermatol 2007; 157: 311-318.

[122] Kim YC, Lee MG, Choe SW, Lee MC, Chung HG, Cho SH. Acral lentiginous melanoma: an immunohistochemical study of 20 cases. Int J Dermatol 2003; 42: 123-129.

[123] Stalkup JR, Orengo IF, Katta R. Controversies in acral lentiginous melanoma. Dermatol Surg 2002; 28: 1051-1059.

[124] Hollmig ST, Sachdev R, Cockerell CJ, Posten W, Chiang M, Kim J. Spindle cell neoplasms encountered in dermatologic surgery: a review. Dermatol Surg 2012; 38: 825-850.

[125] Murali R, Loughman NT, McKenzie PR, Watson GF, Thompson JF, Scolyer RA. Cytologic features of metastatic and recurrent melanoma in patients with primary cutaneous desmoplastic melanoma. Am J Clin Pathol 2008; 130: 715-723.

[126] Chen JY, Hruby G, Scolyer RA, Murali R, Hong A, Fitzgerald P et al. Desmoplastic neurotropic melanoma: a clinicopathologic analysis of 128 cases. Cancer 2008; 113: 2770-2778.

[127] Busam KJ. Desmoplastic melanoma. Clin Lab Med 2011; 31: 321-330.

[128] Kay PA, Pinheiro AD, Lohse CM, Pankratz VS, Olsen KD, Lewis JE et al. Desmoplastic melanoma of the head and neck: histopathologic and immunohistochemical study of 28 cases. Int J Surg Pathol 2004; 12: 17-24.

[129] Manganoni AM, Farisoglio C, Bassissi S, Braga D, Facchetti F, Ungari M et al. Desmoplastic melanoma: report of 5 cases. Dermatol Res Pract. 2009; 2009: 679010.

[130] Chorny JA, Barr RJ, Kyshtoobayeva A, Jakowatz J, Reed RJ. Ki-67 and p53 expression in minimal deviation melanomas as compared with other nevomelanocytic lesions. Mod Pathol 2003; 16: 525-529.

[131] Podnos YD, Jimenez JC, Zainabadi K, Jakowatz JG, Barr RJ. Minimal deviation melanoma. Cancer Treat Rev 2002; 28: 219-221.

[132] Hantschke M, Mentzel T, Kutzner H. Follicular malignant melanoma: a variant of melanoma to be distinguished from lentigo maligna melanoma. Am J Dermatopathol 2004; 26: 359-363.

[133] Hu SW, Tahan SR, Kim CC. Follicular malignant melanoma: a case report of a metastatic variant and review of the literature. J Am Acad Dermatol 2011; 64: 1007-1010.

[134] Ivan D, Prieto VG. An update on reporting histopathologic prognostic factors in melanoma. Arch Pathol Lab Med 2011; 135: 825-829.

[135] Garbe C, Eigentler TK, Bauer J, Blödorn-Schlicht N, Fend F, Hantschke M et al. Histopathological diagnostics of malignant melanoma in accordance with the recent AJCC

classification 2009: Review of the literature and recommendations for general practice. J Dtsch Dermatol Ges 2011; 9: 690-699.

[136] Piris A, Mihm MC Jr, Duncan LM. AJCC melanoma staging update: impact on dermatopathology practice and patient management. J Cutan Pathol 2011; 38: 394-400.

[137] Piris A, Mihm MC Jr. Progress in melanoma histopathology and diagnosis. Hematol Oncol Clin North Am 2009; 23: 467-480.

[138] Garbe C, Peris K, Hauschild A, Saiag P, Middleton M, Spatz A et al. Diagnosis and treatment of melanoma: European consensus-based interdisciplinary guideline. Eur J Cancer 2010; 46: 270-283.

[139] Ohsie SJ, Sarantopoulos GP, Cochran AJ, Binder SW. Immunohistochemical characteristics of melanoma.J Cutan Pathol 2008; 35:433-444.

[140] Puri PK, Forman SB, Ferringer T, Elston D. S100A6 immunohistochemical staining for spindle cell and desmoplastic melanomas. J CutanPathol 2008; 35:256-257.

[141] Prieto VG, Shea CR. Use of immunohistochemistry in melanocytic lesions. J Cutan Pathol 2008; 35 Suppl 2: 1-10.

[142] Hong A, Fogarty G. Role of radiation therapy in cutaneous melanoma. Cancer J. 2012; 18: 203-207.

[143] Larkin JM, Fisher RA, Gore ME. Adjuvant interferon therapy for patients at high risk for recurrent melanoma: An updated systematic review. Clin Oncol. 2012; 24: 410-412.

[144] Kaufman HL. Vaccines for melanoma and renal cell carcinoma. Semin Oncol. 2012; 39: 263-275.

[145] Damian DL, Saw RP. Dramatic regression of cutaneous, nodal, and visceral melanoma metastases. J Am Acad Dermatol. 2011; 65: 665-666.

[146] Schwartzentruber DJ, Lawson DH, Richards JM, et al. gp100 peptide vaccine and interleukin-2 in patients with advanced melanoma. N Engl J Med. 2011; 364: 2119–2127.

[147] Abdelmalek M, Loosemore MP, Hurt MA, Hruza G. Geometric staged excision for the treatment of lentigo maligna and lentigo maligna melanoma: A long-term experience with literature review. Arch Dermatol. 2012; 148: 599-604.

[148] Szabo A, Osman RM, Bacskai I, Kumar BV, Agod Z, Lanyi A, Gogolak P, Rajnavolgyi E. Temporally designed treatment of melanoma cells by ATRA and polyI: C results in enhanced chemokine and IFNβ secretion controlled differently by TLR3 and MDA5. Melanoma Res. 2012 [Epub ahead of print]

[149] Burmeister B, Henderson M, Thompson J, et al. Adjuvant radiotherapy improves regional (lymph node field) control in melanoma patients after lymphadenectomy: results of an intergroup randomized trial. Int J Radiat Oncol Biol Phys. 2009; 75: 1-2.

[150] Arbiser JL, Bips M, Seidler A, Bonner MY, Kovach C. Combination therapy of imiquimod and gentian violet for cutaneous melanoma metastases. J Am Acad Dermatol. 2012; 67: 81-83.

[151] Mohan M, Sukhadia VY, Pai D, Bhat S. Oral malignant melanoma: systematic review of literature and report of two cases. Oral Surg Oral Med Oral Pathol Oral Radiol. 2012. [Epub ahead of print]

[152] Hardin RE, Lange JR. Surgical treatment of melanoma patients with early sentinel node involvement. Curr Treat Options Oncol. 2012. [Epub ahead of print]

[153] Neier M, Pappo A, Navid F. Management of melanomas in children and young adults. J Pediatr Hematol Oncol. 2012; 34: 51-54.

[154] Smalley KS, McArthur GA. The current state of targeted therapy in melanoma: this time it's personal. Semin Oncol. 2012; 39: 204-214.

[155] Mozzillo N, Caracò C, Mori S, Di Monta G, Botti G, Ascierto PA, Caracò C, Aloj L. Use of neoadjuvant electrochemotherapy to treat a large metastatic lesion of the cheek in a patient with melanoma. J Transl Med. 2012; 10: 131.

[156] Falchook GS, Lewis KD, Infante JR, Gordon MS, Vogelzang NJ, Demarini DJ et al. Activity of the oral MEK inhibitor trametinib in patients with advanced melanoma: a phase 1 dose-escalation trial. Lancet Oncol. 2012; 13: 782-789.

[157] Anforth RM, Blumetti TC, Kefford RF, Sharma R, Scolyer RA, Kossard S, Long GV, Fernandez-Peñas P. Cutaneous manifestations of dabrafenib (GSK2118436): A selective inhibitor of mutant BRAF in patients with metastatic melanoma. Br J Dermatol. 2012; 10: 1365-1367.

[158] Kalady MF, White RR, Johnson JL, Tyler DS, Seigler HF. Thin melanomas: predictive lethal characteristics from a 30-year clinical experience. Ann Surg. 2003; 238(4): 528-35.

[159] Krathen M. Malignant melanoma: advances in diagnosis, prognosis, and treatment. Semin Cutan Med Surg. 2012; 31(1): 45-9.

[160] Balch CM, Gershenwald JE, Soong SJ et al. Final Version of 2009 AJCC Melanoma Staging and Classification. J Clin Oncol 2009; 27(36): 6199-206.

[161] Balch CM, Buzaid AC, Soong SJ, Atkins MB, Cascinelli N, Coit DG, Fleming ID, Gershenwald JE, Houghton A Jr, Kirkwood JM, McMasters KM, Mihm MF, Morton DL, Reintgen DS, Ross MI, Sober A, Thompson JA, Thompson JF. Final Version of the American Joint Committee on Cancer Staging System for Cutaneous Melanoma. J Clin Oncol 2001; 19: 3635-3648.

[162] Kruijff S, Bastiaannet E, Francken AB, Schaapveld M, van der Aa M, Hoekstra HJ. Br J Cancer. Breslow thickness in the Netherlands: a population-based study of 40 880 patients comparing young and elderly patients.2012; 24;107(3):570-4.

[163] Pflugfelder A, Weide B, Eigentler TK, Forschner A, Leiter U, Held L, Meier F, Garbe C. Incisional biopsy and melanoma prognosis: Facts and controversies.Clin Dermatol. 2010; 28(3): 316-8.

[164] Owen SA, Sanders LL, Edwards LJ, Seigler HF, Tyler DS, Grichnik JM. Identification of higher risk thin melanomas should be based on Breslow depth not Clark level IV. Cancer. 2001; 1; 91(5): 983-91.

[165] Azzola MF, Shaw HM, Thompson JF, Soong SJ, Scolyer RA, Watson GF, Colman MH, Zhang Y. Tumor mitotic rate is a more powerful prognostic indicator than ulceration in patients with primary cutaneous melanoma: an analysis of 3661 patients from a single center. Cancer. 2003; 15;97(6): 1488-98.

[166] Attis MG, Vollmer RT. Mitotic rate in melanoma: a reexamination. Am J Clin Pathol. 2007; 127(3): 380-4.

[167] Lee S, Margolin K. Tumor-Infiltrating Lymphocytes in Melanoma. Curr Oncol Rep. 2012 Aug 10.

[168] Azimi F, Scolyer RA, Rumcheva P, Moncrieff M, Murali R, McCarthy SW, Saw RP, Thompson JF. Tumor-infiltrating lymphocyte grade is an independent predictor of sentinel lymph node status and survival in patients with cutaneous melanoma. J Clin Oncol. 2012; 20; 30(21): 2678-83.

[169] Wilmott J, Haydu L, Bagot M, Zhang Y, Jakrot V, McCarthy S, Lugassy C, Thompson J, Scolyer R, Barnhill R. Angiotropism is an independent predictor of microscopic satellites in primary cutaneous melanoma. Histopathology. 2012; 30: 1365-2559.

[170] Joosse A, de Vries E, Eckel R, Nijsten T, Eggermont AM, Hölzel D, Coebergh JW, Engel J. Gender differences in melanoma survival: female patients have a decreased risk of metastasis. J Invest Dermatol. 2011; 131(3): 719-26.

[171] Bradford PT, Anderson WF, Purdue MP, Goldstein AM, Tucker MA. Rising melanoma incidence rates of the trunk among younger women in the United States. Cancer Epidemiol Biomarkers Prev. 2010; 19(9): 2401-6.

[172] Bulliard JL, Cox B. Cutaneous malignant melanoma in New Zealand: trends by anatomical site, 1969-1993. Int J Epidemiol. 2000; 29(3): 416-23.

[173] Barnhill RL, Lugassy C. Angiotropic malignant melanoma and extravascular migratory metastasis: description of 36 cases with emphasis on a new mechanism of tumour spread. Pathology. 2004; 36(5): 485-90.

[174] Ryszard M. Pluta, MD, PhD: Melanoma. JAMA 2011;305:2368.

[175] Riker AI, Zea N, Trinh T: The epidemiology, prevention and detection of melanoma. The Ochsner Journal 2010; 10: 56-65.

[176] Halpern AC, Marghoob AA, Sober AJ: Clinical characteristics. In: Cutaneous Melanoma. Balch CM, Houghton AN, Sober AJ, Soong S. Eds. 4th Edition. Canada, Quality Medical Publishing 2003; 7: 135-162.

[177] Jou PC, Feldman RJ, Tomecki KJ: UV protection and sunscreens: what to tell patients. Cleve Clin J Med 2012; 79: 427-436.

[178] Sefton E, Glazebrook C, Garrud P, Zaki I: Educating patients about makignant melanoma: computer-assisted learning in a pigmented lesion clinic. Br J Dermatol 2000; 142: 66-71.

[179] Berwick M, Begg CB, Fine JA, et. al. Screening for cutaneous melanoma by skin self-examination. J Natl Cancer Inst 1996; 88: 17.

[180] Mujumdar UJ, Hay JL, Monroe-Hinds YC, Hummer AJ, Begg CB, Wilcox HB, Oliveria SA, Berwick M: Sun protection and skin-self examination in melanoma survivors. Psychooncology 2009; 18: 1106-1115.

[181] Swetter SM, Geller AC, Kirkwood JM. Melanoma in the older person. Oncology (Williston Park). 2004; 18: 1187-96; discussion 1196-7.

[182] Uliasz A, Lebwohl M: Patient education and regular surveillance results in earlier diagnosis of second primary melanoma. Int J Dermatol 2007; 46: 575-577.

[183] Constantinidou A, Afuwape SA, Linsell L, Hung T, Acland K, Healy C, Ramirez AJ, Harries M: Informational needs of patients with melanoma and their views on the utility of investigative tests. Int J Clin Pract 2009; 63: 1595-1600.

[184] Husson O, Holterhues C, Mols F, Nijsten T, van de Poll-Franse LV: Melanoma survivors are dissatisfied with perceived information about their diagbosis, treatment and foolow-up care. Br J Dermatol 2010; 163: 879-881.

Chapter 5

About Suncare Products

C. Couteau and L. Coiffard

Additional information is available at the end of the chapter

http://dx.doi.org/10.5772/55411

1. Introduction

The prevalence of skin cancer varies greatly according to the geographic location and is developing rapidly in Western countries. This type of cancer is most frequent in fair-skinned people. In Australia, the rate of melanomas increased annually by 6.3% in men and 2.9% in women between 1959 and 1985. This type of cancer is the most frequent one in fair-skinned people. Since 1985, the rate has levelled off, which is reassuring even though the incidence of skin cancer in Australia is the highest in the world [1] (table 1) [2], followed by New Zealand and Norway [3]. As a comparison, we can look at the rate of non-melanoma skin cancer (NMSC) in Japan, which is between 1.2 and 5.4 per 100,000, that is to say a factor of 50 compared to Australia [4]. Skin cancer in children is rare. In teenagers (from 15 to 19 years old) the prevalence in England is 10 cases per million per year for melanomas and 24 cases per million per year for NMSC. The risk factors are: a family history of melanomas, *Xeroderma pigmentosum* [5] and pathologies responsible for states of immunosuppression. Cases of congenital melanomas are extremely rare [6]. Excessive sun exposure has long been recognised as the most important environmental factor to be taken into account; indeed, ultra-violet radiation (UV) is the cause of 90% of NMSC and 67% of melanomas [7]. The high incidence of skin cancer in certain countries of the world is therefore not just down to chance but has a direct link to the population's skin type (fair-skinned, blue-eyed people who burn easily, who never tan and who often have freckles) [8] and to the level of sunshine [9]. Although UV rays only represent 3% of the total radiation which reaches Earth, from a point of view of energy, it is thought that they account for 10% of light energy [10]. Mountainous regions bring a greater risk of developing sunburn, as the quantity of UVB increases by 4% every 300 metres [11], and in a similar way, the position with relation to the equator is of utmost importance, (the risk is greatest around the Tropics). UV radiation (UVA and B) causes alterations in DNA by either direct or indirect actions (by means of an oxidizing stress). The types which react to oxygen can cause either an increase in cell proliferation or their apoptosis, accordingly [12]. The notion of phototypes, put forward by Fitzpatrick as early as 1975 within the framework of the care of patients treated with PUVA therapy, is linked to the concept of sun-reactive skin. This scale enables Caucasian subjects to be classed according to their sensitivity to UV rays. At first, 4 phototypes were established, called I, II, III and IV (Table 2), then this scale was later extended to include phototypes V (brown skin or Asian skin) and VI (black) [13]. A classification concerning Japanese people was also drawn up by Kawada [14]. The three corresponding groups are JI (always burn and rarely tan), JII (burn and tan moderately), JIII (never burn and always tan). These three groups should be linked to the Caucasian phototypes II, III and IV [15]. In the 1990s, JP Césarini introduced the notion of melano-compromised subjects (Phototypes I and II), melanocompetent subjects (Phototypes III and IV) and melanoprotected subjects according to their varying capabilities to protect themselves against skin cancer [16]. The best level of photoprotection is reached by black subjects, who are shown to have a low incidence of skin cancer (1 to 2% of cancers affecting black people are skin cancers compared to 20 to 30% for Caucasians). The phototypes are linked to melanin, which is a biopolymer functioning as a filter and which enables black people to produce an SPF (Sun Protection Factor) of around 13. The dispersion of melanosomes and their lack of degradation throughout the keratinization process forms an effective barrier. A black person's melanin filters twice as much UVB radiation as a Caucasian's melanin. The black epidermis is much more protected than a Caucasian one, as it transmits 7.4% of UVB radiation and 17.5% of UVA radiation compared to 24 and 55% for a Caucasian epidermis. In terms of Minimal Erythemal Dose (MED), it can be observed that this dose is between 6 and 33 times higher in black subjects [17]. It is important to create new classifications on a regular basis because of the interbreeding of races in the population. For example, in 1990, the US Census Bureau registered 6 races and 23 sub-types in the United States; 10 years later, the Census Bureau still counted 6 categories, but the number of sub-types had increased to 67, creating a multiplicity of sensitivities to the sun [18]. It seems that precautions taken by people who work outside to protect themselves from the sun are related to their phototype, as an American study shows that fair-skinned people are more aware in this respect [19]. The current way of life in industrialized countries goes hand in hand with an increase in the frequency of the length of exposure to the sun during leisure time. Contrary to previous centuries where pale skin tones were all the rage, the fashion of having a sun-tan, which began in the Thirties, is still current. The SUVIMAX study which was conducted in France in 1994 showed that in the cohort of 7,822 subjects questioned, 196 (110 women and 86 men) had travelled to a country with high levels of sunshine (high UV index) within the previous year and for a period of at least one month. Women, in particular, appear to be most concerned with daily exposure to sunshine (more than 2 hours per day) and admit that "getting a tan" is very important for them [20]. Sunbathing is still popular. Professor Dubertret is pessimistic and considers that if nothing is done in the way of prevention campaigns, the rate of skin cancer will double every ten years and a child born in 2000, if he behaves in the same way as his parents regarding his exposure to the sun, will have a 1 in 75 risk of developing a melanoma and a 1 in 7 risk of developing basocellular cancer [21]. The behavior of young Europeans tends towards improvement. Indeed, an increase in the use of sun products throughout exposure can be observed. In 10 years (between 1990 and 2000), the use of sun products increased from 52 to 63% in boys and from 80 to 87% in girls. It is a pity

http://dx.doi.org/10.5772/55411

that a minority is still so resistant to using sun products [22]. On the other hand, young Australians (from 12 – 17 years old) largely ignore prevention campaigns and the use of sun products decreased between 1993 and 2000 (going from 54 to 36% for teenagers in general and from 73 to 50% for girls in particular) [23]. A second more optimistic study praises the SunSmart television advertising campaign, which seems to be bearing fruit [24]. Indeed, the slogans are well-chosen and are likely to bring about a change of attitude; as proof: « Leave your hat on » (1991 – 1992), « How to remove a skin cancer » (1996 – 1998) and « No tan is worth dying for: Clare Oliver » (2008). In short, depending on the panels and on the authors, opinions differ [25]. The fact remains that young people in general, and more particularly young Americans (from the south of the USA) are stubborn and are still fond of exposing themselves to the sun. Sunburn at the end of the weekend is not uncommon [26]. A lot of efforts still have to be made, as only 1/3 of parents questioned say that they prefer activities for their children which avoid exposure to the sun and confirm that they apply sun products whilst doing beach-based activities [27]. Public awareness campaigns are necessary, as childhood is a key stage and it is important to understand that people who do not want to use sun products whilst continuing to expose themselves to the sun, do so for aesthetic reasons, in order to have a tan [28]. We set out, therefore, to present a method for topical skin protection: the use of sun products.

Countries	Prevalence
France	7/100000
Sweden	11/100000
US	14/100000
Australia	50/100 000

Table 1. Prevalence of skin cancers - 1995 [2]

Phototypes	Sensitivity to sunlight
I	Always burns, never tans
II	Burns easily, tans minimally
III	Burns moderately, tans gradually to light brown
IV	Burns minimally, always tans well to moderately brown
V	Rarely burns, tans profusely to dark
VI	Never burns, deeply pigmented

Table 2. Phototypes according to the Fitzpatrick classification

2. Topical photoprotection

2.1. Definition

There are many methods of sun protection, such as photoprotection by clothing, systemic photoprotection (medicine and dietary supplements) and topical photoprotection, using sun products with a variety of dosage forms.

Sun products are used to avoid skin damage due to the sun. These products contain molecules which can work through absorption or by reflecting UV rays [29].

The classification of sun products as either cosmetics, or as over-the-counter medicines, differs according to the health authority governing bodies concerned.

The Agence Française de Sécurité Sanitaire des Produits de Santé (AFSSaPS) [The French Agency for Health Safety and Health Products – equivalent to the FDA – Food and Drugs Administration (USA) and the MHRA (UK) remains cautious, saying that "Sun products are effective in the prevention of actinic erythema" It insists, by saying that their preventive effects concerning photo-ageing and skin cancer is yet to be proved [30]. In France, although the Code de la Santé Publique (Public Health Code), defines cosmetics in a general way, it does not, however, give a specific definition for sun products [31].

In the USA, an over-the-counter sunscreen drug product in a form suitable for topical administration is generally recognized as safe and effective and is not misbranded if it meets each condition. Here, we are talking of harmlessness and of efficacy (but without being specific about possible prevention regarding effects of UV radiation) [32]. This notion of harmlessness can be found in the Public Health Code [33], in European directives [34] and more recently in regulation N°1223/2009 [35] which has just been written and whose aim is to suggest a more legible type of legislation bringing together successive directive demands.

2.2. Which regulatory status for sun products?

2.2.1. Different categories of sun products

As we mentioned earlier, the status of sun product is not unique and differs from country to country. We will mention more specifically the two main legislations on suncare products, namely the European and American ones. It should be noted that the indices which may appear on the packaging of sun products are not the same for European products as they are for American ones (Table 3). In Europe, all of the products which have an SPF (Sun Protection Factor) lower than 6 are not considered as sun products (compared to 2 according to American legislation). The number of categories is bigger in Europe than in the USA (4 large categories and 8 indices in Europe compared to 3 large categories and an infinite number of indices which could be seen on the packaging in the USA. In Europe, in order to make the consumer's life easier and to avoid swamping them with too many indices, a standard index system on packaging was established. Therefore, on the market, products with indices of 17, 24, 36, 54 etc. cannot be found. The index value is always rounded down. In Europe, the tendency is to

http://dx.doi.org/10.5772/55411

reduce the number of indices, and the aim of the creation of an index of 50+ concerning all products which have a determined SPF equal to or higher than 60 was to avoid having indices higher than 100 on packaging, as this could have led the consumer to believe that the product provided total protection.

	European regulation	American regulation
Different categories of sunscreens	- Low protection SPF labelled: 6, 10 - Moderate protection SPF labelled: 15, 20, 25 - High protection SPF labelled: 30, 50 - Very high protection SPF labelled: 50+	- Minimal sun protection product (2 < SPF < 12) - Moderate sun protection product (12 ≤ SPF < 30) - High sun protection product (SPF ≥ 30)

Table 3. Different categories of sunscreens

2.2.2. *Authorized filters*

Whichever legislation is considered, a limited number of filters are authorized in the formulation of sun products. In Europe, Appendix VI of the Regulation lists the 26 authorized filters, that is to say 25 organic filters and one screen, titanium dioxide, each one having a maximum concentration of use (% m/m) and perhaps a list of comments which should feature on the packaging. In the USA, the original list was made up of 16 filters (15 filters and 1 screen). In the period from 1997 to 2008, 8 filters recognized safe and effective were gradually added to this list. The FDA gradually authorized a certain number of products which were synthetized and patented in Europe in order to beef up the original list. It should be noted that zinc oxide is not mentioned in Appendix VI of the Regulation (Table 4). The concentration of zinc oxide is therefore not limited. This, however, remains theoretical, as the limit is imposed by its dosage form, as in high percentages of concentration, a paste is obtained, which would be difficult to market. Seventeen filters are currently in common between the European and American legislation.

2.2.3. *The combination of different filters or the combination of filters with active ingredients*

European formulators have a great deal of freedom. They can combine as many filters as they want, as long as the combinations are not already patented, of course. They can also combine filters with active ingredients which have a softening, antioxidizing or soothing effect, etc. They have to check that the raw material they want to incorporate is not banned and they must check to see if the material is on a list if regulated ingredients (Appendix III: substances with restricted use in particular). In the USA, combinations with **protectants** are authorized within the limits of the maximum authorized concentrations (Table 5). **A skin protectant drug product is defined as «a drug product that temporarily protects injured or exposed skin or mucous membrane surfaces from harmful or annoying stimuli, and may help provide relief to such surfaces».**

INCI name/American name (trade name)	C_{max} authorized (Europe)	C_{max} authorized (US)
Aminobenzoic acid	/	15%
Cinoxate	/	3%
Dioxybenzone	/	3%
Meradimate	/	5%
Trolamine salicylate	/	12%
Zinc oxide	/	25%
Camphor benzalkonium methosulfate (Mexoryl SO®)	6%	/
Homosalate (Eusolex HMS, Néohélipan HMS, Parsol HMS)	10%	15%
Oxybenzone (Eusolex 4360, Uvinul M40)	10%	6%
Phenylbenzimidazole sulfonic acid, Ensulizole (Eusolex 232, Parsol HS, Néohéliopan Hydro USP)	8% (in acid form)	4%
Terephtalydene dicamphor sulfonic acid, Ecamsule (Mexoryl SX)	10% (in acid form)	10%
Butylmethoxydibenzoylmethane (Eusolex 9020, Parsol 178)	5%	3%
Benzylidene camphor sulfonic acid (Mexoryl SL)	6% (in acid form)	/
Octocrylene (Uvinul N539T, Eusolex OCR, Parsol 340, Néohéliopan 303 USP)	10% (in acid form)	10%
Polyacrylamidomethylbenzylidene camphor (Mexoryl SW)	6%	/
Ethyl hexyl methoxycinnamate, Octinoxate (Uvinul MC 80, Eusolex 2292, Parsol MCX, Néohéliopan AV)	10%	7.5%
PEG-25 PABA (Uvinul P25)	10%	/
Isoamyl p-methoxycinnamate, Amiloxate (Néohéliopan E1000)	10%	10%
Octyl triazone (Uvinul T150)	5%	5%
Drometrizole trisiloxane (Mexoryl XL)	15%	
Diethylhexylbutamidotriazone (Uvasorb HEB)	10%	3%
4 -methylbenzylidene camphor, Enzacamene (Eusolex 6300, Néohéliopan MBC, Parsol 5000)	4%	4%
3-benzylidene camphor (Unisol S22)	2%	/
Ethylhexylsalicylate, Octisalate (Eusolex OS, Néohéliopan OS, Dermoblock OS)	5%	5%
Octyl dimethyl PABA, Padimate O (Eusolex 6007)	8%	8%
Benzophenone-4 et 5 , Sulisobenzone (Uvinul MS40)	5% (in acid form)	10%
Methylene bis-benzotriazolyl tetramethylbutylphenol, Bisoctrizole (Tinosorb M)	10%	10%
Disodium phenyl dibenzimidazole tetrasulfonate (Néohéliopan AP)	10% (in acid form)	/
Bis-Ethylhexyloxyphenol Methoxyphenyl Triazine, Bemotrizinal (Tinosorb S)	10%	10%
Polysilicone 15 (Parsol SLX)	10%	/
Titanium dioxide	25%	25%
Diethylamino hydroxybenzoyl hexyl benzoate (Uvinul A+)	10%	/

Table 4. Authorized UV-filters in Europe and in US

	US	Europe
1 - Allantoin	0.5 – 2%	/
2 - Cocoa butter	50 – 100%	/
3 - Cod liver oil	5 – 13.56%	/
4 - Dimethicone	1 à 30%	/
5 - Glycerin	20 – 45%	/
6 - Hard fat	50 – 100%	/
7 - Lanolin	12.5 – 50%	/
8 - Mineral oil	50% 30 – 35% in combination with colloidal oatmeal	/
9 - Petrolatum	30%	/
10 - White petrolatum	30%	/
11 - Aluminium hydroxyde gel	0.15 – 5%	Annex III
12 - Calamine	1 - 25%	/
13 - Kaolin	4 – 20%	/
14 - Zinc acetate	0.1 – 2%	Annex Colorant (CI 77950)
15 - Zinc carbonate	0.2 – 2%	Annex III (1% expressed in Zinc)
16 - Zinc oxide	1 – 25%	Annex Colorant (CI 77947)
17 - Colloidal oatmeal	0.007% minimum 0.003% minimum in combination with mineral oil	/
18 - Topical starch	10 – 98%	/
19 - Sodium bicarbonate	/	/

Three ingredient groups in US : group 1 [1 to 10] – group 2 [11 to 16] and group 3 [17]

The active ingredients in each of these groups can be combined only with the other active ingredients in the same group. Active ingredients in different groups cannot be used in the same drug product. For example, cocoa butter can be combined with glycerine, but not with aluminium hydroxide gel.

Table 5. Comparative regulation of ingredients called « protectants » in US

2.2.4. Labelling rules

The comments which must be included on the packaging are presented in Table 6. The same concern for public health governs the labelling rules, no matter which legislation is concerned. It is a pity that at present, on the packaging of European sun products, there is no clear reference to the size of the recommended dose of the product which should be applied on the skin. This lack is currently being studied, and it has to be said that having directions on the packaging as to how much of the product should be used would be very useful, as it is known that consumers do not use as much of the product as they should, on average 4 times less [36]. It is known that the effect is linked to the dose. A good initiative of the Colipa should be noted concerning sun protection cosmetics: this committee has in fact created a logo (Figure 1) which reminds us that the product in question provides protection against UVA rays. A ratio of UVA efficacy/UVB efficacy equal to or lower than 3 was imposed in order to avoid products which only protect against UVB rays.

	EU	Europe
Categories of sunscreens	2 ‹ SPF ≤ 12 : « provides minimal » or « provides minimum » « minimal » or « minimum » « protection against » « sunburn » or « sunburn and tanning » or "for skin that sunburns minimally" 12 ≤ SPF ‹ 30 : « provides moderate » or "moderate" « protection against » « sunburn » or « sunburn and tanning » or "for skin that sunburns easily" SPF ≥ 30 : « provides high » or "high » « protection against » « sunburn » or « sunburn and tanning » or "for skin highly sensitive sunburn"	SPF : 6 – 10 Low protection SPF : 15 – 20 – 15 Moderate protection SPF : 30 – 50 High protection SPF : 50+ Very high protection
Warnings	"When using this product keep out of eyes. Rinse with water to remove" "Sto use and ask a doctor if rash or irritation developps and lasts"	/
Particular allegations	« retains SPF after 40 minutes of activity in the water or sweating or perspiring » « retains SPF after 40 minutes of activity in the water or sweating or perspiring"	Water resistant Very water resistant
Quantity to apply	« apply » « liberally » or « generously » or « smoothly » or « evenly » ""reapply as needed or after towel drying, swimming, or sweating or perspiring"	
Cas of childrens	« children under 6 months of age : ask a doctor »	No sun exposure before 36 months

Table 6. Labelling of sunscreens

http://dx.doi.org/10.5772/55411

Figure 1. UVA logo

2.2.5. Procedures to be followed

In Europe, it is just necessary to draw up a file on cosmetics which should remain relatively short. This is only consulted by authorized personnel from the authorities which are concerned (AFSSaPS or the Répression des Fraudes [Fraud Prevention]) in case of inspection. The status of an over-the-counter medicine is very restricting as solid clinical studies must back up the request for such a status. As an example, we can look at the Anthélios SX® product by the Laboratoires La Roche Posay whose sale is now authorized in the USA following FDA approval. The file was backed up by 28 clinical studies including 2500 patients from 6 months to 65 years of age. It can be said, therefore, that sun products destined for the American market are ones which have sufficient hindsight in Europe (enough time has lapsed to enable clinical studies to be compiled). What is more, very few active ingredients are present in the formula: ecamsule, avobenzone and octocrylene.

2.3. Dosage forms

Sun products come in different dosage forms: liquid forms (oils), thick pasty forms (emulsions which are referred to as milks or creams according to the texture) and solid forms (sticks). The most interesting forms are the systems which contain 2 phases enabling hydro- and liposoluble filters to be incorporated together. The role of the excipient is a minor one, and will have little influence on the SPF measured. However, it will have an important role to play in terms of how the product is spread [36], in terms of its substantivity (a sun product must stay on the surface and the phenomenon of transdermal penetration must be reduced to as little as possible) [37]. Pickering emulsions are interesting as their formula contains titanium dioxide which not only carries out the role of an active sun-protection ingredient but also that of an emulsion stabilizer [38].

2.3.1. Liquid forms: Sun oils and waters

Oils and waters are single-phase systems and are forms which provide minimal sun protection. Generally, they are composed of thermal water to which a hydrophilic filter is added. As for sun oils, they are generally composed of a vegetal oil, such as monoi, for example, or coconut or sesame oil, to which one or more lipophilic filters is added.

2.3.2. Paste forms: Gels and emulsions

Gels, often called "sun jellies", are forms which are not very photoprotective. These are aqueous or hydroalcoholic phases (the latter being quite incompatible with exposure to the sun!) which are thickened using a derivative of cellulose (carboxymethyl cellulose, for example) or a derivative of carboxyvinylic acid and incorporating a hydrophilic filter.

As for emulsions, they are the most commonly used dosage forms in the field of topical photoprotection. According to their viscosity and therefore their use limited to small surface areas (the face for example), or adapted to large areas (the whole body), they are referred to either as milks or creams. Whichever they may be, these forms provide a wide range of SPF values, going up to 50+. As they are two phase systems, (containing a hydrophilic phase and a lipophilic phase), they offer the great advantage of enabling all sorts of combinations of filters (hydro- and lipophilic ones) to which screens (such as zinc oxide and titanium dioxide) can be added. Lipophilic aqueous emulsions (W/O) are to be preferred due to their water-resistant character.

2.3.3. Solid forms: Sticks

The stick is a highly photoprotective cosmetic form which is adapted for application on small surface areas, obviously for the lips, and also for the sides of the nose, for example. A stick is made up of a mixture of waxes (animal wax, such as bees' wax, or vegetable waxes such as carnauba wax) which act as a "spine" for the finished product and give it its hardness, fats (vaseline, shea butter, etc.) and oils (sweet almond, jojoba, etc.). Lipophilic filters and screens are then incorporated into this mixture.

2.4. Determining the efficacy

2.4.1. Efficacy indicators: SPF and UVA-PF

In France, article L 5131-6 of the Public Health Code states that " a cosmetic product can only be put onto the market free of charge or against payment if the manufacturer, or their representative, or the person for whom the cosmetic product is made [...], effectively makes available to the controlling authorities [...] proof of the effects that it is claimed to have, when it is warranted by the nature of the effect or of the product". As for over-the-counter products, clinical trials must have been carried out, of course, in order for the product to be able to be put onto the market, as in this case, it is a medicine.

2.4.1.1. A few words about sun protection factor

The Sun Protection Factor (SPF) is a factor which indicates the efficacy of a sun product regarding erythema, as UVB rays are 1000 times more erythemogenic than UVA rays [39]. If we briefly recount the history of sun products, everything started in the 1930's with the marketing of a certain number of products containing sun filters (such as benzyl salicylate) [40] and claiming to prevent sunburn, without being able to evaluate precisely the level of efficacy. At this time, the product Ambre solaire® by the chemist Eugène Schueller could be found on the market. At the time, no particular attention was paid to the molecules used and a certain number of ingredients used were likely to cause what Freund defined for the first time as Berloque Dermatitis [41]. From the end of the Second World War, the number of companies involved in the field of sun protection (Coppertone, Piz Buin, etc.) increased, and more and more knowledge was gained about efficacy. Some errors were committed, however, such as the Bergasol products (in the 1970's) which were formulated with bergapten, which is a molecule with photosensitizing properties which are nowadays well-known [42]. The efficacy indicators which were initially very low, defined by Blum et al in 1945 [43], gradually increased, eventually reaching the values of 50+ which we know today.

2.4.2. In vivo methods of determination

Currently, whatever the country, protocols can be found which have similar conditions (type of panel, mass of the product applied, type of lamp used, etc.).

2.4.2.1. Definition of the MED

The FDA defines the MED as the "the quantity of erythema-effective energy (expressed as joules per square meter) required to produce the first perceptible, redness reaction with clearly defined borders".

The Colipa [44] gives its own definition, a precision of time, as we know that sunburn is likely to develop over a 24-hour period: "The Minimal Erythema Dose in human skin is defined as the lowest UV dose that produces the first perceptible unambiguous erythema with defined borders appearing over most of the field of UV exposure, 16 to 24 hours".

2.4.2.2. Definition of SPF

An individual Sun Protection Factor (SPF_i) value for a product is defined as the ratio of the MED on product protected skin (MED_p) to the MED on unprotected skin (MED_u) of the same subject:

$SPF = MED_p$ (protected skin) / MED_u (unprotected skin)

The SPF for the product is the arithmetic mean of all valid individual obtained from all subjects in the test, expressed to one decimal place.

2.4.2.3. Information concerning the volunteers

The comparative elements between the Colipa and the FDA concerning the subjects selected are presented in Table 7. As we can notice, the selection conditions are very similar. In Europe, the selection of subjects is made following the visual determining of the phototype of the subjects and by questioning or by instrumental methods using a chromameter which converts the colours into a digital code comprising 3 coordinates (Lab system). Using these coordinates, we can determine the ITA (Individual Typological Angle) which is proportional to the degree of pigmentation of the skin. The darker the skin, the smaller the angle [45, 46]. However, it is regrettable that the minimum number of subjects required by the Colipa in order to obtain valid results is only 10. The FDA demands double that number, which seems more reasonable. No notion of latent period between the tests is mentioned by the FDA. It is a pity that the presence of nevi is not totally unacceptable in the US, indeed, the link between multiple nevi and melanomas is a well-established fact. The risk of developing a melanoma for a person with multiple nevi, that is to say between 100 and 120, is 7 times higher than for someone who only has a few nevi (between 0 and 15) [47, 48, 49]. It would be interesting, therefore, to limit the tests to subjects with a low number of nevi. It also seems absurd to find references to people with phototype I skin, as these subjects are at risk of developing skin cancer [50]. It therefore appears useless to subject them to UV irradiation, whether it be natural or artificial.

	Colipa	**FDA**
Phototype	- Phototype I, II or III according to Fitzpatrick - or ITA°value > 28° by colorimetric methods	- Only fair-skin subjects with skin types I, II, and III using the following guidelines : I – always burns easily; never tans (sensitive) II – Always burns easily; tans minimally (sensitive) III – Burns moderately; tans gradually (light brown) (normal) (Skin type and Sunburn and tanning history based on first 30 to 45 minutes sun exposure after a winter season of no sun exposure)
Medical characteristics	- Exclusion of sensitive subjects (previous history of abnormal response to the sun) - children - pregnant or lactating women - subjects taking medication with photosensitising potential - subjects with dermatological problems - subjects accustomed to using tanning beds - subjects having marks, blemishes or nevi or presenting with existing sun damage	- Exclusion of sensitive subjects (previous history of abnormal response to the sun) - the presence of nevi, blemishes, or moles wille be acceptable if the physician's judgement they will not interfere with the study results.
Written consent	- Informed, written (signature) consent	- Legally effective written informed consent
Number of volunteers	- minimum 10 (10 valid results) - maximum 20	- minimum 20 (20 subjects must produce valid data for analysis) - maximum 25
Frequency of participation in tests	- Latence time of 2 months	/

Table 7. Characteristics of the panel

http://dx.doi.org/10.5772/55411

A test will be considered as valid if "confidence limits (95% Confidence Interval) for the mean SPF should fall within the range of ± 17% of the mean SPF". In the case of a high level of uncertainty, the subject(s) having generated over-large standard deviation are excluded from the study.

2.4.2.4. The conditions of the test

2.4.2.4.1. Test area

The irradiation sites are similar whether it be for the Colipa or the FDA: between the scapula line and the waist. The minimum surface area required according to the FDA is one of 50cm² for an area, and of 4 to 5 cm² for a subsite area. For the Colipa, the minimum area for a product application site shall be 30 cm² and the maximum shall be 60 cm².

The dose of the product applied on the skin is **2 mg/cm²** (this dose is universally recognized). The Colipa specifies that the quantity of the product applied on the skin before spreading should be 2 mg/cm² ± 2.5% (the sensitivity of the scales should be at least 0.0001 g, ie. with at least 4 decimal places). The product should be applied with a finger-cot and can be deposited with a syringe for liquid products, or for products which can be made into liquids after being warmed slightly. The Colipa states a quantity of 15 drops of the product for 30 cm² in order to obtain a homogenous distribution of the product. The application time is also measured and should be between 20 and 50 seconds according to the surface area in question. The products are applied in a randomized way.

The Colipa makes a clarification regarding the proximity of the test sites: there must be a minimum distance of 1 cm between the borders of adjacent product application sites.

A variable latent period is respected between application and irradiation: 15 minutes (FDA) or 15 to 30 minutes (Colipa).

The lack of information concerning the quantity of the product present on the skin after spreading is also regrettable. No *in vivo* method states the quantity of the product which remains on the finger-cot, a quantity which varies according to the nature of the product which is applied (a product which is either fluid or pasty, with either sticky or, on the contrary, film-forming ingredients).

The conditions of temperature of the room in which the tests are carried out are drawn up by the Colipa. It is recommended to use rooms with air-conditioning. However, the temperature range is quite wide (18 to 26°C).

2.4.2.4.2. The characteristics of the lamp used

The characteristics in terms of quality of emitted UV rays, of total irradiance and the uniformity of the beam are similar in Europe to the United States. The characteristics are the following: a solar simulator used for determining the SPF of a sunscreen product should be filtered so that it provides a continuous emission spectrum from 290 to 400 nm similar to sunlight at sea level from the sun at a zenith. No emission fluctuations should be seen through time and the intensity of irradiation should be as uniform as possible. The material should be subjected to frequent radiometric controls.

The source of illumination should be either a tungsten light bulb or a warm white fluorescent light bulb that provides a level of illumination at the test site within the range of 450 to 550 lux (FDA) or a xenon arc solar simulator with a filtering system.

2.4.2.4.3. Determining the MED in practice

A series of UV radiation exposures expressed as joules per square meter is administered to the each subject with an accurately-calibrated solar simulator.

A Colipa – FDA comparison is presented in Table 8. The FDA suggests some examples for SPF from 8 to 15.

	Colipa	**FDA**
Unprotected skin	- a minimum of **5** sub-sites centred on the estimated MEDu shall be exposed with incremental UV doses using a recommended geometric progression of either **1.12** or **1.25**.	- a series of **5** exposures should be administered to the untreated skin. The doses selected shall be a geometric series represented by (1.25^n), wherein each exposure time interval is **25%** greater than the previous time .
Protected skin	- The centre of the UV dose range is that of the unprotected MED multiplied by the expected SPF of the product. - a minimum of **5** sub-sites centred on the estimated MEDu shall be exposed with incremental UV doses using a recommended geometric progression of either **1.12** or **1.25**	- **7** exposures - the doses selected shall consist of a geometric series of five exposures where the middle exposure is placed to yield the expected SPF plus two other exposures placed symmetrically around the middle exposure.
Measure	- 24 h after exposure	- 24 h after exposure

Table 8. MED determination

For a product with an SPF of 8, given that the MED must correspond to the dose or to the median time, it will be surrounded with values obtained according to a geometric sequence at a rate of 1.25:

0.64 x MED – 0.80 x MED – 1 MED – 1.25 Med – 1.56 MED

Furthermore, 2 doses placed symmetrically in relation to the median dose are added, here:

0.9 x MED and 1.10 x MED

Sometimes, we speak in terms of SED (Standard Erythema Dose) which corresponds to the efficient erythemogenic exposure. For human beings, an SED corresponds to an exposure of 100 j/m^2. Caucasian subjects have an MED of between 150 j/m^2 (or 1.5 SED) and 600 j/m^2 (or 6.0 SED) according to the phototypes (as the Caucasian type includes phototypes which differ as much as phototypes I and IV) [51]. We can speak indifferently either in terms of dose or time.

2.4.2.5. Determining the UVA protection factor (UVA-FP)

2.4.2.5.1. Introduction

Although the protocol of determining the SPF is very clearly defined, both in Europe and in America, this is not the case concerning the UVA protection factor [52]. The two most frequently used methods are the IPD (Immediate Pigment Darkening) and PPD (Persistent Pigment Darkening) methods. Since 2007, taking the UVA protection in a sunscreen into account has become a necessity in Europe, with the establishing of 5 categories corresponding to no, low, medium, high and highest UVA protection [53].

2.4.2.5.2.- IPD and PPD methods

These methods are based on the evaluation of the Meirowski phenomenon consecutive to the action of UVA rays. To do this, a halide lamp or a xenon arc lamp equipped with UVB filters is used. The subjects who are recruited have phototypes III and IV because they are likely to develop a tan in the evening. If the reading takes place at a maximum of 2 hours after irradiation, we refer to the IPD (immediate pigment darkening) method. If the reading is taken later, we can refer to it as the PPD (persistant pigment darkening) method [54, 55, 56].

The UVA-PF is defined according to:

$$UVA\text{-}PF = MIPDD_{\text{protected skin}} / DMIPDD_{\text{unprotected skin}}$$

with MIPDD, Minimum Immediate Pigment Darkening Dose

or :

$$UVA\text{-}PF = MPPDD_{\text{protected skin}} / MPPDD_{\text{unprotected skin}}$$

with MPPDD, the Minimal Persistent Pigment Darkening Dose.

2.4.3. In vitro methods of determining the efficacy of sun products

2.4.3.1. Determining the SPF in vitro

There is no official method in this field. All the methods which are proposed are spectrophotometric methods based on the Beer Lambert law which links the absorbance of a sample to its concentration of active molecules. The principal of determining the SPF *in vitro* is based on measuring the transmittance of a sun product applied on various kinds of support. In the 1980's, Sayre and Agin studied different spectral light sources enabling them to correlate the results obtained respectively by *in vitro* and *in vivo* methods [58]. The first trials were carried out on supports such as certain animal skins (mice and pigs) or even on human skin. In 1989, Diffey and Robson tested a new substrate called Transpore® (3M, St Paul, US), a cheap adhesive system [59]. Its supple texture means that it must be placed on a rigid plate (such as quartz). The main disadvantage for its use is that it has varying sizes of pores depending on the part of the roll of the material which is used (which means that the first and last 60cm of the roll must be discarded and that the pores vary in size from one roll to the next. It is interesting for testing simple formulas, however, the results obtained are very different from those observed *in vivo* for formulas including complex mixtures of filters [60]. The quartz plates can also be used alone. They have 2 disadvantages: they are expensive and as they are not disposable, they must be rigorously cleaned between 2 series of measurements. Even though they are able to be used in research, they seem to be quite unsuitable for industrial use [61]. Skin substitutes (Vitroskin®) provide an interesting analogy with real skin, but they are expensive and they have a limited length of use once they have been rehydrated [62]. Different synthetic substrates are currently used, such as polyvinylchloride film (Saran Wrap®), Teflon [63] and polymethylmethacrylate (PMMA) [64, 65]. Whatever support is chosen, its efficacy in UVB light is determined by calculation, by effecting the convolution product of the spectrum of the source, of the spectrum transmitted through the sample and of the spectrum of the erythemogenic efficacy (figure 2) [66] and by integrating the area under the curve in the following formula:

$$SPF = \frac{\sum_{290}^{400} E_\lambda S_\lambda \Delta\lambda}{\sum_{290}^{400} E_\lambda S_\lambda T_\lambda \Delta\lambda}$$

with E_λ being the spectral erythemogenic efficacy (International Committee on Illumination), S_λ being solar spectral irradiance and T_λ being the spectral transmittance of the sample.

2.4.3.2. In vitro determination of the UVA-PF

The Colipa published guidelines in 2007 for determining the UVA index *in vitro*. The initial UVA-PF is calculated using the UV absorbance spectrum which was adjusted to the labelled SPF. Sunscreen samples were then exposed to a single UV dose of 1.2 times the initial UVA-PF (in joules/m^2). The final UVA-PF values for the samples were calculated from the adjusted absorbance spectrum after irradiation [67]. Other calculations made are those of the SPF/UVA-PF ratio, which must be lower than 3, and the critical wavelength λ_c (the wavelength under which the product is 90% effective) which must be above or equal to 370 nm according to the recommendations of the AFSSaPS.

At the same time, the FDA suggested an *in vitro* method for determining the efficacy in UVA rays. The *in vitro* UVA proposed is based on measurement of UV transmission through a sunscreen film. The absorbance curve was obtained, in this case after pre-irradiation with a UV dose specified as two thirds of the SPF in Minimal Erythemal Doses (MEDs) (1 MED = 20 SED), and the mean absorbance in the UVA1 range from 340 to 400 nm and the entire UV range from 290 to 400 nm were determined. The ratio of mean UVA1 absorbance to mean absorbance

http://dx.doi.org/10.5772/55411

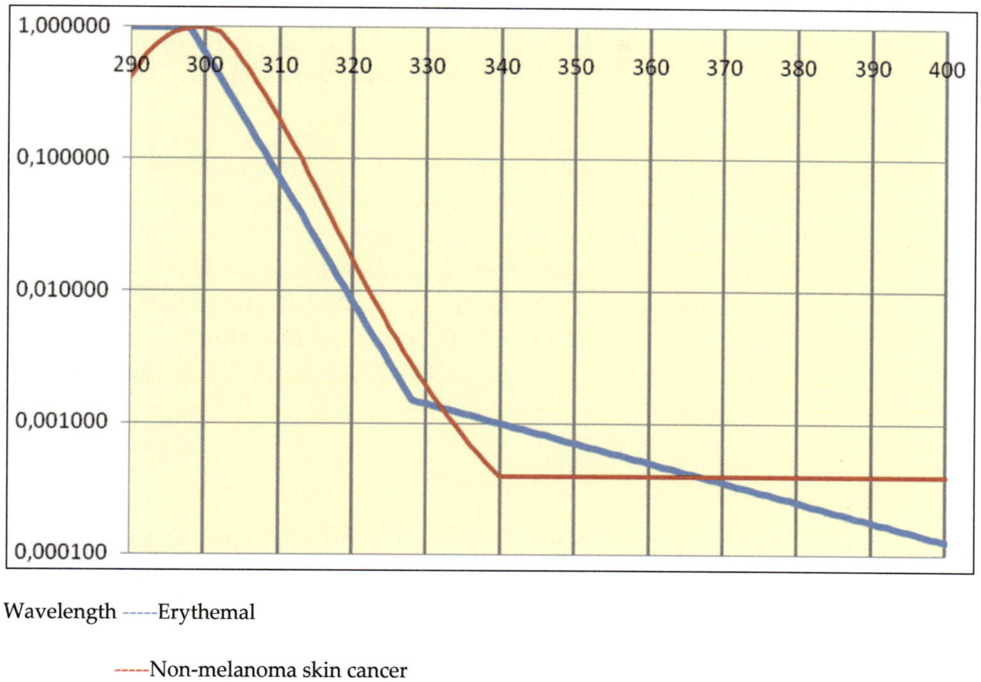

Figure 2. Variations of weighting coefficients for each wavelength concerning erythema and non-melanoma skin cancer (Norme CEI 60335-2-27, 2002)

determines the rating. There are 4 categories (ratio ≥ 0.2 "low – 1 star" ; ratio ≥ 0.4 "medium – 2 stars" ; ratio ≥ 0.7 "high – 4 stars" ; ratio > 0.95 "highest – 4 stars") [68].

2.5. Determining water-resistance and photostability

2.5.1. Determining water-resistance

The technique and the quantity of the product applied on the skin play an important role in the obtained level of photoprotection. The same applies to the water-resistance of products [69] which is an important element to take into account when choosing a product which is going to be used on the beach.

2.5.1.1. In vivo methods of determining water-resistance

The FDA and the Colipa propose protocols for determining the water-resistance of sun products [70, 71].

The principal is the same in both cases. The subjects are immersed in a swimming pool or a jacuzzi, etc. On the other hand, the way of interpreting the results is not done in the same way in Europe and in the United States.

In the United States, a product can display the words "water resistant" on the packaging and the SPF mentioned is the SPF obtained after 2 successive baths of 20 minutes. For the product to qualify as being "very water resistant", it must have undergone a test of 4 successive baths of 20 minutes.

In Europe, a certain number of pre-requisites must be checked before the test is carried out to ensure that the incertitude is less than 17% of the average SPF. A percentage of water resistance is calculated by comparing the SPF obtained after 2 successive baths of 20 minutes and the initial SPF. If the percentage is higher than or equal to 50% of the initial SPF, then the product is declared as being "water resistant". In the same way, a product is declared as being "very water resistant" if after 80 minutes of immersion (4 periods of 20 minutes) the percentage of water resistance is higher than or equal to 50%. In both cases, the SPF displayed is the initial one (obtained before immersion).

2.5.1.2. In vitro method of determining water resistance

Very few studies exist concerning the development of *in vitro* techniques. Work by Choquenet et al can be quoted, which, by analogy with the Colipa method, provide the necessary conditions for distinguishing water resistant products from products which can be washed away with water [72]. The authors recommend immersing the PMMA plates, coated with the product which is to be tested, in a bath of distilled water, shaken gently (5 $L.min^{-1}$) and at a temperature of 29 ± 2°C. The creams are applied to the PMMA plates and their SPF is measured using an integrating sphere spectrophotometer (Labsphère UV1000S) before and after immersion. As in the *in vivo* method, the product is deemed "water resistant" if the SPF after the bath is at least 50% of the initial SPF.

2.5.2. Determining the photostability of sun products

The photostability of sun products is an important criterion for two reasons: if the product is not photostable, its efficacy will decrease rapidly over time and the subject will thus no longer be sufficiently protected. Furthermore, the production of photo-oxidation products can lead to problems of skin tolerance [73]. It is advisable therefore to study the photodegradation profile of the filters incorporated into the excipients and to determine efficacy kinetics over time. Certain filters such as PABA [74] or benzophenones [75] are reputed to be very photostable. Other filters which are not very photostable, such as avobenzone, have a varying degree of stability according to the composition of the medium [76]. The filters can be studied alone or in a mixture, they can be irradiated after being placed on a glass plate in the UVB/UVA field and their photostability can be assessed by the dose of HPLC [77] or they can be studied *in vivo*. L'Oréal carried out an *in vivo* study in 2008 on 5 subjects. This study consisted in applying a product (SPF 15 ; FP-UVA 15) onto the volunteers' skin, formulated with 3 organic filters, octocrylene, avobenzone and Mexoryl SX®, irradiating them at doses ranging from 64 to 200% of the SPF, in retrieving the product from the skin and then dosing the filters. There was no significant difference between the rate of filters before and after irradiation, even for the high doses (200% SPF ie. 30 MED) [78]. A systematic study of the 18 UVB filters which are authorized in Europe enabled the filters to be ranked in ascending order of photostability. The filters which

http://dx.doi.org/10.5772/55411

retain more than 90% of their efficacy after irradiation in a solar simulator are deemed to be photostable. Eight filters (PABA, Oxybenzone, Phenilbenzimidazole sulfonic acid, Octocrylene, Diethylhexylbutamidotriazine, 4-methylbenzylidene camphor, Benzophenone-5 and Methylene bis-benzotriazolyl tetramethylbutylphenol) appear to be interesting and likely to stabilize the formulas they are incorporated into [79].

2.6. Active ingredients

There are two categories of active ingredients, inorganic filters, also known as screens, and organic filters.

2.6.1. Inorganic filters or screens

Two screens could be used: titanium dioxide and zinc oxide which act by reflecting the ultraviolet rays. Both take the form of an inert, particularly photostable white powder [80, 81]. They were used for a long time in pigmentation, but were considered not to be very effective and were not very aesthetic due to the fact that they leave a white film on the skin sometimes called the "Pierrot's mask". The micronization of powders brought a solution to these 2 disadvantages [82, 83]. The reduction of the size of the particles from 200 nm to 15 nm makes the products more acceptable and coating them makes them disperse more easily in the chosen excipient. However, the reduction of the size of the particles raises certain questions, namely as to whether they can cross the skin barrier. Studies on pig skin show that micro-thin zinc oxide and titanium dioxide powders do not penetrate into the skin [84]. Similar results were obtained *in vivo* by the stripping method and showed that zinc oxide (Z-Cote Max® BASF) was restricted to the superficial layers of the epidermis, namely the *Stratum corneum* [85]. As for harmlessness, the results contrast. Some people argue that a risk exists, zinc oxide could have potentially genotoxic effects on human epidermal cells [86] and titanium dioxide could be cytotoxic and genotoxic on cell cultures (hamster ovary cells) [87]. For others, these ingredients are totally safe [88, 89]. Concerning efficacy, titanium dioxide proves to be the most efficient, as it gives an SPF value of 10 (Eusolex TS®) as opposed to 5 for zinc oxide (Z-Cote Max®) for the same incorporation percentage of 10%. It can be noted, however, that zinc oxide has a wider spectrum as it proves to be as efficient in the UVA field as in the UVB field, contrary to titanium dioxide which is 2.5 times less efficient in UVA rays as in UVB rays [90].

2.6.2. Organic filters

2.6.2.1. Introduction

It is a question of molecules which have one or more aromatic cycles associated with a substituent electron donor and/or an unsaturated hydrocarbon chain. These molecules are characterized by a chromophoric group which absorbs the incident photons' energy at certain wavelengths. It is said that the filters are selective, as they only absorb energy in a well-defined range of the UV spectrum. Each filter is thus characterized by its wavelength of maximum absorption (λ_{max}).

2.6.2.2. The main families and their characteristics

PABA (λ_{max} = 309 nm) is now banned in Europe due to the fact that it is highly allergenic [91]. Its derivatives (PEG-25 PABA and Octyldimethyl PABA) are less allergenic and are still authorized in Europe. They are some examples of the few hydrosoluble filters available. According to the grafting which was carried out, the efficacy is variable. Octyldimethyl PABA (Padimate O) enables an SPF value of 9 to be attained for 8% of incorporation, and PEG-25 PABA gives an SPF of 4 for 10% [92].

Cinnamates are the most widely used UVB filters. As an example, we can give octylmethoxycinnamate (OMC) (λ_{max} = 310 nm). Indeed, it is found in a large number of products on the market. Cinnamates are well tolerated, even though they are linked with the notion of being endocrine disruptors. It should be remembered however, that OMC has 140,000 times less affinity for α receptors and 500,000 times less affinity for β oestrogen receptors than βestradiol, the standard oestrogen [93] and that its uterotrophic effects in animals is judged to be very low [94]. Cinnamic esters are quite efficient filters as they generate approximately 1 SPF unit per percentage of use [92].

Salicylates are poor photoprotectors. We can mention in particular homomenthyl salicylate or homosalate (λ_{max} = 306 nm) which, when incorporated into the recommended excipient at 8%, constitutes the FDA standard and which enables an average SPF of 4.47 (4.47 ± 1.279) to be reached. It is practically non-existent in European products. Certain publications report that octisalate (or octyl salicylate) has a proliferative effect on MCF-7 cells in breast cancer [95].

Benzophenones are wide spectrum filters which give 2 maxima of absorption in UV rays, one of 285 nm and the other close to 325 nm. As examples, we can mention benzophenone-3 (or oxybenzone) and benzophenone-4 and 5. Although they are not very efficient filters (SPF of 3 to 10% for oxybenzone and 4 to 5% for benzophenone-4), they are interesting, however, because they are very stable. Their low substantivity is a disadvantage, as is their poor tolerance (frequent allergic reactions for oxybezone) [96, 97]. Questions are being raised in other respects, as there could be a potentialization of the transdermic penetration of oxybenzone by a frequently associated repellent, DEET (NN diethyl-m-toluamide) but opinions are divided [98, 99]. What is certain is that oxybenzone is a filter which is found in the organism after topical application. It is known that 1 to 2% of the oxybenzone contained in a formula is absorbed after 10 hours. It is advised that these products should not be applied over large surfaces and that repeated applications should be avoided [100]. As for formulation, certain ingredients such as Transcutol® (diethylene glycol monoethyl ether) could be looked for, which increase substantivity without favouring crossing the skin barrier [101]. These are not therefore filters that should be rejected, but rather filters that should be used with care.

Triazines and derivatives (Bemotrizinal or Tinosorb S® -305 and 360 nm- and Bisoctrizole or Tinosorb M® -310 et 340 nm) are safe from a toxicological point of view [102]. They are marketed by a company called Ciba and are synergic. It is thus particularly interesting to combine them in the same formula. Bisoctrizole is both the best UVB and the best UVA filter on the market [92].

Mexoryls® and more precisely Mexoryl SX® are derivatives of camphor. The latter is the only Mexoryl® of the series to be authorized in the United States. It is presented as an interesting filter regarding protection from skin damage caused by UVA rays both *in vitro* and *in vivo* [103, 104].

Concerning UVA filters, avobenzone is widely used and its lack of stability can be compensated for by combining it with other filters. Encapsulation, although fuelling many publications, has not enabled any industrial application so far [105, 106]. Neoheliopan AP® and Uvinul A+® are not authorized in the United States yet.

It is a pity that 3-benzylidene camphor (limited to 2%) is still authorized in Europe, as at this dose it is almost inefficient and it is also suspected of being an endocrine disruptor [107, 108].

2.6.3. Molecules of interest

Although a certain number of authors claim that the toxicity of organic filters is irrefutable, the same cannot be said for the others. The potential endocrine effect of certain filters is not conclusive and the controversy concerning parabens which has shaken the scientific community [109] lead us to believe that in the field, it is necessary to be prudent and indispensable ingredients for photoprotection should not be too hastily discredited. However, confronted with these threats, it would be advisable to find new filters, especially using plants as a source, as well as ingredients which could complete the action thanks to their original properties.

We could mention, for example, boldine, an alkaloid from the boldo tree, which has been known for a long time for its antioxidant properties [110] and more recently for a potential photoprotective effect [111]. Aromatic compounds contained in certain lichens [1 chloropannarine, epiphorelic acid I and II, calicine) prove *in vitro* to be of a level of efficacy comparable to that of OMC [112]. Flavonoids, natural colorants of many plants prove to be an interesting family too with chlorogenic acid in particular (SPF = 10), baicaline (SPF = 8), luteoline (SPF = 7), apigenine (SPF = 7), puerarine (SPF = 6) for a usage dose of 10% [113]. Coming from the sea, mycosporine-like aminoacids seem to be interesting in particular with a potential photoprotective effect in the UVA field [114, 115, 116].

3. Care products and make-up with SPF

Recently, there has been a wave of care products and make-up with SPF on the market, their SPF being mainly around 15. The justification for this is found in publications which state that there is a beneficial effect of using filters on a daily basis in order to prevent skin ageing and in particular using a mixture of avobenzone (1.5%) - ecamsule (1.5%) - octocrylene (4%) [117]. Even if we know very well that UV rays are responsible for actinic ageing, the daily use of products containing filters does not seem to be a good thing. It appears that filters, even though they are active, sometimes have adverse effects. They must be kept, therefore, for use in sun care products, all the more so as these other care products are not sun care products, so do not have to obey the same rules, namely those concerning the SPF / UVA-PF ratio and the critical wavelength [118].

4. Conclusion

Given the consequences for the skin of exposure to the sun, it seems necessary to ensure effective photoprotection. We have seen the various dosage forms, which offer a wide range of products adapted to the site of application. According to the quality-quantity of the product, the level of efficacy can vary greatly. The status of the products in itself is not unique, on one side of the Atlantic or the other, as cosmetics, medical devices and OTC medicines can be found. On the other hand, the methods for determining the efficacy of these products are almost universal.

Author details

C. Couteau and L. Coiffard

Université de Nantes, Nantes Atlantique Universités, MMS, Faculté de Pharmacie, Nantes, France

References

[1] Garvin, T., Eyles, J. (2001). Public health responses for skin cancer prevention: the policy framing of Sun Safety in Australia, Canada and England Social Science & Medicine, 53, 1175-1189.

[2] Bressac-de-Paillerets, B., Avril, M.F., Chompret, A., Demenais, F. (2002). Genetic and environmental factors in cutaneous malignant melanoma Biochimie, 84, 67-74.

[3] Medhaug, I., Olseth, J.A., Reuder, J. (2009). UV radiation and skin cancer in Norway. Journal of Photochemistry and Photobiology B: Biology, 96, 232-241.

[4] Nagano, T., Ueda, M., Suzuki, T., Naruse, K., Nakamura, T., Taguchi, M., Araki, K., Nakagawa, K., Nagai, H., Hayashi, K., Watanabe, S., Ichihashi, M. (1999). Skin cancer screening in Okinawa, Japan. Journal of Dermatological Science, 19, 161-165.

[5] van Steeg, H., Kraemer, K.H. (1999). Xeroderma pigmentosum and the role of UV-induced DNA damage in skin cancer. Molecular Medicine Today, 5, 86-94.

[6] de Vries, E., Steliarova-Foucher, E., Spatz, A., Ardanaz, E., Eggermont, A.M.M.,W.W. Coebergh W.W. (2006). Skin cancer incidence and survival in European children and adolescents (1978–1997). Report from the Automated Childhood Cancer Information System project. European Journal of Cancer, 42, 2170-2182.

[7] Hiom, S. (2006). Public awareness regarding UV risks and vitamin D—The challenges for UK skin cancer prevention campaigns. Progress in Biophysics and Molecular Biology, 92, 161-166.

[8] De Gruijil, F.R. (1999). Skin cancer and solar UV radiation. European Journal of Cancer, 35, 2003-2009.

[9] Armstrong, B.K., Anne Kricker, A. (2001). The epidemiology of UV induced skin cancer. Journal of Photochemistry and Photobiology B: Biology, 63, 8-18.

[10] Meunier, L., Raison-Peyron, N., J Meynadier, J. (1998). Immunosuppression photo-induite et cancers cutanés. La Revue de Médecine Interne, 19, 247-254.

[11] Jean, D. (2008). L'enfant en montagne : dangers de l'altitude, du froid et du soleil. Journal de Pédiatrie et de Puériculture, 21, 349-352.

[12] Ichihashi, M., Ueda, M., Budiyanto, A., Bito, T., Oka, M., Fukunaga, M., Tsuru, K., Horikawa, T. (2003). UV-induced skin damage. Toxicology, 189, 21-39.

[13] Tsukahara, K., Sugata, K., Osanai, O., Ohuchi, A., Miyauchi, Y., Takizawa, M., Hotta, M., Kitahara, T. (2007). Comparison of age-related changes in facial wrinkles and sagging in the skin of Japanese, Chinese and Thai women. Journal of Dermatological Science, 47, 19-28.

[14] Kawada, A. (2000). Risk and preventive factors for skin phototype Journal of Dermatological Science, 23, S27-S29.

[15] Kaneko, F., Nakamura, K., Furukawa, H., Oyama, N., Nakamura, T., Zheng, X. (2008). Biological characteristics of the sensitive Japanese skin, International Journal of Cosmetic Science, 27, 66-67.

[16] Turberg-Romain, C. (2003). Médecine de l'enfant et de l'adolescent. Paris : Elsevier.

[17] Gloster Jr., H.G., Kenneth Neal, K. (2006). Skin cancer in skin of color. Journal of the American Academy of Dermatology, 55, 741-760.

[18] Wendy E. Roberts, W.E. (2009). Skin Type Classification Systems Old and New Dermatologic Clinics, 27, 529-533.

[19] Pichon, L.C., Mayer, J.A., Slymen, D.J., Elder, J.P., Lewis, E.C., Galindo, G.R. (2005). Ethnoracial differences among outdoor workers in key sun-safety behaviors American Journal of Preventive Medicine, 28, 374-378.

[20] Ezzedine, K., Guinot, C., Mauger, E., Pistone, T., Receveur, M.C., Galan, P., Hercberg, S., Malvy, D. (2007). Travellers to high UV-index countries: Sun-exposure behaviour in 7822 French adults. Travel Medicine and Infectious Disease, 5, 176-182.

[21] Dubertret, L. (2000). Peau et environnement. Comptes Rendus de l'Académie des Sciences - Series III - Sciences de la Vie, 323, 629-632.

[22] Peacey, V., Steptoe, A., Sanderman, R., Wardle, J. (2006). Ten-year changes in sun protection behaviors and beliefs of young adults in 13 European countries Preventive Medicine, 43, 460-465.

[23] Livingston, P.M., White, V., Hayman, J., Dobbinson, S.J. (2007). Australian adolescents' sun protection behavior: Who are we kidding? Preventive Medicine, 44, 508-512.

[24] Dobbinson, S.J., Wakefield, M.A., Jamsen, K.M., Herd, N.L., Spittal, M.J., John Lipscomb, E., Hill, D.J. (2008). Weekend Sun Protection and Sunburn in Australia: Trends (1987–2002) and Association with SunSmart Television Advertising. American Journal of Preventive Medicine, 34, 94-101.

[25] Keeney, S., McKenna, H., Fleming, P., McIlfatrick, S. (2009). Attitudes, knowledge and behaviours with regard to skin cancer: A literature review European Journal of Oncology Nursing, 13, 29-35.

[26] Reynolds, K.D., Blaum, J.M., Jester, P.M., Weiss, H., Soong, S., DiClemente R.J. (1996). Predictors of sun exposure in adolescents in a southeastern U.S. population. Journal of Adolescent Health, 19, 409-415.

[27] Robinson, J.K., Rigel, D.S., Rex A. Amonette, R.A. (2000). Summertime sun protection used by adults for their children. Journal of the American Academy of Dermatology, 42, 746-753.

[28] Eid, M. (2004). Sun Exposure and Skin Cancer Prevention International Encyclopedia of the Social & Behavioral Sciences, 15278-15281

[29] González, S., Fernández-Lorente, M., Yolanda Gilaberte-Calzada, Y. (2008). The latest on skin photoprotection. Clinics in Dermatology, 26, 614-626.

[30] AFSSaPS, Recommandations concernant les conditions d'étiquetage des produits de protection solaire, 2006.

[31] Code de la Santé Publique. 23ème édition, Dalloz, 2009, 2856 p.

[32] FDA – PART 352-Sunscreen drug products for over-the-counter human use (stayed indefinitely) – Subpart A – General provisions

[33] Directive 76/768/CEE du Conseil, du 27 juillet 1976, concernant le rapprochement des législations des Etats membres relatives aux produits cosmétiques.

[34] Règlement (CE) n°1223/2009 du parlement européen et du Conseil du 30 novembre 2009 relatif aux produits cosmétiques.

[35] Kim, S.M., Oh, B.H., Lee, Y.L., Choe, Y.B., Ahn, K.J. (2010). The relation between the amount of sunscreen applied and the sun protection factor in Asian skin. Journal of the American Academy of Dermatology, 62, 218-222.

[36] Salka, B.A. (1997). Choosing emollients: four factors will help you decide. Cosmetics and toiletries, 112, 10, 101-104.

[37] Lafforgue, C., Marty, J.P. (2007). Absorption percutanée. Annales de dermatologie et de Vénéréologie, 134, S18-S23.

[38] Stiller, S., Gers-Barlag, H., Lergenmueller, M., Pflücker, F., Schulz, J. Wittern, K.P., Daniels, R. (2004). Investigation of the stability in emulsions stabilized with different surface modified titanium dioxides. Colloids and Surfaces A: Physicochemical and Engineering Aspects, 232, 261-267.

[39] Rosen, C.F. (1999). Photoprotection. Seminars in Cutaneous Medicine and Surgery, 18, 307-314.

[40] Urbach, F. (2001). The historical aspects of sunscreens. Jouranl of Photochemistry and Photobiology B, 64, 99-104.

[41] Albert, M.R.,Ostheimer, K.G. (2003). The evolution of current medical and popular attitudes toward ultraviolet light exposure. Journal of American Academy of Dermatology, 19, 1096 – 1106.

[42] Bakkali, F., Averbeck, S., Averbeck, D., Idaomar, M. (2008) Biological effects of essential oils – a review. Food and Chemical Toxicology 46, 446–475.

[43] Blum, H., Eicher, M., Terus, W. (1945). Evaluation of protective measures against sunburn. American Journal of Physiology, 146, 118–125.

[44] Colipa, (2003). International Sun Protection Factor (SPF) test method.

[45] Pierard, G.E. (1998). Ageing in the sun parlour. International Journal of Cosmetic Science, 20, 251–259.

[46] Wei, L., Xuemin, W., Wei, L., Li, L., Ping, Z., Yanyu, W., Ying, L., Yan, L., Yan, T., Yan, W., Li, C. (2007). Skin color measurement in Chinese female population : analysis of 407 cases from 4 major cities of china. International Journal of Dermatology, 46, 835– 839.

[47] Gandini, S., Sera, F., Cattaruzza, M.S., Pasquini, P., Abeni, D., Boyle, P., Melchi, C.F. (2005). Meta-analysis of risk factors for cutaneous melanoma: I. Common and atypical naevi. European Journal of Cancer, 41, 28-44.

[48] Woolley, T., Buettner, P.G., Lowe, J. (2004). Predictors of sun protection in northern Australian men with a history of non melanoma skin cancer. Preventive Medicine, 39, 300-307.

[49] Richtig, E., Santigli, E., Fink-Puches, R., Weger, W., R. Hofmann-Wellenhof, R. (2008). Assessing melanoma risk factors: How closely do patients and doctors agree? Public Health, 122, 1433-1439.

[50] Kawada, A. (2000). Risk and preventive factors for skin phototype Journal of Dermatological Science, 23, S27-S29.

[51] Narbutt, J., Lesiak, A., Sysa-Jedrzejowska, A., Boncela, J., Wozniacka, A., Norval, M. (2007). Repeated exposures of humans to low doses of solar simulated radiation lead to limited photoadaptation and photoprotection against UVB-induced erythema and cytokine mRNA up-regulation. Journal of Dermatological Science, 45, 210-212.

[52] Curtis, C., Skilman, N.J., Chen, T., Appa, Y. (2008). A primer for understanding and communicating UVA protection in sunscreens. Journal of the American Academy of Dermatology, 58, AB112.

[53] Osterwalder, U., Herzog. B., Dueva-Koganov. O. (2010). Understanding sunscreens: The proposed FDA rule on UVA assessment and labeling will drive US sunscreens towards a uniform UVB/UVA protection profile. Journal of the American Academy of Dermatology, 62, AB24.

[54] Routaboul, C., Denis, A., Vinche, A. (1999). Immediate Pigment Darkening: description, kinetic and biological function. European Journal of Dermatology, 9, 439-445.

[55] Moyal, D., Chardon, A., Kollias, N. (2000). Determination of UVA protection factors using PPD as the end point (Part 1). Calibration of the method. Photodermatology, Photoimmunology & Photomedicine, 16, 245- 249.

[56] Moyal, D., Chardon, A., Kollias, N. (2000). UVA protection efficacy can be determined by persistent pigment darkening (PPD) method (Part 2). Photodermatology, Photoimmunology & Photomedicine, 16, 250-255.

[57] Sayre, R.M., Agin, P.P. (1984) Comparison of human sun protection factors to predicted protection factors using different lamp spectra. Journal of the Society of Cosmetic Chemist, 35, 439–445.

[58] Diffey, B.L., Robson, J.A. (1989). A new substrate to mesure sunscreen protection factors throughout the UV spectrum. Journal of the Society of Cosmetic Chemist, 40, 127–133.

[59] Springsteen, A., Yurek, R., Frazier, M., Carr, K.F. (1999). In vitro measurement of sun protection factor of sunscreens by diffuse transmittance. Analytica Chimica Acta, 380, 155-164.

[60] Arkman, J., Kubac, C., Bendova, H., Jirova, D., Kejlova, K. (2009). Quatrz plates for determining sun protection factor in vitro and testing photostability of commercial sunscreens. International Journal of Cosmetic Science, 31, 119–129.

[61] Garoli, D., Pelizzo, M.G., Nicolosi, P., Peserico, A., Tonin, E., Alaibac, M. (2009). Effectiveness of different substrate materials for *in vitro* sunscreen tests Journal of Dermatological Science, 56, 89-98.

[62] Garoli, D., Pelizzo, M.G., Bernardini, B., Nicolosi, P., Mauro Alaibac, M. (2008).Sunscreen tests: Correspondence between *in vitro* data and values reported by the manufacturers. Journal of Dermatological Science, 52, 193-204.

[63] El-Boury, S., Couteau, C., Boulande, L., Paparis, E., L.J.M. Coiffard, L J.M. (2007). Effect of the combination of organic and inorganic filters on the Sun Protection Factor (SPF) determined by *in vitro* method International Journal of Pharmaceutics, 340, 1-5.

[64] Osterwalder, U., Mueller, S., Giesinger, J., Herzog, B. (2008). Understanding sunscreens—In vitro SPF determination requires correction for in vivo photo degradation. Journal of the American Academy of Dermatology, 58, AB29.

[65] Diffey, B.L., Robson, J. (1989). Sun Protection Factor in vitro. Journal of the Society of Cosmetic Chemist, 40, 127-132.

[66] Colipa (2007). Recommendation N°20 In vitro UVA test method.

[67] Wang, S.Q., Stanfield, J.W., Osterwalder, U. (2008). In vitro assessments of UVA protection by popular sunscreens available in the United States Journal of the American Academy of Dermatology, 59, 934-942.

[68] Diffey, B. (2001). Sunscreen isn't enough. Journal of Photochemistry and Photobiology B: Biology, 64, 105-108.

[69] FDA Part 352- Sunscreen drug products for over-the-counter human use – Subpart D - Testing procedures

[70] Colipa (2006). Recommandation N°16 Water resistance labelling

[71] Choquenet, B., Couteau, C., Paparis, E., Coiffard, L.J.M. (2008). Development of an in vitro test to determine the water-resistance of sunscreens. Pharmazie, 63, 525–527.

[72] Gaspar, L.R., Maia Campos P.M. (2006). Evaluation of the photostability of different UV filter combinations in a sunscreen. International Journal of Pharmaceutics, 307, 123-128.

[73] Flindt-Hansen, H., Nielsen, C.T., Thune, J.P. Measurements of the photodegradation of PABA and some PABA derivatives. Photodermatology, 1988, 5, 257–260.

[74] Kiguchi, M., Evans, P.D. (1998). Photostabilisation of wood surfaces using a grafted benzophenone UV absorber. Polymer Degradation and Stability, 61, 33-45.

[75] Cantrell, A., David J. McGarvey, D.J. Photochemical studies of 4-*tert*-butyl-4′-methoxydibenzoylmethane (BM-DBM). Journal of Photochemistry and Photobiology B: Biology, 64, 117-122.

[76] Venditti, E., Spadoni, T., L. Tiano, L., P. Astolfi, P., L. Greci, L., G.P. Littarru, G.P., Damiani, E. (2008). *In vitro* photostability and photoprotection studies of a novel 'multi-active' UV-absorber. Free Radical Biology and Medicine, 45, 345-354.

[77] Auteur (2008). Evaluation of photostability of a suncare product under UV exposure in humans. Journal of the American Academy of Dermatology, 58, AB112.

[78] Couteau, C., Faure, A., Fortin, J., Paparis, E., Coiffard, L.J.M. (2007). Study of the photostability of 18 sunscreens in creams by measuring the SPF *in vitro*. Journal of Pharmaceutic and Biomedicals Analusis, 44, 270-273.

[79] Allen, N.S., Edge, M., Ortega, A., Christopher M. Liauw, C. John Stratton, Robert B. (2002). Behaviour of nanoparticle (ultrafine) titanium dioxide pigments and stabilisers on the photooxidative stability of water based acrylic and isocyanate based acrylic coatings. Polymer Degradation and Stability, 78, 467-478.

[80] Pinnell, S.R., Madey, D.L. (1999). New and Improved Daily Photoprotection: Microfine Oxide (Z-Cote®)' Aesthetic Surgery Journal, 19, 260-263.

[81] van der Molen, R.G., Hurks, H.M.H., Out-Luiting, C., Spies, F., van't Noordende, J.M., Koerten, H.K., Mommaas A.M. Efficacy of micronized titanium dioxide-containing compounds in protection against UVB-induced immunosuppression in humans in vivo. Journal of Photochemistry and Photobiology B: Biology, 44, 143-150.

[82] Wolf, R., Wolf, D., Morganti, P., Ruocco, V. (2001). Sunscreens. Clinics in Dermatology, 19, 452-459.

[83] Gamer, A.O., Leibold, E., van Ravenzwaay, B. (2006). The in vitro absorption of microfine zinc oxide and titanium dioxide through porcine skin Toxicology in Vitro, 20, 301-307.

[84] Szikszai, Z., Kertész, Z., Bodnár, E., Major, I., Borbíró, I., Kiss, Á.Z., Hunyadi J. (2010) Nuclear microprobe investigation of the penetration of ultrafine zinc oxide into intact and tape-stripped human skin. Nuclear Instruments and Methods in Physics Research Section B: Beam Interactions with Materials and Atoms (In Press)

[85] Sharma, V., Shukla, R.K., Saxena, N., Parmar, D., Das, M., Dhawan, A. (2009). DNA damaging potential of zinc oxide nanoparticles in human epidermal cells. Toxicology Letters, 185, 211-218.

[86] Di Virgilio, A.L., Reigosa, M., Arnal, P.M., Fernández Lorenzo de Mele, M. 2010). Comparative study of the cytotoxic and genotoxic effects of titanium oxide and aluminium oxide nanoparticles in Chinese hamster ovary (CHO-K1) cells. Journal of Hazardous Materials, 177, 711-718.

[87] Theogaraj, E., Riley, S., Hughes, L., Maier, M., David Kirkland, D. (2007). An investigation of the photo-clastogenic potential of ultrafine titanium dioxide particles Mutation Research/Genetic Toxicology and Environmental Mutagenesis, 634, 205-219.

[88] Hackenberg, S., Friehs, G., Froelich, K., Ginzkey, C., Koehler, C., Scherzed, A., Burghartz, M., Hagen, R., Kleinsasser, N. (2010). Intracellular distribution, geno- and cytotoxic effects of nanosized titanium dioxide particles in the anatase crystal phase on human nasal mucosa cells. Toxicology Letters, In Press.

[89] Couteau, C., Chammas, R., El-Bourry, S., Choquenet, B, Coiffard, L.J.M. (2008). Combination of UVA-filters and UVB-filters or inorganic UV-filters – Influence on the Sun Protection Factor (SPF) and the PF-UVA determined by *in vitro* method. Journal of Dermatological Science, 50, 159-162.

[90] de Groot, A.C. (1998). Fatal attractiveness: The shady side of cosmetics. Clinics in Dermatology, 16, 167-1790.

[91] Couteau, C., Pommier, M., Paparis, E., Coiffard, L.J.M. (2007). Study of the efficacy of 18 sun filters authorized in European Union tested *in vitro*. Pharmazie, 62, 449-452.

[92] Seidlová-Wuttke, D., Christoffel, J., Rimoldi, G., Jarry, H., Wolfgang Wuttke, W. (2006). Comparison of effects of estradiol with those of octylmethoxycinnamate and 4-methylbenzylidene camphor on fat tissue, lipids and pituitary hormones. Toxicology and Applied Pharmacology, 214, 1-7.

[93] Seidlová-Wuttke, D., Jarry, H., Christoffel, J., Rimoldi, G., Wuttke, W. (2006). Comparison of effects of estradiol (E2) with those of octylmethoxycinnamate (OMC) and 4-methylbenzylidene camphor (4MBC) — 2 filters of UV light – on several uterine, vaginal and bone parameters. Toxicology and Applied Pharmacology, 210, 246-254.

[94] Hexsel, C.L., Bangert, S.D., Hebert, A.A., Lim, H.W. (2008). Current sunscreen issues: 2007 Food and Drug Administration sunscreen labelling recommendations and combination sunscreen/insect repellent products. Journal of the American Academy of Dermatology, 59, 316-323.

[95] Agin, P., Anthony, F.A., Hermansky, S. (1998). Oxybenzone in sunscreen products. The Lancet, 351, 525.

[96] Nedorost, S.T. (2003). Facial erythema as a result of benzophenone allergy Journal of the American Academy of Dermatology, 49, 259-261.

[97] Kasichayanula, S., House, J.D., Wang, T., Gu, X. Simultaneous analysis of insect repellent DEET, sunscreen oxybenzone and five relevant metabolites by reversed-phase HPLC with UV detection: Application to an in vivo study in a piglet model. Journal of Chromatography B, 822, 271-277.

[98] Kasichayanula, S., House, J.D., Wang, T., Gu, X. (2007). Percutaneous characterization of the insect repellent DEET and the sunscreen oxybenzone from topical skin application. Toxicology and Applied Pharmacology, 223, 187-194.

[99] Hayden, C.G.J. (1997). Skin absorption of oxybenzone in humans. Food and Chemical Toxicology, 35, 1232.

[100] Godwin, D.A., Kim, N., Felton, L.A. (2002). Influence of Transcutol® CG on the skin accumulation and transdermal permeation of ultraviolet absorbers. European Journal of Pharmaceutics and Biopharmaceutics, 53, 23-27.

[101] Ashby, J., Tinwell, H., Plautz, J., Twomey, K., Lefevre, P.A. (2001). Lack of Binding to Isolated Estrogen or Androgen Receptors, and Inactivity in the Immature Rat Utero-

trophic Assay, of the Ultraviolet Sunscreen Filters Tinosorb M-Active and Tinosorb S. Regulatory Toxicology and Pharmacology, 34, 287-291.

[102] Hansenee, I., Marrot, L., Belaidi, J.P., Meunier, J.R. (2008). Prevention of genotoxic damage afforded by three sunscreen products having the same SPF: Beneficial effect of Mexoryl SX. Journal of the American Academy of Dermatology, 58, AB111.

[103] Hansenee, I., Bernerd, F., Lejeune, F. (2008). Daily photoprotection afforded by two sunscreen products having/with the same SPF: Beneficial effect of Mexoryl SX. Journal of the American Academy of Dermatology, 58, AB114.

[104] Yang, J., Wiley, C.J., Godwin, D.A., Felton, L.A. (2008). Influence of hydroxypropyl-β-cyclodextrin on transdermal penetration and photostability of avobenzone. European Journal of Pharmaceutics and Biopharmaceutics, 69, 605-612.

[105] Scalia, S., Tursilli, R., Sala, N., Iannuccelli, V. (2006). Encapsulation in lipospheres of the complex between butyl methoxydibenzoylmethane and hydroxypropyl-β-cyclodextrin. International Journal of Pharmaceutics, 320, 79-85.

[106] Schlumpf, M., Jarry, H., Wuttke, W., Ma, R., Lichtensteiger, W. Estrogenic activity and estrogen receptor β binding of the UV filter 3-benzylidene camphor: Comparison with 4-methylbenzylidene camphor. Toxicology, 199, 109-120.

[107] Søeborg, T., Ganderup, N.C., Kristensen, J.H., Bjerregaard, P., Ladegaard, K., Pedersen, Bollen, P., Hansen, S.H., Halling-Sørensen, B. (2006). Distribution of the UV filter 3-benzylidene camphor in rat following topical application. Journal of Chromatography B, 834, 117-121.

[108] Revuz, J. (2009). Vivent les parabènes. Annales de Dermatologie et de Vénéréologie, 136, 403-404.

[109] Hidalgo, M.E., Farah, M., Carrasco, L., Fernández, E. (2005). Photostability and photoprotection factor of boldine and glaucine. Journal of Photochemistry and Photobiology B: Biology, 80, 65-69.

[110] O'Brien, P., Carrasco-Pozo, C., Speisky, H. Boldine and its antioxidant or health-promoting properties. Chemico-Biological Interactions, 159, 1-17.

[111] Rancan, F., Rosan, S., Boehm, K., Fernández, E., Hidalgo, M.E., Quihot, W., Rubio, C., Boehm, F., Piazena, H., Oltmanns, U. Protection against UVB irradiation by natural filters extracted from lichens. Journal of Photochemistry and Photobiology B: Biology, 68, 133-139.

[112] Choquenet, B., Couteau, C., Paparis, E., Coiffard, L.J.M. (2009). Flavonoids and polyphenols, molecular families with sunscreen potential: determining effectiveness with an *in vitro* method. Natural Product Communications, 4, 227-230.

[113] Zhang, L., Li, L., Wu, Q. (2007). Protective effects of mycosporine-like amino acids of Synechocystis sp. PCC 6803 and their partial characterization. Journal of Photochemistry and Photobiology B: Biology, 86, 240-245.

[114] Conde, F.R., Churio, M.S., Previtali, C.M. (2000). The photoprotector mechanism of mycosporine-like amino acids. Excited-state properties and photostability of porphyra-334 in aqueous solution. Journal of Photochemistry and Photobiology B: Biology, 56, 139-144.

[115] Zudaire, L., Roy, S. Photoprotection and long-term acclimation to UV radiation in the marine diatom Thalassiosira weissflogii. Journal of Photochemistry and Photobiology B: Biology, 62, 26-34.

[116] Seité, S., Anny M.A. Fourtanier, A.M.A. (2008). The benefit of daily photoprotection. Journal of the American Academy of Dermatology, 58, S160-S166.

[117] Stoebner, P.E., Meunier, L. (2008). Photo-vieillissement du visage. Annales de Dermatologie et de Vénéréologie, 135, 21-26.

[118] Sehedic, D., Hardy-Boimartel, A., Couteau, C., Coiffard, L.J.M. (2009). Are cosmetic products which include an SPF appropriate for daily use? Archives of Dermatological Research, 301, 603-608.

Chapter 6

Malignancy in Relation to Autoimmune Blistering Dermatoses: Molecular and Clinical Aspects

Paweł Pietkiewicz, Justyna Gornowicz-Porowska, Monika Bowszyc-Dmochowska and Marian Dmochowski

Additional information is available at the end of the chapter

http://dx.doi.org/10.5772/55240

1. Introduction

Autoimmune blistering dermatoses (ABD) are a group of relatively rare autoantibody-driven diseases affecting primarily skin and/or multiple mucosa. They comprise of two main subdivisions: ABD with autoimmunity to enzymes (dermatitis herpetiformis only) and ABD with autoimmunity to mostly structural proteins (anti-desmosomal autoimmunity circle, anti-dermal-epidermal junction autoimmunity circle and others). As both coexistent development of organ specific autoimmunity (e.g. myasthenia gravis) and transition between ABD groups are possible, ABD seem to be a part of pathological multiorgan autoimmunization syndrome [1]. The replacement of physiological autoimmunity by pathological autoimmunity and triggering blister formation in ABD still remain unexplored and essential issues. It is suggested that malignancy may be a triggering factor inducing the development of pathological autoimmunity. On the other hand, the development of malignancies during chronic immunosuppressive therapy may be observed [2].

In this chapter, we discuss an important and interesting area of research, focused on identifying the relationships, on both clinical and molecular level, between ABD and malignancy. Collectively, the literature data and our own experience indicate that ABD may be associated with different malignant tumors, both cutaneous and affecting internal organs. However, the issue if it is a mere coincidence or true pathogenetic relationship remains to be resolved. It is known that in a state of perpetual activation of immune system, as in ABD, proinflammatory molecules (e.g. cytokines) may cause tissue damage leading to chronic inflammation and subsequently increase the risk of carcinogenesis [3]. At both clinical and molecular level ABD and malignancy-associated ABD (MAABD) may seem similar; nevertheless, the pathogenesis of those entities plausibly is fundamentally distinct. However, broadly observed associations between ABD and cancer indicate that various molecular pathways may contribute to elevated risk of malignancy in these patients. Most importantly, the coexistence of malignancy with ABD changes the management of such patients compared to patients with ABD alone. For a long months and years, many cases of ABD and MAABD are undiagnosed, misdiagnosed and subsequently mistreated due to relative rarity and therefore low awareness of autoimmunity-driven blistering dermatoses among practitioners. The time period elapsed between the first symptoms and diagnosis, makes the time-onset relation between ABD and cancer usually uncertain.

Molecular abnormalities of desmosomal proteins are observed in ABD and epithelial malignancies. A key function of desmosomal proteins is the maintenance of adhesion. However, in malignancy, where cells may separate, detach and metastasize, it is possible that alterations in their expression may be the reason of carcinogenesis process. Interestingly, the altered desmosomal protein expression and subsequent changes in cell-cell cohesion are often associated with signal pathways (e.g. epidermal growth factor – EGF in squamous cell carcinoma).

2. Autoimmune blistering dermatoses

ABD form a group of autoimmunity-driven diseases, where bullous lesions arise on the skin and/or multiple mucosa. Diverse ABD are evoked by different triggering mechanism and are characterized by different clinical onset, course and prognosis. Two main subdivisions can be separated: ABD with autoimmunity to enzymes and ABD with autoimmunity to structural proteins. The entities may be commonly distinguished by clinical, histopathological (presence or absence of acantholysis and differences of its localization, level of blistering and the composition of inflammatory infiltrate), immunohistochemical (localization and patterns of deposits and autoantibody immunoglobulin class) and molecular examination (ELISA, immunoblotting).

2.1. ABD with autoimmunity to enzymes

The entity is represented only by dermatitis herpetiformis (DH), also known as Duhring's disease - chronic, intensely itchy, blistering skin manifestation of the gluten sensitive enteropathy [4]. It affects symmetrically extensor surfaces of limps and the trunk – mainly buttocks and sacral area, where tiny vesicles, papules or even urticarial plaques occur in groups. The onset age is 20-60 years with peak about 35, and incidence ranging from 10 to 39 per 100,000 persons, depending on world region [1,5]. Patients have IgA autoantibodies to transglutaminases (TGs), that are considered major autoantigens in DH, yet other antigens were also reported (antiendomysial, antireticulin, antithyroid and antinuclear antibodies) [5]. It is thought that granular/fibrillar IgA deposits in tips of dermal papillae provoke neutrophile-mediated destruction of the dermal-epidermal junction (DEJ) and forming subepidermal vesicle [1,4,5] Histopathologically, microabscesses in dermal papillae with neutrophile infiltration are seen in bioptate, obtained preferably of perilesional skin of the affected buttocks [5,6].

2.2. ABD with autoimmunity to structural proteins

This large group consists of several distinct circles of diseases with autoimmunity to different antigens – desmosomal, hemidesmosomal and others.

2.2.1. Anti-desmosomal autoimmunity circle / pemphigus group

Anti-desmosomal autoimmunity circle or pemphigus group refers to a group of chronic ABD characterized by the presence of autoantibodies (IgG or/and IgA) binding desmosomal structures and keratinocyte cell-surface antigens, leading to acantholysis and intraepithelial blister formation. The main antigens for pemphigus circle are desmoglein 1 (DSG1) and desmoglein 3 (DSG3), yet there are forms of pemphigus without anti-desmoglein immunization [7]. The commonest subcircle is characterized by IgG-mediated autoimmunity and is composed of:

- pemphigus foliaceus (PF) circle (PF, endemic PF, sebaceous PF, and PF herpetiformis, paraneoplastic pemphigus, drug-mediated PF showing PF-indicative autoantibody profile),
- pemphigus vulgaris (PV) circle (mucosal-dominant PV, mucocutaneous PV, pemphigus vegetans, and paraneoplastic pemphigus, PV herpetiformis, drug-mediated PV showing PV-indicative autoantibody profile),
- pemphigus as a part of multiorgan autoimmunity syndrome,
- pemphigus shifting inside one circle or between circles,
- PV/PF-coexistence cases,
- paraneoplastic pemphigus (PNP) with neither anti-DSG3 nor anti-DSG1 antibodies [1].

A model disease for pemphigus circle and the commonest clinical type of pemphigus is PV. This life-threatening chronic/acute ABD affects the mucocutaneous surfaces significantly debilitating quality of life [5]. The onset age is 40-60 years, and incidence ca. 0.7 per 100,000 persons [5,8]. Blistering in PV appears at suprabasal level as an effect of tissue-bound and serum IgG-driven autoimmunity against keratinocyte cell-surface antigens of aforelisted cadherin superfamily [9], with desmoglein 3 (DSG3) as the main autoantigen. The disease starts initially affecting oral mucosa (50-70%), that may remain the only site involved, yet extraoral lesions may occur simultaneously. Intraepithelial blisters evolve into aching erosions and ulcers. Predilection sites include face, parietal region of the scalp, sternal and interscapular regions of the trunk, intertriginous sites (umbilicus, interdigital spaces, scrotum, inguinal and axillary folds), scars and skin appendages – nail apparatus, hair follicles [1] and areas with transitional epithelium, what could be explained by the change of desmoglein expression pattern.

Histologically, suprabasilar blistering may be observed, whereas direct immunofluorescence study (DIF) of perilesional skin/mucosa depicts IgG (mainly IgG4) pemphigus-type deposits of fishing net pattern in intercellular spaces of the lower epidermis [1]. With virtually no invasiveness, direct immunofluorescence study on a plucked scalp hair (hDIF) may serve as a good alternative for DIF, visualizing pemphigus IgG, IgG1 and IgG4 deposits in outer root sheath of hair follicle even in patients without cutaneous lesions [10]. Still used, indirect immunofluorescence (IIF) test for presence of pemphigus IgG circulating autoantibodies is regarded historical method and is widely replaced with molecular studies e.g. ELISA, enabling assessment in serum, saliva or blister fluid [11].

PF, the less common pemphigus circle condition, usually affects the skin of the face, scalp and trunk, but may generalize. The disease is characterized by autoantibodies binding DSG1, that participate in blister formation at superficial level (granular layer). Although blister is a primary PF lesion, it is hardly ever seen, as it rapidly evolves into crust-covered erosions [1,5]. Interestingly, as main PV DSG3-antigen (130kDa) and PF DSG1-antigen (160kDa) differ, that corresponds with different blistering subtype and clinical features [5].

Concerning association with malignancy, PNP resembles clinically and histologically features of PV and erythema multiforme [5]. However, it differs in autoantibody profile. PNP autoantibodies may target simultaneously multiple antigens – desmoplakin I and II, BP230, periplakin, envoplakin, plectin, 170kDa protein, desmoglein 1 and 3, desmocolin familly, and many yet unknown proteins. PNP-type intercellular deposits can be visualized in IIF on transitional epithelium of rat bladder. Circulating autoantibodies affects not only mucocutaneus epithelium, but may bind organ-specific antigens of gastrointestinal tract or bronchioli – e.g. causing non-reversible and life-threatening constrictive bronchiolitis. Although rare, PNP is characterized with very high mortality [12].

2.2.2. Subepidermal autoimmune blistering dermatoses

Subepidermal ABD circle consists of chronic bullous diseases with autoantibodies binding mostly structural proteins forming DEJ:

- Bullous pemphigoid (BP) circle (urticarial BP, BP herpetiformis, sebaceous BP, erythrodermic BP, BP vegetans, pretibial BP, prurigo-nodularis-like BP, trauma-induced BP, pemphigoid gestationis (PG), lichen planus pemphigoides (LPP), lamina lucida-type linear IgA bullous dermatosis),
- Mucous membrane pemphigoid (MMP)/cicatrical pemphigoid,
- Pemphigoid Brunsting-Perry,
- Epidermolysis bulosa acquisita (EBA) circle (EBA, bullous systemic lupus erythematosus, sublamina densa-type linear IgA bullous dermatosis),
- Linear IgA bullous dermatosis (LABD) (non-EBA circle LABD, non-BP circle LABD),
- anti-laminin gamma1 pemphigoid (former anti-p200 pemphigoid) [1].

BP circle, the commonest ABD, is characterized by heterogeneous clinical patterns. However, it has common molecular feature – autoimmunity to extracellular, non-collagenous NC16A domain of BP180 antigen (BPAG2, collagen XVII alpha1) [1,5,13] and less often BP230 (BPAG2e, protein belonging to plakin family) [1,5]. It begins as a moderate pruritus, papular lesions or urticarial plaques developing in months into chronic bullous eruption characterized by well-tense blisters containing either serous or sanguineus fluid. The localized/generalized lesions may be oval or round, and rupture easily over time [5]. The arciform or serpiginous pattern they present is sometimes described as string of beans or cluster of jewels. Diverse symptoms are consequence of targeting different epitopes of these components of hemidesmosome adhesion complex. It affects often elderly people in their 60's-90's [1,5] with incidence of ca. 4.3 per 100,000 persons [8].

2.2.3. Other, vaguely characterized, autoimmune blistering diseases

There are also other autoimmune blistering diseases e.g. ABD with autoimmunization to IQGAP1 protein, erythema multiforme with anti-desmoplakin 1 and anti-desmoplakin 2 antibodies, linear IgM gestationis dermatosis, linear IgM dermatosis with IgM gammapathy and others that cannot be fitted into above categories, yet these are isolated cases with unknown relation to malignancy.

2.3. Malignancies associated with ABD

The issue of association of malignancy and ABD causes much controversy among researchers. WHO reports from 2008 indicated, that the 13% of death worldwide is caused by cancer, being the major cause of death with toll of 7.6 million people per year [14]. Neoplasms are heterogeneous group of entities characterized by rapid creation of abnormal cells that grow beyond their usual boundaries, and which can then invade adjoining parts of the body and spread to other organs [14]. The leading malignancies worldwide are lung, breast, colon, stomach and prostate cancers [15]. Several malignant tumors were reported in association with ADB, including lymphoproliferative disorders (Castleman's tumor, non-Hodgkin's lymphoma, chronic lymphocytic leukemia), lung, gastrointestinal, prostate, ovarian, endometrial, breast, bladder, renal, laryngeal, pancreatic cancers, thymoma and follicular dendritic cell sarcoma [16–22].

As ABD are relatively rare/regarded as rare conditions, there is limited data covering the association with other diseases. Japanese retrospective study on malignancy in patients suffering from pemphigus and pemphigoid observed incidence of 5.0% and 5.8% respectively [17], whereas lesser studies set these numbers as 11.2% and 10.4% [16]. The association ratio of malignancy with pemphigus increases by age, while no such correlation is found in pemphigoid. No gender-predisposition in ABD was reported in these patients [16]. Interestingly, lung cancer was most common in pemphigus and gastrointestinal tumors (gastric cancer in particular) in bullous pemphigoid [17]. Moreover, age-dependent malignancy-association in PV patients under (6.5%) and above 60 years (15%) should not be omitted [15]. Studies on BP and malignancy did not reveal age-correspondence [23].

As far as anti-enzyme ABD is concerned, association of DH with subsequent development of lymphoma seems well-documented [18,24,25]. It is possible that gluten intolerance is the factor associated with malignancies. Some data suggested, that following a strict gluten-free diet is protective against malignancy [26]. Moreover, researchers postulate that the risk of malignancy decreases with time from diagnosis of gluten-sensitive enteropathy to nearly the same as occurs in the general population. In light of above, it is postulated that the increased risk of malignancy in patients with DH may be the result of a polyclonal stimulation of lymphocytes by gluten that causes transformation into a malignant clone [18]. Still, in our over 20 years of clinical/laboratory experience as a clinician/clinical researchers we do not recall a DH-associated lymphoma patient.

There is a wide group of malignancies concomitant with ADB. Lung cancer has been reported in coexistence with wide range of ABD: PV [17,27,28], PNP [29], pemphigus vegetans [30,31], pemphigus herpetiformis [32], IgA pemphigus [33], BP [34] and MMP [35]. In some BP cases, tumor resection led to complete recovery [36] supporting the thesis of close interrelation of the diseases. Gastrointestinal tumors have been reported in association with BP [17,37], PNP [38], pemphigus vegetans [39], PV [40–45] and MMP [46] sometimes with post-excisional remission [47,48]. Both chronic leukemia and lymphoma have been reported with DH [49–51] and PNP [52–54]. Based on few case reports, MMP [55–57] is not rare finding in leukemia. There has been only one case of BP reported in patient with leukemia [58]. Thymoma and PV appears in numerable patients [43] with post-excisional remissions not uncommon [59]. Among reported thymoma-related ABD, there are also cases of PF [60,61], BP [62] and MMP [63]. Malignant tumor of the pancreas seem to be generally connected to MMP [64,65] and sometimes PNP [66]. Renal neoplasm has been reported to occur in with BP [67–70] and occasionally with MMP [71], PNP [72] and PF [73]. Ovarian cancer was incidentally described in relation with BP [74], anti-laminin gamma1 pemphigoid [75] and MMP [76]. Concerning prostatic cancer, single cases of PNP [77], pemphigus herpetiformis [78], PF [79] and MMP [80] were described in literature. There are numerous case reports on ABD and breast cancer including predominantly BP [20,81–85] and PV [86,87] with well-documented BP-lesion induction with radiotherapy.

3. Endogenous factors leading to breakage of self-tolerance in malignancy

Endogenous factors seem to be crucial for development of autoimmunity, as they form the organism reaction to external threat.

3.1. Development of paraneoplastic immunity

The autoimmunity in cancer is developed by distortion of immune system, arising from central tolerance disruption, peripheral immunity rearrangement and altering of self-antigens. Cancer-associated impairment of the function of immune system may take place at many stages. Rearrangement of T-cell receptor (TCR) genes proceeding in thymus cortex promotes T-cell education to recognize major histocompatibility complex (MHC) molecules of self-cells. It is a necessary condition for a T-cell to pass the positive selection process. The negative selection, being the following stage, is conducted in thymus medulla, where T-cells are exposed to plethora of tissue specific self-antigens (TSAs) by medullary thymic epithelial cells. Self-antigens presented to T-cells are previously processed, thus some T-cells expressing TCR with high affinity to poorly presented antigens may evade negative selection achieving maturation [88]. The process is controlled by autoimmune regulator (AIRE) transcription factor [89]. Autoaggressive thymocytes are being terminated in apoptosis. Impairment of any of these stages – positive selection, negative selection, antigen processing, antigen presentation by malignancy, might have impact on T-cell set and scope of activity in periphery. Thymoma is the most common neoplasm of thymus, outrunning lymphomas, germ cell tumor, thymic carcinoma, carcinoid tumors and others [90]. One of the syndromes in relation to thymoma is paraneoplastic pemphigus, where diverse autoantibodies target diverse structural autoantigens. While pemphigus vulgaris (PV) and paraneoplastic (PNP) pemphigus may both target the same antigen, the difference is within the range of them and difference in epitopes bound (e.g. mucocutaneus PV preferably targets DSG3 N-terminal determinant, while PNP binds multiple epitopes). Another distinctive feature is IgG subclass – predominant PV IgG autoantibody subclass is IgG4, while in PNP – subclass is IgG1 and IgG2 [1].

Some authors hypothesized that tumor cells alone may produce the autoantibodies [91,92]. The thesis of in-tumor immature T-cell improper maturation, without negative selection, leading to autoaggression may be supported by findings in patient with follicular dendritic cell sarcoma [93]. Malignancy is based on breakage of cell cycle guarding and dysregulation of gene expression resulting in over- or underexpression of proteins. Via gene mutation, the neoplastic cell changes the antigen suit, by exposing altered self-antigens or "hiding" those already known. The reaction of immune system to cancer growth is immune cells recruitment (T-cells, NK cells, mast cells) and inflammation by various mediators causing apoptosis of both neoplastic and non-neoplastic cells. One T-cell can recognize many antigens presented by different MHC molecules. The condition of recognition is the compatibility of antigen fragment with lymphocyte TCR. Along with antigen sequestration theory, the determinants of cell proteins released in tumor necrosis can be exposed by antigen presenting cells to matured T-cells that migrate to lymph nodes. B-cells in response start to produce polyclonal antibodies against novel tumor epitopes. However, T-cells may also react with cancer antigens starting the chain of events leading to production of certain antibody cross-binding both neoplastic antigens and self-antigens [90].

The role of immune system protection against malignancy can be exemplified by noticeable higher cancer incidence in patients given immunosuppressive drugs impairing self/foreign-antigens recognition. Hence hypothetically, the distortion in immune system function in ABD may contribute to further susceptibility to the development of malignancy. Naive T-cell activation in the periphery alone is thought to be insufficient for autoimmunity induction and co-stimulation by CD28, a co-stimulatory molecule activating T-cells, seem to be necessary [94]. CD28 is able to bind CD80 molecule and CD86 molecule, constitutionally expressed on B-cells, subsequently enhancing IgG antibody production [95]. CD80 molecule appear also scantly on other antigen-presenting cells (APC – primarily B-cells, macrophages and dendritic cells) and is upregulated after APC activation. Active APC present CD40, a ligand for CD40L expressed on active T helper cells. Ligation of CD40 on APC cells leads to increase co-stimulatory capacity and antigen presentation ability enhancement. It is worth noticing that, CD80/CD86 is also expressed on cells of diverse lymphomas (e.g. non-Hodgkin lymphoma and chronic lyphocytic leukemia), that can act on behalf of APC, evading being recognized by the immune system. It was suggested that T-cells may omit the "APC guarding stations" in lymph nodes and directly infiltrate the tumor. Thus, the tumor itself may act as a "T-cell kidnapper" and support naive T-cell infiltration, activation and differentiation into effector cells [96], hypothetically programming or "indoctrinating" T-cells to achieve autoimmune potential. Moreover, the study based on collective incubation of non-malignant regulatory and cytotoxic T-cells with chronic lymphocytic leukemia cells showed non-malignant T-cells cytoskeleton remodeling decrease and vesicle trafficking decrease resulting in impaired synapse formation [97,98].

Fc receptors (FcRs) play essential role in the activation/inhibition of various cells in antibody-mediated immune responses. Thus, FcRs function may be a key purpose in the treatment with monoclonal antibodies (mAbs) therapy. Probably, FcRs may be a molecular link between ABD and malignancies [99,100]. FcRs-targeting therapies are used for ABD and cancer, e.g. rituximab, which is used in ABD and is the first anti-tumor mAb drug admitted by the US Food and Drug Administration. It was demonstrated that Fc-receptor-dependent mechanisms contribute substantially to the action of cytotoxic antibodies against tumors and indicated that an optimal antibody against tumors would bind preferentially to activation Fc receptors and minimally to the inhibitory partner FcγRIIB [101]. Interestingly, rituximab – the chimeric monoclonal IgG1antibody specific for the B-cell marker CD20 – was recently approved for the treatment of B-cell lymphoma. In vitro studies with rituximab have indicated that a direct pro-apoptotic activity may be associated with this antibody [102].

3.2. Genetic predisposition

There seems to be a causative relation between HLA-association and autoimmunity in ABD, especially in pemphigus [103–109] and pemphigoid [110], yet these observations may vary geographically. HLA-DQB1*0301 allele, associated with MMP [111–114], was reported in patients with esophageal squamous cell carcinoma [113], gastric cancer [115], HPV-associated cervical neoplasia [116]. It was hypothesized, that the gene may have a role in T-cell recognition of basement membrane antigens resulting in production of IgG autoantibodies binding basement membrane antigens [117]. It is also possible, that the link exists between certain malignancies and HLA or autoimmunity predisposition connected to defective apoptotic genes. Nonetheless, there are few studies covering that field, so coexistence may also be purely coincidental.

3.3. The role of cytokines

There is eventuality of oversecretion of certain cytokines regulating the mRNA expression and polarization of certain T helper (Th) cell population [118,119], as the most common neoplasms in relation to ABD seem to be lymphoproliferative malignancies. It has been reported that qualitative as well as quantitative alterations in cytokine production can result in activation of inefficacious effector mechanisms and therefore, complex and severe impairment in immune functions [119]. Polarization to Th1-mediated immunity via IL-1, IL-4, IL-5, IL-6 IL-8 and IFN-gamma was observed in BP [120], while Th2-mediated reaction via IL-10 and IL-4, in conjunction with decrease in IL-2 and IFN-gamma levels, were shown in PV [119]. The cytokines that promote cancer growth (e.g IL-8 for colon and gastric cancer) [121,122] may collaterally initiate Th population shift to the profile promoting ABD. Likewise, a proliferation inducing ligand (APRIL) of TNF family plays an important role in several autoimmune diseases, including ABD, and in several malignancies. Soluble APRIL level was reported to be raised in e.g. lung, thyroid, lymphoid and gastrointestinal tumors [123,124], thus supposedly contribute to dysregulation of immunity in cancer. B-cell activating factor (BAFF/BLyS), belonging to TNF family, regulates B-lymphocyte proliferation and survival, also in B-cell lymphoproliferative disorders [125]. Interestingly, serum of BP-, but not PV-patients, showed high titers of BAFF [126]. It seems rational, that molecular mechanisms leading to increase of BAFF level in BP patients may favor pathological lymphoproliferation.

3.4. Sex hormones

As some entities of ABD have sex-predisposition, just as some malignancies, the role of sex hormones on development of MAABD need to be investigated. Certain tumors prevail in female (breast cancer, non-Hodgkin lymphoma), in man (gastrointestinal tumor, laryngeal cancer, Hodgkin lymphoma or kidney cancer) or are typical for one sex for anatomical reasons (prostate cancer, ovarian cancer) [15]. Sex-associated distribution of PV and BP seems equal with slight female dominance, while other ABD promote males (DH – 2:1) or are exquisitely female domain (PG) [5,127]. Both T and B cells have estrogen, testosterone and prolactin receptors. Furthermore, androgens and estrogens have an impact on the Th1/Th2 balance [128]. Therefore, menopause may be followed by change in cytokine profile affecting immune response. Interestingly, studies on endocrine hormones in PV- and BP-patients have revealed increased serum levels of both adrenocorticotropic hormone (ACTH) and hydrocortisone [129]. It was hypothesized, that slight female predominance of women in PV may be contributed to hormone replacement therapy (HRT) [130]. HRT is known risk factor for ovarian cancer, yet the impact on neoplasm induction in breast cancer and endometrial cancer is uncertain [131].

4. Exogenous factors: Epitope spreading and bystander effect

Multiple exogenous factors of diverse origin may contribute to trigger MAABD, e.g. drug-induction of malignancy in ABD patients and, contrarily, self-antigen drug/virus/bacteria-induced alteration. Drug-induced immunosuppression in ABD (e.g. with methotrexate) was considered a prospective triggering factor for lymphoproliferative disorders [132]. Viral/microbial factors could serve both as a trigger for autoimmunity and risk factor for malignancy. It was hypothesized, that foreign antigens (e.g. viral, fungal, bacterial) may act as a superantigen in ABD induction or take part in epitope spreading phenomenon [133,134]. HBV, HCV, H. pylori, T. gondii and CMV were reported to contribute to elicit ABD [135]. Viral infection (TTV, HSV2, HHV6, HHV8, HSV1, HSV2, EBV, HBV, HIV-1, Coxsackie virus) [136–143] has been put forward as a causative agent of ABD-type autoimmunity in PV, PF, BP and pemphigus vegetans. There has been multiple factors suspected of prostatic cancerogenesis, including viruses (BK, HSV2, HSV6, HSV11, HSV16, HSV18, HSV31, HSV33, HHV8, XMRV, CMV) and microbial agents (Chlamydia trachomatis, Mycoplasma hominis, Ureaplasma urealyticum, Neisseria gonorrhoeae and Treponema pallidum), yet data was inconclusive or supported no relation [144–151]. Surprisingly, Epstein-Barr virus infection has been found statistically associated with increased breast carcinoma risk [152]. It was speculated that the virus itself may play a role in ABD induction [153,154]. The data covering the issue of exogenous factors contributing to both malignancy and ABD is yet generally inconclusive.

Constant activation of immune system in ABD sustains chronic inflammation leading to tissue degeneration by proinflammatory molecules. As a result, the risk of the neoplasy increases [3]. However, that relation could be two-sided. Inflammation in tumor nest stimulates and modifies the immunity mechanisms. Furthermore, there is a hypothesis that the multiplicity of target antigens in ABD may result from intra- and intermolecular epitope spreading. The effect of epitope spreading in ABD is well-known fact and it seems to be a constitutional compound of autoimmunity. Structural similarities between autoantigen epitope and to-be-autoantigen epitope may lead to production of autoaggresive cross-reacting immunoglobulins [9,155]. This phenomenon, which represents a broadening of the immune response from a single epitope to additional epitopes, is also described in cancer and recent findings suggests that epitope spreading may be a more significant predictor of effective immunity [156].

The initial anti-cancer immunity may ricochet to autoaggresion by epitope spreading and bystander effect alike [157]. Local inflammation in the course of malignant tumor or chemotherapy/radiotherapy treatment may result in enhanced autoantigen presentation that causes T-cell priming, activation and expansion of additional specificity [158]. Therefore, in situations where immunosuppressive/anti-cancer treatment is absent or ceased, anti-cancer response may be responsible for development of autoimmunity to self-antigens characteristic for ABD.

5. Molecular mechanisms: The possible connection between malignancies and ABD

ABD are characterized by autoantibodies against structural proteins of the skin, including molecules of dermal-epidermal junction and desmosomes. Cancer progression is a complex and multi-step process in which components of DEJ as well as a desmosomal molecules play a pivotal role in the development of metastasis. Probably, more than 90% of human cancers are of epithelial origin [159] and the autoimmunity against epidermal structures may play important role in those carcinogenesis. Thus, probably DEJ/desmosomes is the first barrier in tumor cells invasion. In light of this, understanding the molecular basis of pathological autoinflammation induction in autoimmune blistering dermatoses in relation to the mechanisms of malignant transformation is paramount for early detection and treatment of epithelial-derived cancers [160]. However, the precise molecular mechanisms underlying the association of malignancy with ABD still remain unknown. Nevertheless, understanding the link between the production of pathogenic autoantibodies in ABD and the development of the associated neoplasy should facilitate the development of more specific diagnostic tests and therapeutic strategies [160].

5.1. Malignancy in relation to the autoimmunity in pemphigus group: The role of desmosomes components

Pemphigus group is characterized by presence of autoantibodies against desmosomal cadherins. Research on human and animal models indicated that alternation in desmosomes components may lead to tumor progression and metastasis. However, little is known about the role of desmosome during cancer development [161]. It is clear, that the origin and maintenance of epidermis requires the coordinated regulation of proliferation, adhesion, migration and differentiation. Conceptually, desmosome complexes form when desmosomal cadherins – DCs (desmogleins – DSGs and desmocollins – DSCs) participate in heterotypic interactions that bring the plasma membranes of adjacent cells in close apposition [161]. The cytoplasmic tails of these cadherins interact with plakoglobin and plakophilins.

The data describing desmosome protein expression during human cancer progression are conflicting [161–163]. Molecular abnormalities of desmosomal proteins (DPs) are observed in ABD and epithelial malignancies. However, in malignancy, where cells may separate, detach and metastasize, it is possible that alterations in DPs expression may be the reason of carcinogenesis process. Several studies demonstrated that downregulation of DCs occurs during the progression of cancers and is often correlated with and predictive of tumor metastasis [161,162]. On the other hand, other studies reported overexpression of DCs during the cancer progression, and this pattern is associated with poor prognosis [163]. The regulatory mechanism controlling DCs expression are scanty explained. As known, gene expression may be modulated by genetic and/or epigenetic mechanisms and in this way may contribute to the development of pathologic autoimmunity or malignancies. Genetic changes as mutation, deletion, and gene rearrangement of DCs have been poorly found in cancer and ABD. Possible mechanism may also involve post-translational modification of protein, like phosphorylation, acetylation or methylation. In light of this, some data reported methylation of DCs, e.g. methylation of DSC3 in breast cancer. It was showed, that DSC3 is downregulated in colorectal cancer by DNA methylation [164]. Thus, further analysis of methylation status of DCs DNA may be useful to predict clinical outcomes in patients with malignancy.

Alternatively, the possible link between desmosomal components and malignancy may be the Perp protein. The Perp tetraspan membrane protein was originally identified as a transcriptional target of the p53 tumor suppressor upregulated during apoptosis [161,165]. However, Perp may have function as a target of the p53-related transcription factor (p63) involved in maintaining epithelial integrity by promoting desmosomal cell-cell adhesion. Electron microscopy and biochemical analyses showed that the blistering phenotype observed in the Perp-deficient epithelia is accounted for by both a reduction in desmosome number and compromised desmosome complex formation. It is suggested, that pemphigus autoantibodies may trigger internalization of Perp, which enhances adhesion defects [166]. Perp's position downstream of p63 and p53, as well as its essential role in normal desmosome function, suggest that it may be a target for mutation in human blistering diseases or cancer [167]. An interesting issue remains why a p53 target would play such a prominent role in adhesion in the skin. It was suggested [167], that this role relates to Perp being a key component of the transcriptional program for stratified epithelial development and maintenance specified by the p53 family member p63. Perp is a transcriptional target of p63 during development and in mature mouse skin [168]. Beyond a role in epithelial function, Perp's status as a p53 target involved in apoptosis may suggest a potential role as a tumor suppressor. Given that loss of both p53 and p63 cooperate in tumorigenesis, loss of Perp similarly may be expected to promote cancer development in some context. The future analysis of Perp will provide new insight into the role of desmosomes in epithelial homeostasis and cancer [167]. It was disputed, that Perp-deficiency promotes cancer by enhancing cell survival, desmosome loss and inflammation, and fundamental role for Perp and desmosomes in tumor suppression [161]. Interestingly, it seems that DSC3 is a p53 response gene and addition of wild-type p53 was found to be sufficient to induce expression of DSC3 in breast cancer [169]. Thus, it was of great interest to investigate whether this pathway is also active in tumor cells. In light of above, the induction of p53 may have impact on expression of DCs [164].

Malignancy may be also associated with pemphigus group via pemphigus-antibodies-induced signaling pathways. Thus, cadherins expression can function as a tumor and invasion suppressor due to its participation in processes such as morphological differentiation and contact inhibition of growth and motility. Several different molecular mechanisms for perturbation of cadherin function in epithelial tumors are reported: (i) transcriptional or genomic regulation of cadherin expression, (ii) mutations (e.g. deletion, insertion) of cadherin or catenin genes and (iii) regulation of adhesive function by signaling pathways. A signaling cascade initiated by pemphigus vulgaris antibodies may results in reduced availability of plakoglobin and abrogation of its function as transcriptional repressor of the proto-oncogene c-Myc. This in turn results in accumulation of c-Myc. Moreover, c-Myc expression is commonly upregulated in tumors. There is also evidence, that etiology of some skin cancer (e.g. BCC) may be dependent on several signaling pathways [170], which can be shared with pathological autoimmunity induction in pemphigus group. Other signaling pathways may engagement of Src, Wnt, hedgehog, epidermal growth factor receptor (EGFR) kinase (EGFRK), cAMP, protein kinases A and C (PKC), phospholipase C, mTOR, p38 MAPK, JNK [166]. Especially, it is postulated that DSG3 is a key player in Src signaling and overexpression of DSG3 elicited a phenotype similar to this with increased Src activity. Interestingly, this phenotype may be observed in some kind of cancers (e.g. SCC) [171]. Moreover, it is estimated that 35% of cancers show increased MAPK activity [172]. On the other hand, MAPK is involved in the process of acantholysis in pemphigus group.

Furthermore, some data [173,174] demonstrated possibility that switching of DCs could play an important role in the development of some kind of cancer. Tumor development is in part characterized by the ability of cells to destruct of cell-cell adhesion and invade the surrounding tissue. Perhaps, the disturbances in desmosomal cadherin (as DSCs) expression could affect beta-catenin signaling [174]. It is known, that increased beta-catenin signaling is a common causative event in some kind of cancer (e.g. colorectal cancer), thus desmocollin switching could play a contributory role in the initiation of early stages of cancer. In light of this, the evidence that altered expression of desmosomal proteins in various human malignancies has been accumulating.

5.2. Malignancy in relation to the autoimmunity in subepidermal blistering dermatoses: The role of the DEJ proteins

Pathogenesis of blister formation in subepidermal blistering dermatoses is associated with destruction of dermal-epidermal junction and anchoring fibers. Recent studies shown interesting function of the hemidesmosome (HD) components in signal transduction, involving effect on cell behavior in tumor invasion [175]. Data indicated altered expression of DEJ proteins at different stages of carcinogenesis, what may suggest the association between tumor progression. Aberrant expression of DEJ proteins, which are associated with subepidermal blistering dermatoses (e.g. BP180, BP230, alfa6beta4 integrin, laminin-322) in epithelial cancers was demonstrated, what may indicate their role in tumor development and invasion [175]. Reduced expression of HD components may results in the detachment of cells from the basement membrane, facilitating piling or migration of cells [176]. On the other hand, carcinoma cells may upregulate the expression of HD molecules to enhance the attachment capacity of metastatic cells to the DEJ at the metastatic site in order to establish metastatic growth.

The aberrant expression of DEJ component may reflect dysfunction of HD, that occurs as an early event in multistep carcinogenesis of epithelium [177]. Downregulation of BP180 – one of the major autoantigen in bullous pemphigoid – was found in basal cells in mild dysplasias, upregulation of BP180 in suprabasal keratinocytes in moderate and severe dysplasis as well as in the central cells of squamous cell carcinomas (SCC; G2 and G3) using immunohistochemical (IHC) and in situ hybridization (ISH) methods [175]. Furthermore, this group of researchers indicated that overexpression of BP180 was found at the invasive front of the tumors. Authors suggested that reduced BP180 expression at the early step of carcinogenesis may reflect disturbed keratinocyte adhesion to the basement membrane. BP180 gene expression is significantly induced by a tumor promoter PMA [175]. Previous findings obtained by the same authors revealed reduced BP180 expression in the peripheral cells of carcinoma islands in solid and keratotic basal cell carcinomas (BCC) and in the basal cells of invading buds in superficial BCCs [178]. The altered expression of DEJ proteins is likely to coincide with the disassembly of HD, which is an essential step in keratinocyte migration and carcinoma cell invasion [175]. Moreover, downreguation of BP180 and other hemidesmosome components was previously detected in vivo in prostate cancer and in the invasive cells of ductual mammary carcinoma [179,180]. On the other hand, upregulation of HD components has been reported in a variety of SCCs [177,181]. It was argued that BP180 upregulation in carcinoma cells at the invasive front of malignant tumors is important in the carcinoma cell migration [175]. Other study described upregulation and altered distribution of BP230 and alfa6beta4 integrin in the areas of invasive growth of head and neck SCCs [181]. PMA is a potent tumor promoter capable of inducing several genes that have a role in carcinogenesis and tumor invasion [182]. It is known, that laminin-332 gamma2 chain gene promoter is one of the targets of PMA activation, occurring via interaction with the activator protein 1 complexes [183]. The relationship of BP180 to malignancy is discussed. BP180 has possible phosphorylation sites and may by phosphorylated in SCC [177]. Enhanced expression and abnormal distribution of BP180 in various precancerous and cancerous tissues was revealed, including e.g. SCCs and Bowen's disease [177].

As it was demonstrated that expression of BP180 was decreased or absent in cutaneous neoplasms [184], some authors speculated that some type of carcinomas itself might expose BP180 antigenic epitope, which would normally be hidden, thus inducing the production of autoantibodies that lead to the onset of BP [185]. It was proposed that BP180 neoexpression could be associated with early/malignant transformation of keratinocytes as widely expression of BP180 was demonstrated in SCC in contrast to normal skin, where this protein is restricted to basal keratinocytes [186].

Laminin-322 (previously named laminin-5) is the main autoantigen in anti-epiligrin cicatricial pemphigoid, mucouse membrane pemphigoid. Laminin-332 and alfa6beta4integrin may play an important role in tumor progression via activation of phosphatidylinositol-3 kinase signaling (PI3K) [187]. There was shown, that it is highly expressed in several types of squamous and other epithelial tumours [188]. Moreover, in these tumors, laminin-322 shows tendency to accumulate at the interface of the tumor with the surrounding stroma, and expression of this proteins correlates with tumor invasiveness [188]. Interestingly, keratinocytes from patients with junctional epidermolysis bullosa, that did not express laminin-322 or beta4integrin, showed a lack of tumorigenecity in immunodeficient mice after transformation [188]. Perhaps, the binding of collagen VII to laminin-322 may be essential for tumorigenesis [188]. Furthermore, the laminin-322-derived signaling is an important component of tumorigenesis. As mentioned above, constitutive activation of the PI3K pathway leading to RAC1 GTPase activation may be the triggering factor inducing tumor invasion.

6. Case reports of MAABD

As the association between ABD and malignancy is noted in many case reports, the question of causal connection is raised. There are three situations possible concerning the relation: i) malignancy preceding ABD, ii) malignancy coexisting with ABD, iii) malignancy following ABD. For a long months and years, many cases of ABD are undiagnosed, misdiagnosed and subsequently mistreated due to relative rarity and therefore low awareness of ABD and its symptoms. The time period elapsed between the first symptoms and diagnosis, makes the time-onset relation between ABD and cancer usually uncertain.

Here, based on our personal clinical/laboratory/research experience, we present a dozen of memorable/representative patients with association of malignancy, both cutaneous and internal, and ABD over the last decade. Unfortunately, usually there is no experimental data indicating if it is a random coincidence or cause-and-effect relationship in individual patient. Still, the diagnosis of such a concurrence increases mortality.

6.1. Anti-desmosomal autoimmunity circle / pemphigus group cases

6.1.1. Case 1 — Mucocutaneous pemphigus vulgaris / lung cancer

An elderly female with painful oral erosions, flat white-speckled infiltrations, mucosal edema and enlarged submandibular lymph nodes was admitted to oncology center outpatients. Histopathological examination of the retromolar mucosa of the left alveolar process of maxilla showed paraepidermoid epithelium with focal high-grade dysplasia and few neoplastic cells.

Due to improper biopsy technique full examination of the material was impossible. Therefore, the patient was readmitted to the oncology ward, with tentative diagnosis of carcinoma planoepitheliale with bilateral metastases to neck lymph nodes, for bilateral selective lymphadenectomy and probational excision of the lesions at right buccal region and left soft palate. Histopathological examination on probational biopsy showed mucous membrane fragments with features of basement membrane disruption and acantholysis. There was abundant infiltration consisting of lymphoid cells with plasmocyte prevalence and presence of granulocytes. The overall image did not support the diagnosis of carcinoma planoepitheliale, yet suggested pemphigus. Chest x-ray showed left-sided pleural effusion with costodiaphragmatic recess filling. At the posterolateral side of the lung, thin layer of liquid reaching 7th rib in the posterior axillary line was observed. Ultrasonography of the neck showed non-enlarged thyroid gland (10 ml of volume) with hypoechogenic node (11 mm x 8 mm) and 3 lesser hypoechogenic nodes of diameters up to 4 mm in the left lobe. Enlarged lymph nodes, with narrow lymph sinuses (up to 15 mm x 8 mm) and unclear character, were seen bilaterally in the upper part of the neck vessels beyond mandibular angles.

The patient was directed to dermatological ward for further diagnostics. Laboratory tests showed increased sedimentation rate. DIF of perilesional skin of the vulva revealed IgG(+), IgG1(++) and C3(+) deposits in the intercellular spaces of the spinous layer of epidermis. hDIF on pulled-out hair revealed IgG(+), IgG1(+) and IgG4(+) deposits in the intercellular spaces of the outer root sheath. DIF of larynx mucosa showed fragmented specimen, mainly without epithelium. There was fragmented epithelium consisting of several cells at the specimens margin (evident acantholysis) with surrounding noticeable IgG(+/-) and C3(+/-) deposits. IIF study on monkey esophagus revealed circulating IgG class of pemphigus-type autoantibodies against desmosomal proteins of keratinocytes – titer above 1/80. On the basis of abovementioned tests the diagnosis of mucocutaneous PV was reached.

After amelioration of the lesions, due to pulse steroid treatment, she was dismissed from the ward. Two months later, she suffered from aggravation of mucosal erosions, haematopnoe and dyspnoe. The woman was admitted to oncology center, where chest computed tomography (CT) scan visualized solid mass in the left lung (Fig. 1A). Via bronchofiberoscopy, carcinoma planoepitheliale of the left lung (G4) with hepatic metastases was diagnosed. Palliative radiotherapy (20 Gy/T) of the mediastinal/left pulmonary region led to aggravation of mucocutaneous PV (Fig. 1B).

6.1.2. Case 2 — Mucocutaneous pemphigus vulgaris / oropharyngeal cancer

A middle-aged man observed blisters localized in the interscapular region and the posterior aspect of the neck (Fig. 2B, C). Simultaneously, he suffered from excruciating sore throat and dysphagia. He was consulted by ENT-specialist and subsequently was directed to oncology center for further diagnosis and treatment. Histological material obtained during laryngological diagnostics revealed carcinoma planoepitheliale keratodes invasivum of the right palatine tonsil, soft palate and uvula (T3N2M0) with metastatic focus in lymph node (Fig. 2A). Therefore, the patient underwent excision of the lesion with bilateral modified cervical lymphadenectomy. Neck ultrasound imaging visualized hypoechogenic polycyclic tumorous mass (43 mm x 25 mm) associated with lower pole of parotid gland with numerous small satellite nodules of diameter up to 6 mm and dissolved reactive lymph nodes up to 7 mm of length. The patient was treated with Intensity Modulated Radiation Therapy (IMRT) – 6 MeV photons for 34 cycles (68 Gy/t). Due to lesions regarded as notable cutaneous radiation syndrome of the neck (II* according to EORTC/RTOG scale), the few last cycles were diminished by 1 fraction and postradiative topicals were applied. Interestingly, the bullous lesions exacerbated (Fig. 2D) and appeared on the thorax, abdomen and limbs (Fig. 2E). No mucosal involvement was present at that time.

Due to above symptoms, he was consulted by the dermatologist. Histology of the skin revealed suprabasilar separation and acantholysis in the upper epidermis (Fig. 2F). IIF on monkey esophagus revealed circulating IgG class pemphigus-type antibodies against desmosomal proteins of keratinocytes – titer 1/320. DIF on the perilesional skin of the back showed IgG(+), IgG1(+), IgG4(+++) and C3(+) deposits in intracellular spaces of lower layers of epidermis (Fig. 2G). DIF of the plucked hair showed IgG4(+++), IgG1(++), IgG(++) and C3(+/-) deposits in intracellular spaces of outer hair sheath (Fig. 2H). Performed tests supported the diagnosis of mucocutaneous PV.

Four months later, patient was admitted to dermatological ward with numerous blisters and erosions on the skin of the thorax, back, limbs and head. Reddish postradiative aggravated PV lesions, which healed later with aggressive immunosuppressive treatment, with marginal blistering notably limited to the anterior surface of the neck, showed no visible reepithelialization. Numerous painful erosions presented on oral mucosa disabling patient's feeding and resulting in 10 kg weight loss. ELISA study revealed the presence of anti-desmoglein 1 (DSG1) IgG of titer 130.34AU/ml (cut-off point 41AU/ml) and anti-desmoglein 3 (DSG3) IgG of titer >150AU/ml (cut-off point 40AU/ml). IIF performed on rat bladder did not reveal serum antibodies of paraneoplastic pemphigus (PNP) type. Consulting laryngologist described numerous erosions of buccal and oral mucosa, yet noticed no features of recurrence of malignancy. The case was reported in literature [189].

6.1.3. Case 3 — Pemphigus foliaceus / pseudomyxoma peritonei

An elderly female was admitted to dermatological ward with numerous erythematous plaques, blisters and non-healing erosions covered with crusts – on the scalp, trunk and limbs (Fig. 3A, B). Her medical history was significant for angina pectoris, angioplasty (PTCA) with

http://dx.doi.org/10.5772/55240

stent implantation due to myocardial infarction, hypertension, hypercholesterolemia, diabetes mellitus type 2, hiatal hernia and epigastric hernia.

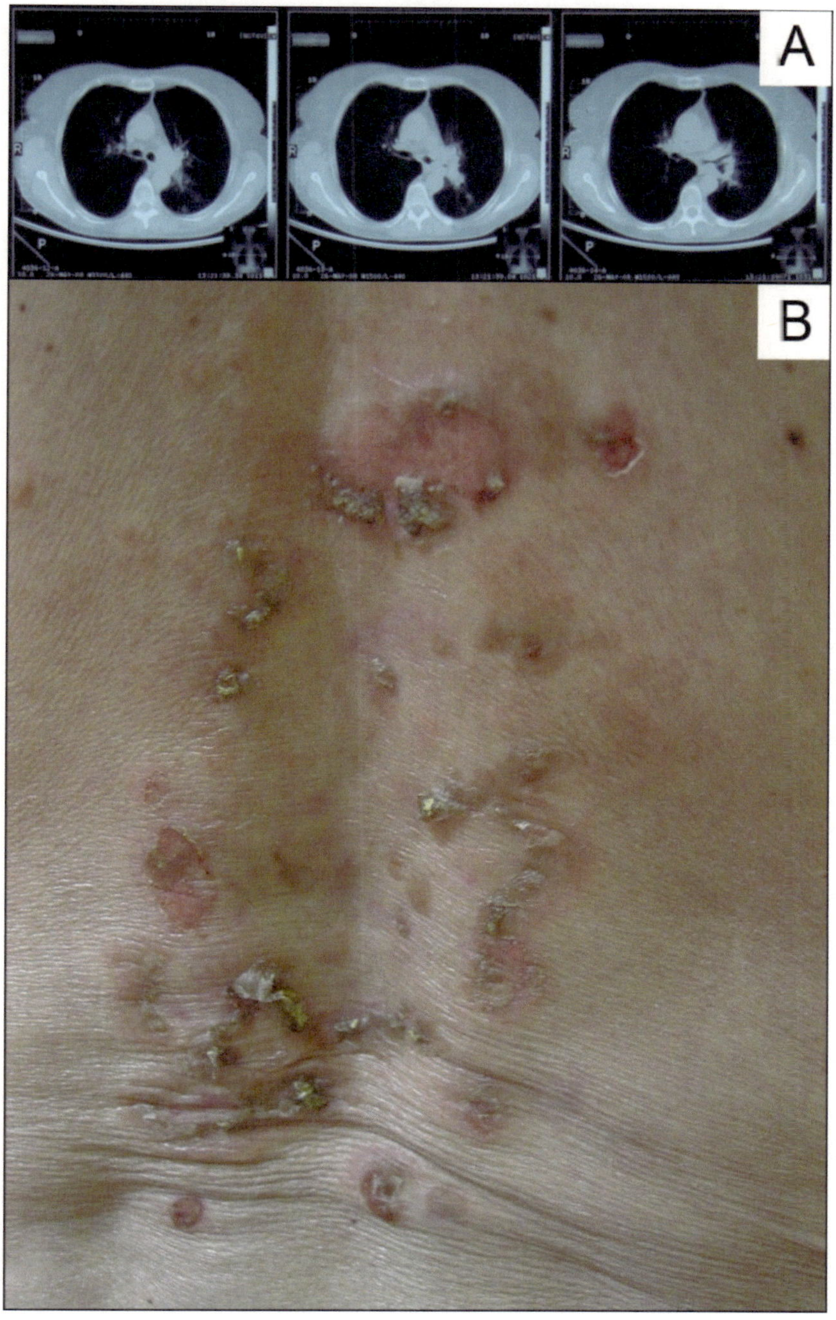

Figure 1. A. Chest CT of an elderly PV patient showing tumor in the left lung. B. Aggravation of mucocutaneous PV after palliative radiotherapy (radiotherapy-induced PV lesions).

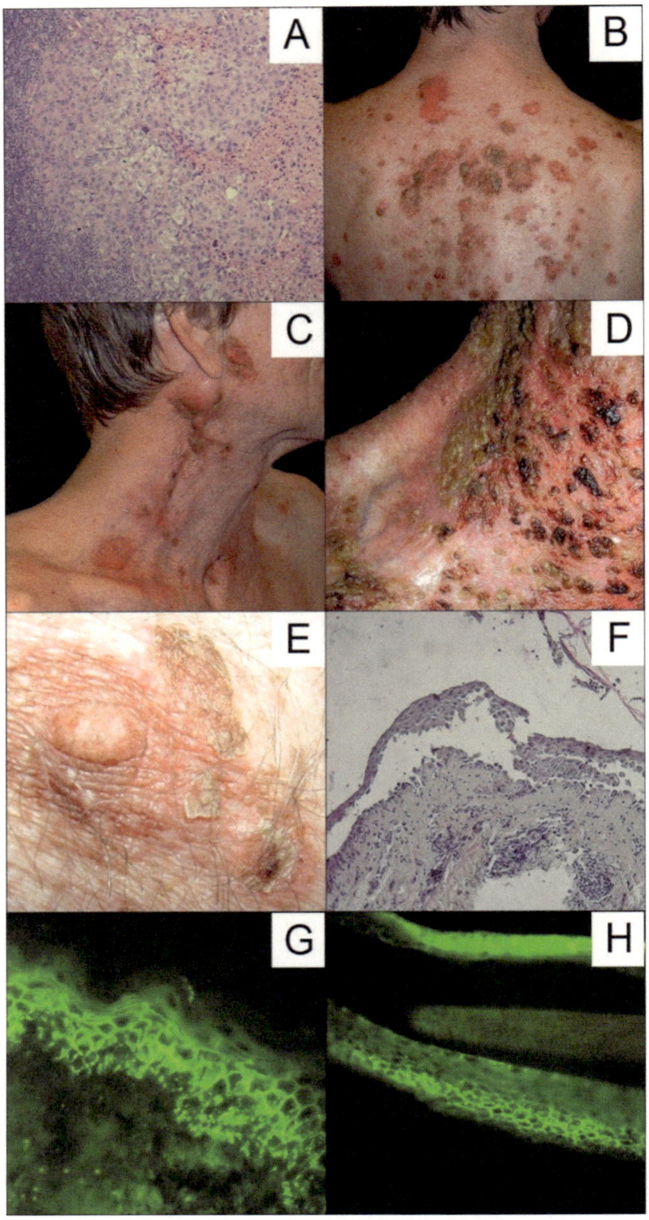

Published in [189]

Figure 2. A. Carcinoma planoepitheliale keratodes invasivum in lymphoid tissue. H+E staining. Courtesy of Prof. J. Bręborowicz. B. Numerous erosions on non-inflammatory skin of the back, some of them covered with brownish-greenish crusts. C. Erosions on non-inflammatory skin of the face and neck. Scar after the surgical excision of the cancer. D. Numerous merging erosions, some covered with bloody and greenish crusts on the skin of the neck area subjected to radiotherapy. E. Erosions covered with crusts around the nipple (a natural body orifice area). F. Suprabasilar separation and acantholytic blister in the upper epidermis. H+E staining. G. DIF of perilesional skin of the back: pemphigus IgG4 deposits in lower epidermis. H. DIF of plucked scalp hair: pemphigus IgG4 deposits in outer root sheath.

Initially, lesional skin sample examined by the cutaneous pathologist showed thin epidermis with fissures and flat vesicles in upper layer with slight acantholysis. Perivascular inflammatory infiltrates with prevalence of lymphocytes and eosinophils, focally involving the epidermis, were seen in the dermis. DIF test revealed deposits of IgG(+), IgG4(++) and C3(++) in intercellular spaces of epidermis. Marked acantholysis was visible and upper layers of epidermis were absent. Serum IgG, but not IgG4, autoantibodies of pemphigus type against desmosomal proteins of keratinocytes were present in IIF on rabbit labial mucosa and normal human skin, of titers respectively 1/40 and 1/160. The diagnosis of PF was made. She was treated with oral steroids and cyclophosphamide achieving remission before dismissal.

Six years later she was readmitted to dermatological ward due to aggravation of PF. IIF study on monkey esophagus showed serum IgG4 autoantibodies of pemphigus type against desmosomal proteins of keratinocytes – titer 1/80 (Fig. 3C). Abdominal ultrasonography revealed oval hyperechogenic solid mass (12 mm x 14 mm) in the middle part of the right kidney medulla suggesting kidney tumor. Two-phased abdominal CT scan visualized hypodensic well-delineated lesion (transverse diameter ca. 10 mm) in right renal medulla (suggestive of angiomyolipoma) characterized by density of adipose tissue, without contrast intensification.

The patient was supervised for years by dermatology practitioner. Due to increase of waist circumference, she was suggested to visit gynecologist. In gynecological control, the physician found right adnexal mass. The patient was directed urgently to gynecologic ward with tentative diagnosis of ovarian cancer, where she underwent hysterectomy with adnexotomy, omentectomy and appendectomy. The tumor was described by the histopathologist as low grade appendiceal mucinous neoplasm (pseudomyxoma peritonei) with metastasis to right ovary and omentum. Since then, she regularly visited gynecological oncologist

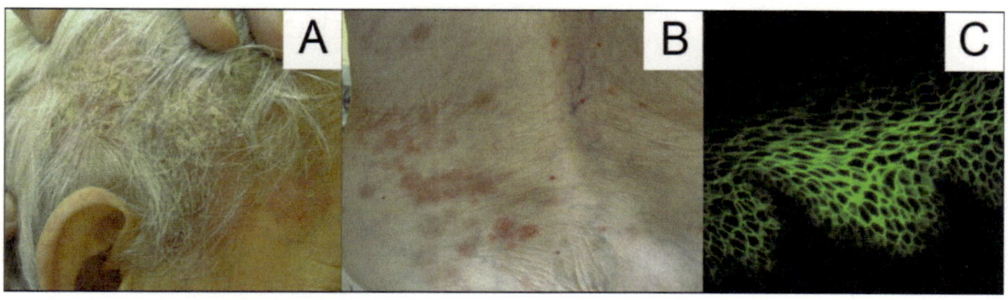

Figure 3. A. Erythematous plaques and crusts on the scalp of the head. B. Erosions and blisters on the back. C. IIF on monkey esophagus: pemphigus IgG4 autoantibodies. PF recurrence in the course of ACE-inhibitor treatment for myocardial infarction.

6.1.4. Case 4 — Pemphigus foliaceus / squamous cell carcinoma of the thorax

A middle-aged man was consulted by dermatological specialist due to disseminated erythematous plaques. The lesions were preceded by three months of uncomfortable itching on hands and feet. He was not diagnosed beforehand and was solely treated with topical steroids.

Therefore, he was directed do dermatological ward with tentative diagnosis of pemphigus/PNP for further diagnostics and treatment.

On admission, he presented erythroderma (Fig. 4A) and notable exophytic tumor on anterior surface of the thorax (c.a. 13 cm of diameter), clinically carcinoma verrucosum (Fig. 4B). Laboratory tests showed anemia, increased sedimentation rate and CRP. Histology of the perilesional skin showed marked acantholysis (Fig. 4C). Tumor margin bioptate showed clustered isles of atypic cells with fine keratin pearls giving overall image of highly differentiated squamous cell carcinoma (SCC) G1 (Fig. 4D). IIF on monkey esophagus proved the presence of serum IgG pemphigus-type antibodies against desmosomal proteins of keratinocytes – titer 1/160, yet IIF on rat bladder for serum PNP-type IgG was negative. ELISA test showed serum anti-DSG1 IgG level >200 RU/ml (cut-off point 20 RU/ml), yet did not revealed serum anti-DSG3 IgG – level 0 RU/ml (cut-off point 20 RU/ml). DIF of the perilesional skin visualized IgG(+), IgG1(++) and IgG4(++) deposits in the intercellular spaces of higher layers of epidermis and C3(+ +) deposits in the intercellular spaces of lower layers of epidermis (Fig. 4E). hDIF showed IgG(+), IgG1(+) and C3(+) deposits in the intercellular spaces of outer root sheath (Fig. 4F). With clinical and histological findings and molecular findings, the diagnosis of PF was made. After achieving dermatological improvement with doxycycline, antihistamine drugs and oral/topical steroids, patient was directed to oncology ward for SCC therapy.

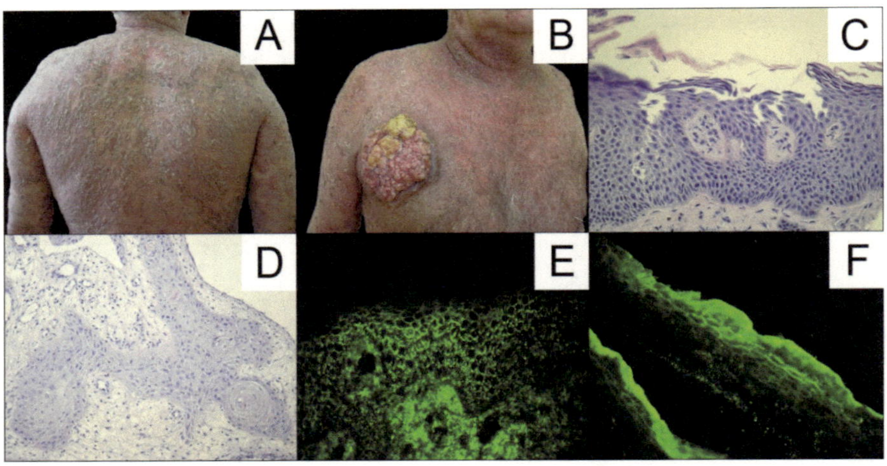

Figure 4. A. Disseminated erythematous plaques and crusts on the back. B. Exophytic tumor on anterior surface of the chest. C. Histology of the perilesional skin: Acantholysis. H+E staining. D. Histology of the tumor margin: Clustered isles of atypical cells with fine keratin pearls. Highly differentiated SCC. H+E staining. E. DIF of perilesional skin: IgG4(++) deposits in the intercellular spaces of higher layers of epidermis. F. hDIF of plucked scalp hair: IgG(+) deposits in the intercellular spaces of outer root sheath.

6.1.5. Case 5 — Mucocutaneous pemphigus vulgaris shifting from mucosal dominant form / lower lip squamous cell carcinoma

An elderly man treated for lower lip squamous cell carcinoma (SCC planoepitheliale keratodes; G2) that developed in lesions showing histological features of PV (Fig. 5E, F) suffered from painful erosions on oral mucosa dating back several months (Fig. 5A). Subsequently, the blistering lesions and oozing erosions appeared on the skin (Fig. 5B, C). He called the dermatology professional and was directed to dermatological ward for diagnosis and treatment.

His laboratory tests showed increased sedimentation rate. Chest x-ray revealed fine atelectasis in the inferior aspect of the right lung. Ultrasonography of the abdomen showed non-echogenic area (16 mm x 18 mm) with intramural calcification and features of a cyst within VII segment and hypoechogenic lesion (dia. of 12 mm), probably angioma, in VI/VII segment of the of the right lobe of the liver. Two lesser cysts (up to dia. 5 mm) were found in left lobe. Gallstone (dia. 18 mm) was depicted in gall bladder, while right kidney showed sonographic features of hydronephrosis. An intravenous urogram (IVU) proved the presence of renal stone in right ureteropelvic junction, causing obstruction and dilatation of the pelvicalyceal system. In Tzanck test rounded acantholytic cells were present (Fig. 5D). Skin bioptate was characterized by the pathologist as PV material. hDIF showed IgG(++) and IgG4(+) deposits in intercellular spaces of outer root sheath (Fig. 5G). DIF on skin lesion margin showed IgG(+), IgG4(++) and C3(+) deposits in intercellular spaces of the lower spinous layer of epidermis (Fig. 5H). IIF on monkey esophagus revealed circulating IgG pemphigus-type antibodies against desmosomal proteins of keratinocytes – titer 1/320. ELISA test with patient's serum revealed serum anti-DSG1 and anti-DSG3 IgG class autoantibodies – levels respectively 133.81 RU/ml (cut-off point 41 RU/ml) and > 150 RU/ml (cut-off point 40 RU/ml). The diagnosis of mucocutaneous PV (shifting from mucosal dominant PV) was established. He was treated with pulses of high dose intravenous steroids combined with oral/topical steroids and doxycycline as a fundamental therapy with satisfactory effect.

6.1.6. Case 6 — Mucosal dominant pemphigus vulgaris / breast cancer

An elderly female, five years after right-side mastectomy due to breast cancer (invasive ductal carcinoma; G1; pT1cpN1Mx), was admitted to dermatological ward with painful non-healing erosions of oral and tongue mucosa. Her medical history was significant for diabetes mellitus type 2, arterial hypertension, diverticulosis, hemorrhagic gastritis and past episodes of deep vein thrombosis in the legs and thrombosis of the right central retinal vein. hDIF revealed IgG (+++), IgG1(++), IgG4(+++) and C3 deposits in intercellular spaces of outer root sheath (Fig. 6A). DIF on the perilesional mucosa showed IgG(+), IgG1(++), IgG4(+)and C3 deposits in intercellular spaces of lower layers of oral epithelium (Fig. 6B). IIF on monkey esophagus showed circulating IgG pemphigus-type antibodies binding spinous layer desmosomal proteins of keratinocytes – titer 1/160. Serum PNP-type autoantibodies were absent in IIF study on rat bladder transitional epithelium. ELISA study revealed elevated anti-DSG3 IgG level: 112.83 AU/ml (cut-off point 40 AU/ml), while IgG anti-DSG1 level was normal: 34.49 AU/ml (cut-off point 41AU/ml). Both laboratory tests and immunopathological findings supported the diagnosis of mucosal dominant PV. She was treated with oral methyloprednisolone, doxycycline and cyclophosphamide.

Because of her medical history, she was gradually deprived of methyloprednisolone, that resulted in an aggravation of PV within a month and need for urgent hospitalization. She was admitted with diffused erosions and blisters both on the skin and oral mucosa. Laboratory

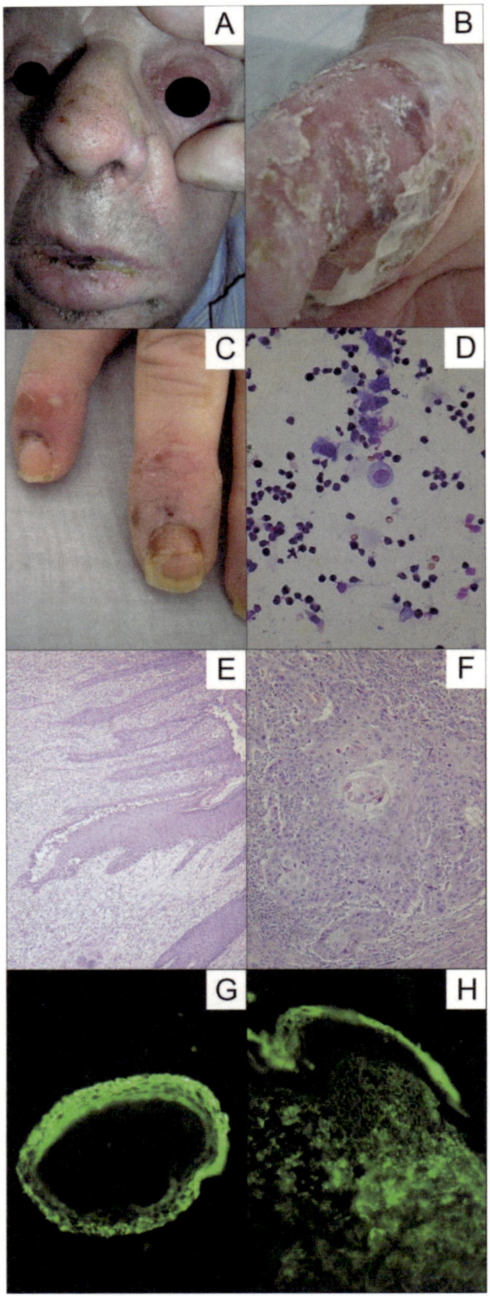

Published in [190].

Figure 5. A. Mucosal erosions in patient with lower lip SCC and mucocutaneous PV. B. Fragile blister on the hand. C. Pemphigus vulgaris imitating paronychia. D. Positive Tzanck test: rounded acantholytic cells suggestive for PV. E. Suprabasilar cleft with acantholysis in the lower lip specimen showing also features of SCC. H+E staining. F. Lower lip SCC. H+E staining. Courtesy of Prof. J. Bręborowicz. G. hDIF: pemphigus IgG deposits in intercellular spaces of outer root sheath. H.DIF showing IgG pemphigus-type deposits.

tests revealed elevated CEA level – 8.05 ng/ml (cut-off point 5 ng/ml) with normal levels of other cancer biomarkers (CA19-9, Ca125, AFP). She was treated with cyclophosphamide, doxycycline and high doses of both intravenous and oral steroids.

She was readmitted to the ward six months later with erosions on buccal mucosa, base of the mouth, soft palate and epiglottis. Laboratory tests revealed elevated CA19-9 level: 843.8 U/ml (cut-off point 37 U/ml). After achieving remission of lesions, she was directed to oncology outpatients to screen for malignancy.

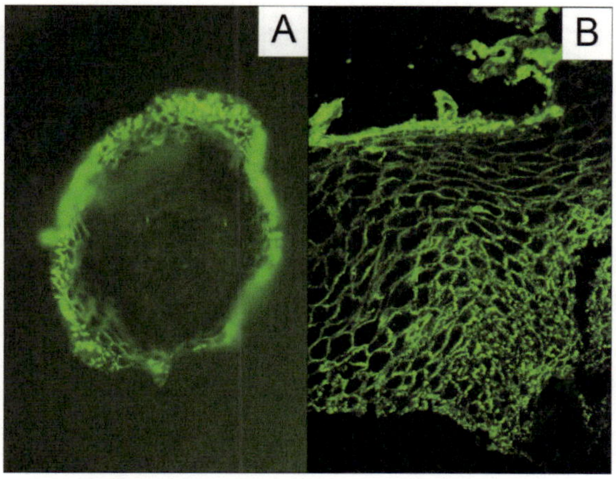

Figure 6. A. hDIF visualizing IgG1(++) deposits in the outer root sheath. B. DIF of perilesional mucosa revealing IgG1(++) deposits in intercellular spaces of lower layers of oral epithelium.

6.1.7. Case 7 — Pemphigus foliaceus / squamous cell carcinoma of external nose and upper lip

A middle-aged man with exophytic ulcerative nasal tumor was diagnosed with paranasal sinuses roentgenogram revealing massive shade of polycyclic outline. Surgical excision of the external nose tumor infiltrating upper lip was performed in oncology center (Fig. 7A). Exophytic lesion was described by a pathologist as carcinoma planoepitheliale keratodes (G2). The patient was frequently monitored in oncology outpatients finding no features of tumor recurrence.

Two years afterward, erythemous plaques with flaccid serous blisters, oozing erosions and crusts appeared on lower limbs. It took several weeks until lesions generalized and occupied trunk, limbs, head and intertriginous regions forming vast desquamative surfaces of flaky puff pastry-like appearance (Fig. 7B). Mucous membranes remained free of lesions. Due to ineffective ambulatory management, he was directed to dermatological ward with tentative diagnosis of PF.

Histological features of perilesional skin supported PF diagnosis. IIF on monkey esophagus revealed serum IgG pemphigus-type antibodies against desmosomal proteins of spinous layer of epidermis – titer 1/320, yet IIF on rat bladder epithelium as a substrate did not detected circulating PNP-type autoantibodies. DIF of perilesional skin visualized well-defined IgG(+++) and IgG4(+++) deposits in intercellular spaces of lower layers of epidermis and linear C3(+) deposits alongside DEJ (Fig. 7C). Serum anti-DSG1 IgG ELISA was positive – level >150 AU/ml (cut-off point 41 AU/ml), whereas serum anti-DSG3 IgG ELISA proved negative – level 6.20 AU/ml (cut-off point 40 AU/ml). The molecular tests confirmed the PF diagnosis. He was treated with oral/intravenous steroids and cyclophosphamide, azathioprine and doxycycline as adjuvant treatment. The compliance in ambulatory care was poor as the patient repeatedly was treated in dermatological ward with IIF IgG pemphigus-type antibody titer reaching 1/2560.

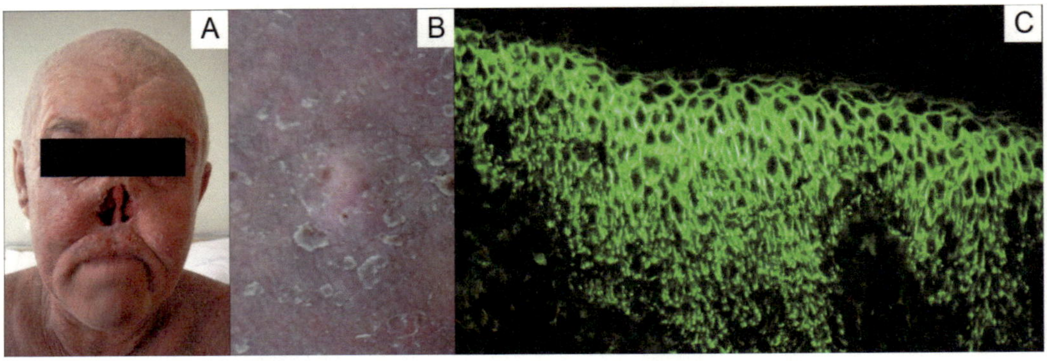

Figure 7. A. Nose stump after tumor excision. Courtesy of S. Stusek MD. B. Flaky puff pastry-like desquamative lesions on the trunk. Courtesy of S. Stusek MD. C. DIF of perilesional skin: intense pemphigus IgG4(+++) deposits.

6.2. Subepidermal autoimmune blistering diseases

6.2.1. Case 8 — Bullous pemphigoid / colon cancer

An elderly man was directed to chirurgical ward due to ileus. He underwent left hemicolectomy and forming of colostomy because of appendicitis, chronic peritonitis and colon cancer. Histopathological examination of the excised material revealed partially gelatinous tubular adenocarcinoma (G2; T4N0M0) infiltrating pericolic adipose tissue (Fig. 8B).

After the surgery, eczematous vesicular oozing eruption appeared on the surrounding of the stomy (Fig. 8A), while itchy well-tense bullae occurred on the skin of the back covering trunk and limbs in a few weeks. Histopathological and immunopathological tests were performed in dermatological outpatient ward two years after operation. Histology of the perilesional skin showed subepidermal vesicle filled with inflammatory cells with predominance of eosinophils (Fig. 8C). Perilesional skin DIF revealed linear deposits of IgG4(++) and C3(+++) along dermal-epidermal junction (DEJ) (Fig. 8D). IIF, performed on monkey esophagus as a substrate, was negative for IgG serum autoantibodies against desmosomal proteins of keratinocytes and basement membrane antigens. ELISA anti-BP180NC16a examination was positive for serum IgG antibodies against BP180 – titer 60.47 U/ml (cut-off point 9 U/ml), that enabled the diagnosis of trauma-induced and paraneoplastic BP at the molecular level. Control chest X-ray and ultrasonography of the abdomen did not showed neoplasm.

BP tend to manifest in natural and iatrogenic orifices featured by transient epithelium (e.g. the scar or the stomy site). It may be possible, that malignant tumor causing pathological immunization triggered the onset of this subepidermal dermatosis. The case is a hallmark of literature data [191–193].

6.2.2. Case 9 — Bullous pemphigoid / family history of renal cancer

A middle-aged female was directed to dermatological ward for diagnostics and treatment of disseminated itchy blisters and vesicles on erythematous skin (Fig. 9A, B) dating back two months. Her family history was significant for renal cancer coexisting with a subepidermal IgG-mediated bullous dermatosis, most likely BP, in grandmother. Her laboratory test were noncontributory. Immunohistochemical study showed subepidermal blister with neutrophil elastase (NE) deposits (Fig. 9C). IIF on monkey esophagus was positive for serum IgG pemphigoid-type antibody against DEJ proteins – titer 1/80. DIF of the perilesional skin revealed IgG1(+), IgG4(+) and C3(++) deposits along DEJ (Fig. 9D). Direct immunofluorescence test on salt-split skin (ssDIF) showed IgG4(+) and C3 deposits on epidermal side of the split. Aforementioned methods made it possible to diagnose BP and begin treatment with oral/ topical steroids, cyclophosphamide, doxycycline and antihistamines. Because of family history of autoimmune blistering dermatosis coexistent with cancer, the patient was advised to undergo meticulous follow-up to reveal any signs of malignancy as soon as possible.

6.2.3. Case 10 — Mucous membrane pemphigoid / hodgkin lymphoma

An elderly female, with swollen left supraclavicular lymph nodes, weight loss, fatigue, low grade fever and night sweats, was admitted to internal diseases ward for diagnostics. Both clinical symptoms, laboratory tests and histological examination of lymph node supported the diagnosis of Hodgkin lymphoma (IIB). She was treated with ABVD chemotherapy regimen (adriamycin, bleomycin, vinblastine, dacarbazine) and COPP regimen (cyclophosphamide, vincristin, procarbazine, prednisone) - due to bad tolerance of anthracyclines, achieving lymphoma remission.

Six years later, she called ENT professional due to dysphagia, oral itching and numerous painfull erosions on oral mucosa covered with whitish coating (Fig. 10A). The lesions were diagnosed mycologically as oral candidiasis (Candida famata, Candida glabrata). Antimycological treatment seemed ineffective and another erosive lesion (3 cm in diameter) appeared in umbilical region (Fig. 10B). She was directed to dermatological ward for further diagnostics and treatment six months later. Her medical history was also significant for total hysterectomy and episode of upper gastrointestinal bleeding (diffused intestinal metaplasia of the stomach mucosa; coagulated). Laboratory blood tests showed increased sedimentation rate and CRP. IIF on monkey esophagus did not revealed circulating IgG antibodies against desmosomal proteins of keratinocytes and basement membrane antigens (Fig. 10C). DIF of the perilesional skin from the umbilical region showed linear deposits of IgG(+/-), IgG1(+), and C3(+) along dermal-epidermal junction (Fig. 10D). In natural blister, autoantibody deposits were seen on epidermal side of the split. The diagnosis of MMP was based on clinical and DIF findings fulfilling the criteria of this dermatosis.

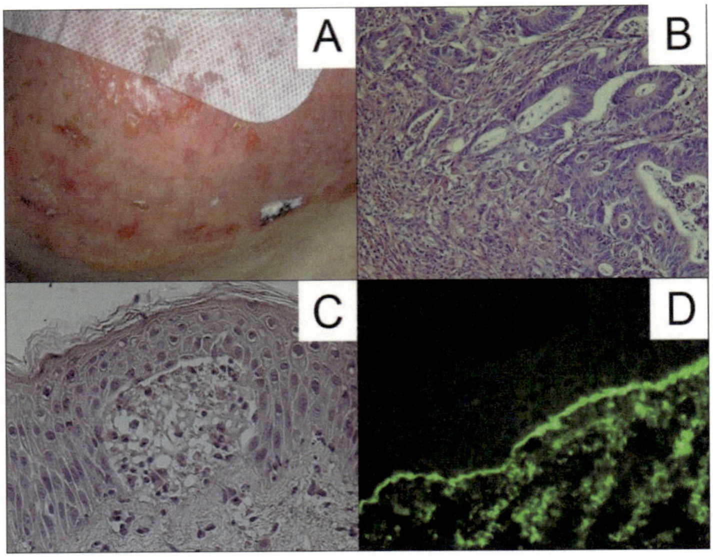

Published in [191].

Figure 8. A. Blisters and their evolutionary lesions on inflamed skin around colostomy. B. A part of neoplastic infiltrate in the wall of large intestine showing cramped glandular ducts with irregular shapes. Epithelium cells with high-grade atypical cells. Inflammation of the periphery. H+E staining. Courtesy of I. Turczuk-Bierła MD. C. Histology of perilesional skin: Subepidermal vesicle with admixture of eosinophils within it. H+E staining. D. DIF of the blister skin margin: linear IgG4(++) deposits along DEJ.

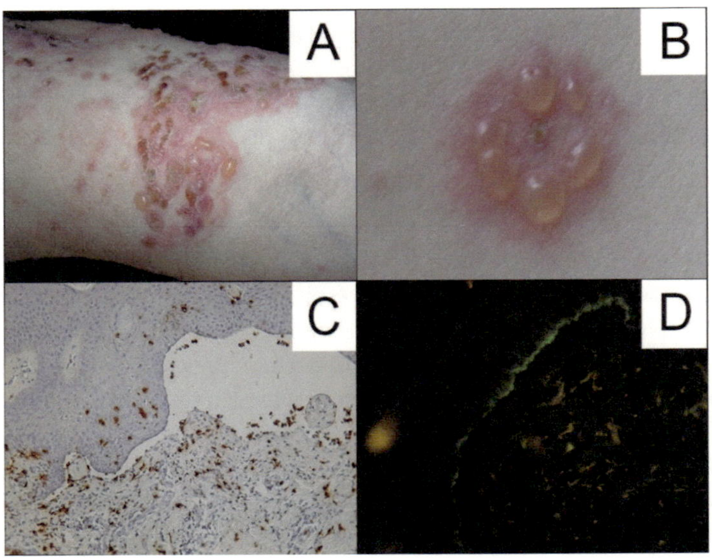

Figure 9. A. Erosions and bullae on erythematous skin forming "string of beans". B. Group of small blisters forming "cluster of jewels". C. Immunohistochemical study of the lesional skin. Visualization of neutrophil elastase (NE) deposits in the subepidermal blister. D. DIF on the perilesional skin: linear IgG4(+) deposits along DEJ.

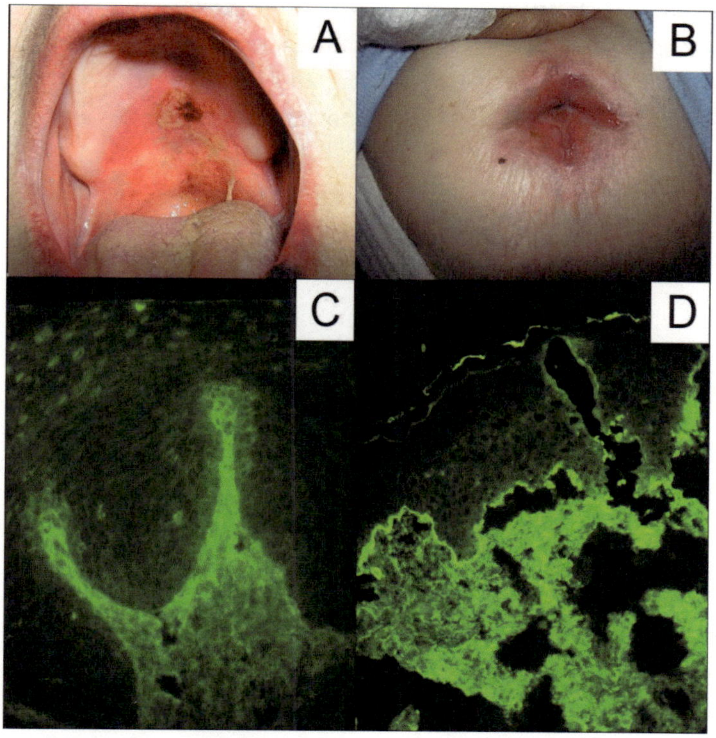

Figure 10. A. Mucosal erosions in oral cavity. B. Erosion in the navel. C. IIF study revealing no IgG antibodies binding either desmosomal proteins of keratinocytes or basement membrane antigens. D. DIF of the perilesional navel skin: linear IgG1(+) deposits alongside DEJ. Autoantibody deposits on epidermal side.

6.2.4. Case 11 — Bullous pemphigoid / renal cancer / prostate cancer

An elderly man visited the dermatologist due to disseminated erythematous itchy lesions, papules, erosions and a few well-tensed blisters filled with serous exudate on the forearms, arms and trunk (Fig. 11A, B). He was treated without clinical effect with antibiotics, antihistamine drugs and oral steroids. After a month, he was directed to dermatological ward for further diagnostics.

His medical history was significant for nephrectomy because of carcinoma clarocellulare, prostate adenocarcinoma (Gleason 1+3=4) treated with brachytherapy (HDR 20 Gy) and radiotherapy, two hypermetabolic abdominal foci at level of kidney vessels in PET (supposedly metastatic lymph nodes), thyroid nodule and testis hydrocele. Laboratory tests revealed increased CRP levels, monocytosis, eosinocytosis, hypertriglyceridemia.

Histology of the perilesional skin showed subepidermal blistering and inflammatory mixed infiltrate with neutrophils and eosinophils (Fig. 11C). DIF of the perilesional skin of gluteal region showed linear deposits of IgG1(+), IgG4(++) and C3(+) along DEJ. DIF performed on vesicle margin skin showed linear deposits of IgG(+), IgG1(+), IgG4(+++) and C3(++) along dermal-epidermal junction. (Fig. 11D). IIF on monkey esophagus did not revealed circulating IgG antibodies against desmosomal proteins of keratinocytes and basement membrane antigens. ELISA test revealed increased serum anti-BP230 IgG level – 81.356 RU/ml (cut-off point 20 RU/ml), yet circulating anti-BP180 IgG level was normal – 8.037 RU/ml (cut-off point 20 RU/ml). Vesicular and paraneoplastic BP was confirmed at the molecular level.

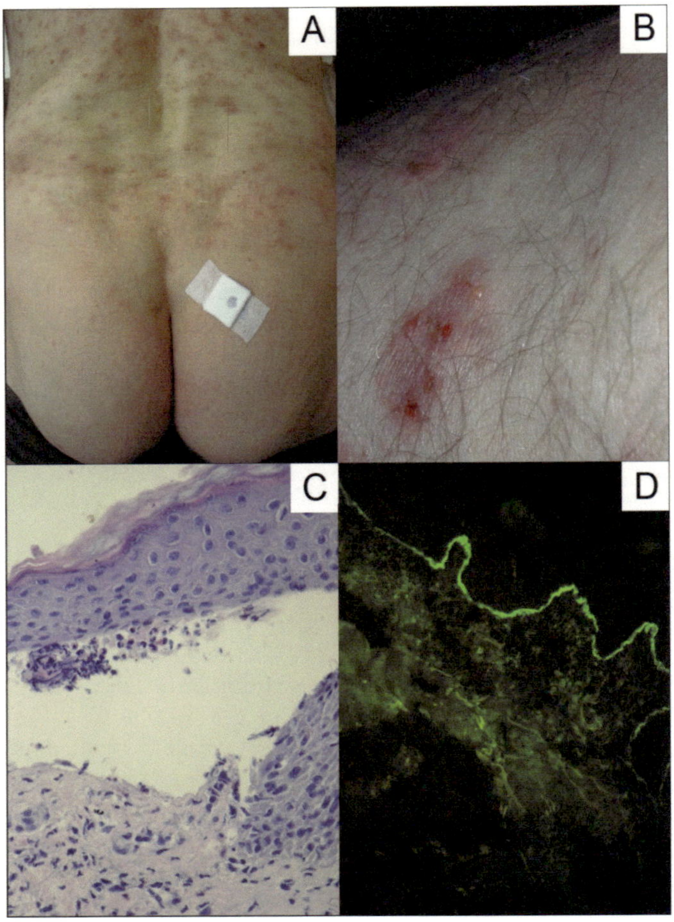

Published in [220].

Figure 11. A. Erythemous/oedematous lesions and erosions on the back in patient with vesiculous form of BP. Sticking plaster marks the site of biopsy. B. Vesicular lesions on posteriomedial surface of the left arm. C. Histology of subepidermal blister. Inflammatory mixed infiltrate with neutrophils and eosinophils. H+E staining. D. DIF on perilesional skin: IgG4 deposits along DEJ.

6.2.5. Case 12 — Bullous pemphigoid / lung cancer

A middle-aged heavy smoker visited dermatologist because of disseminated eruption of well-tensed painful blisters (Fig. 12A). Histological examination was suggestive of BP (Fig. 12B).

DIF of perilesional skin revealed linear deposits of IgG4(+) and C3(++) along dermal-epidermal junction (Fig. 12C). IIF on monkey esophagus did not revealed circulating IgG antibodies against either desmosomal proteins of keratinocytes or basement membrane antigens. The patient was directed to dermatological ward for further diagnostics. Laboratory tests showed leukocytosis, increased sedimentation rate and CRP. Apart of slightly increased CEA (6.79 ng/ml; cut-off for non-smokers 5.00 ng/ml, for smokers 6.50 ng/ml), other cancer biomarkers (AFP, CA19-9, Ca125, PSA) were negative. ELISA study was positive for serum anti-BP180 IgG – 19.50 RU/ml (cut-off point 9 RU/ml), yet negative for serum anti-BP230 IgG – 0.00 RU/ml (cut-off point 9 RU/ml). The diagnosis of BP was established. Abdominal ultrasound displayed enlarged liver without visible focal changes. Chest x-ray revealed a tumorous mass (7.0 cm x 6.6 cm), in middle lobe of the right lung, infiltrating lower root (Fig. 12D). Chest CT showed heterogeneous tumor of the right lung with consequent emphysema and metastatic mediastinal lymph nodes.

Consulting pulmonologist ordered further diagnostics and treatment in pulmonological ward, where bronchofiberoscopy was performed. With the histological diagnosis of carcinoma planoepitheliale akeratodes (G3; T4N2M0; IIIB) the patient began chemotherapy (cisplatin/vinorelbine regimen), yet he died within months.

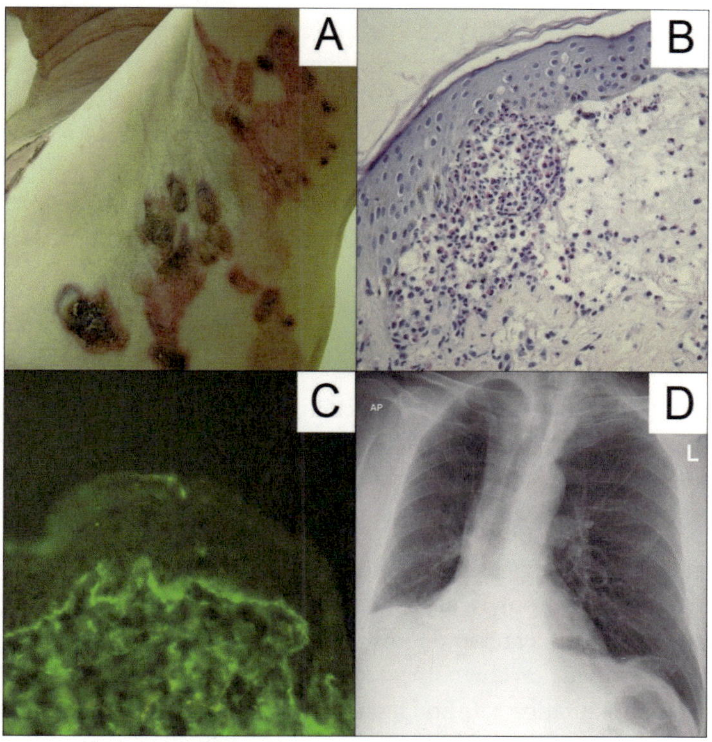

Figure 12. A. Painful well-tensed blisters, crusts and erosions on erythematous skin of the axillary area. B. Histology: subepidermal vesicle with abundant eosinophil infiltrate. H+E staining. C. DIF: linear deposits of IgG4 along DEJ. D. Chest x-ray: solid mass in middle lobe of the right lung, Tumor infiltration of lower lung root.

6.2.6. Case 13 — Bullous pemphigoid / prostate cancer

An elderly man consulted dermatology outpatient clinic due to itchy and painful well-tense blisters on the legs and subsequently on flexural surfaces of the forearms dating back four months (Fig. 13A). Perilesional skin bioptate and patient's blood sample were obtained for diagnostic purposes. Histology showed subepidermal blister. Major basic protein was visualized with immunohistochemical method marking eosinophil infiltrate (Fig. 13B). DIF study revealed linear deposits of IgG1(+), IgG4(+) and C3(++) along DEJ (Fig. 13C). IIF on monkey esophagus revealed circulating pemphigoid-type IgG, IgG1 and IgG4 antibodies against basement membrane antigens, of titers respectively 1/320, 1/160 and 1/160 (Fig. 13D). He was treated with limecycline, antihistamine drugs and incidental intramuscular steroids and was directed to dermatological ward, with tentative diagnosis of BP, for further diagnostics and treatment.

On admission he presented oozing erosions and well-tensed blisters filled with serosanguineous exudate on the right forearm. His medical history was significant for prostatic cancer (treated for 8-year-period with hormonal therapy) and orchidectomy. He was treated by urologist with tamsulosin, cyproterone, finasteride, flutamide, leuprorelin and goserelin. Several months before lesions' appearance, the urologist ceased the hormonal treatment, finding it purposeless. Laboratory tests revealed erythrocytopenia, increased sedimentation rate and PSA (17.49 ng/ml; cut-off 4.00). Other cancer biomarkers (CEA, AFP), FOBT and stool examination for parasite infestation were negative. ELISA test performed on patient's serum and blister fluid showed increased anti-BP180 IgG level: 14.01 RU/ml and 13.21 RU/ml respectively (cut-off 9 RU/ml) and increased anti-BP230 IgG level: 90.66 RU/ml and 75.85 RU/ml respectively. The diagnosis of BP as a paraneoplastic syndrome was made. Due to previous oncologic history, patient was urgently directed to urologist. Leuproreline readministration with immunosuppressive and anti-inflammatory treatment enabled remission of cutaneous lesions.

6.2.7. Case 14 — Ocular mucous membrane pemphigoid / endometrial cancer

A middle-aged woman was admitted to dermatological dispensary due to erosive lesions on oral mucosa lasting for 2 years. She was treated by stomatologist, but without effect. Moreover, due to involvement of conjunctivae two months earlier, she called the ophthalmologist, yet the administered treatment seemed insufficient.

She was directed to dermatological ward for diagnostics. Her medical history was significant for hysterectomy and adnexotomy with fistula and colon partial resection and transversostomy due to endometrial adenocarcinoma infiltrating colon, causing recto-vaginal fistula (G2; pT3aNx). She was planned for chemotherapy by gynaeco-oncologist. Her laboratory tests showed increased sedimentation rate and increased antinuclear antibodies (ANA) titer. IIF on monkey esophagus was negative for serum IgG autoantibodies against both desmosomal proteins of keratinocyte and basement membrane antigens. DIF on oral mucous membrane bioptate revealed scant linear C3 deposits along DEJ. Both clinical and immunopathological findings supported the diagnosis of ocular MMP.

http://dx.doi.org/10.5772/55240

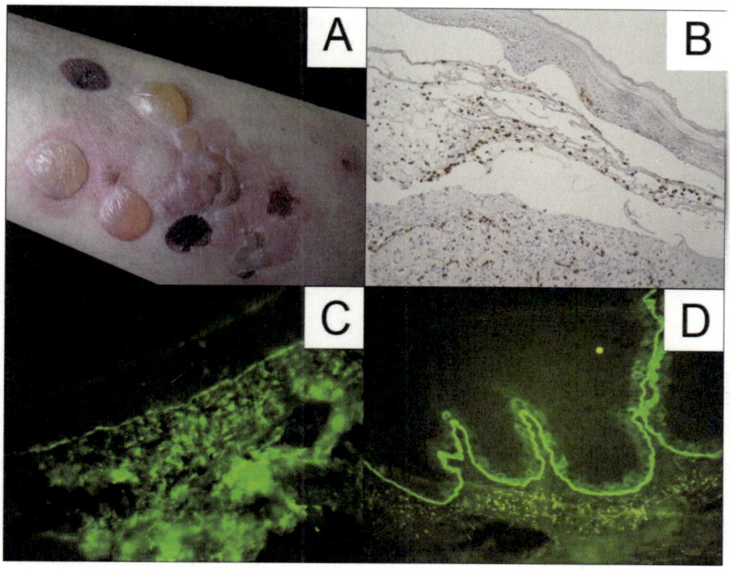

Published in [21].

Figure 13. A. Blisters and their evolutionary lesions on urticarial skin on the flexural surface of a forearm. B. Eosinophil major basic protein (MBP) deposits in lesional skin. Immunohistochemistry of subepidermal blister showing histological features of regeneration. C. DIF of perilesional skin: linear IgG1(+) deposits along DEJ. D. IIF on monkey esophagus: IgG4 antibodies against epithelial basement membrane antigens.

6.2.8. Case 15 — Bullous pemphigoid / breast cancer

An elderly female with itchy bullous eruption on acral parts of the limbs visited the dermatological outpatient clinic. The lesions dated back four months and suggested BP. Her medical history was significant for mastectomy due to breast cancer (infiltrating desmoplastic ductal and intraductal carcinoma of intermediate grade of malignancy; G2 according to Bloom-Richardson Grading System). DIF study of the perilesional skin sample revealed linear IgG4(+/-) and C3(++) deposits along DEJ. IIF, on monkey esophagus as a substrate, revealed neither serum IgG nor IgG4 antibodies against desmosomal proteins of keratinocytes and basement membrane antigens. ELISA study defined serum anti-BP180 IgG level as >200 RU/ml (cut-off point 20 RU/ml), yet serum anti-BP230 IgG level was normal – 3.182 RU/ml (cut-off point 20 RU/ml). With molecular methods, the tentative clinical diagnosis of BP was confirmed. The patient remained in control of both dermatology and oncology outpatient clinics.

6.3. Discussion on MAABD cases

ABD can insidiously don the masks of other diseases imitating e.g. ulcerative carcinomas, paronychia, eczema or pruritus. Generalized or localized, the eruption may remain disguised for many months and years until the diagnosis is reached. In the light of contemporary data, ABD circle shift in one patient by acquiring autoimmunity to new epitopes (via epitope spreading or bystander effect) is possible. It should be concluded, that every circle is not a coherent group of diseases, yet forms a continuum of autoimmune blistering dermatoses within autoimmune multiorgan syndrome. The causative relation between ABD and cancer is difficult to establish, as both malignancy and ABD develops and stay undiagnosed over some time period.

In review based on PubMed, Scopus and EMBASE literature data, SCC has been found responsible of projection the majority of paraneoplastic syndromes, with pemphigus being one of the commonest dermatological conditions among them [194]. Case 1 and 2 both presented carcinoma planoepitheliale/SCC with PV. The latter entity, by imitating mucosal neoplastic process, presumably confused the clinicist and elongated the onset-diagnosis period. Interestingly, both cases showed recrudescence of their pemphigus lesions after radiotherapy. It seems to be a common finding in ABD, thus supports the role of radiotrauma-induced denudation of formerly hidden epitopes in disease pathogenesis. The issue of SCC driving autoimmunity is still enigmatic, yet change in DSG profile promoting tumor cell migration may play a role in autoaggresion [177]. Similar cases to abovementioned ones were reported in literature [17,195]. As pseudomyxoma peritonei classification still causes controversy [196], the association between PF and ovarian/appendiceal tumor in case 3 is disputable. Some researchers speculated on the role of HPV16 and bacteria in development of this tumor of appendiceal origin [197,198]. A single case of PNP, breast tumor and pseudomyxoma peritonei was mentioned in literature [53]. To our best knowledge, case 3 is the first report on coexistence of these two conditions. The concomitance of exophytic thoracic SCC-tumor and PF (case 4) seem to be well-defined, yet behavior of the patient is difficult to comprehend since his stinky tumor was present for years. Apparently, his PF lesions finally prompted him to seek dermatological advise, but not the tumor itself. Apart of that, the case 5 is no less enigmatic. PV may imitate multiple conditions and it should be noted, that his lip lesion (described correctly as SCC by general pathologist) coexisted at the same site with the lesion of PV initially missed by general pathologist but diagnosed as such by cutaneous pathologist by reevaluation of initial specimen. Both above cases are portrayal of suspicious association of SCC preceding pemphigus, whereas case 5 features additionally shifting PV phenotype, supposedly because of active long-term pathological autoimmunization syndrome involving epitope spreading phenomenon. Case 5 was mentioned in literature [190]. CA19-9 marker is tumor-associated, but not tumor-specific marker. It is used as a screening test for gastrointestinal adenocarcinomas (colorectal, hepatic, lung, ovarian carcinoma and few non-malignant conditions), first of all for pancreatic cancer [199]. Association of PV with breast cancer (case 6) or potential gastrointestinal tract adenocarcinoma is disputable. The case may be considered a model for post-cancer ABD eruption and stands as an evidence for strong need of regular screening for malignancy in ABD patients. As far as case 7 is concerned, once again we find it questionable whether excised nasal/labial tumor was assessed properly as a cancerous or was it just a limited exophytic lesion heralding PF – chancre of pemphigus [200]. There is limited data concerning SCC, second commonest skin cancer coexistent with PF [201]. The negative correlation between DSG1 expression and degree of dysplasia in SCC is an interesting issue indicating contribution of desmosomal adhesion glycoproteins in cancerogenesis [202].

BP tends to manifest in natural and iatrogenic orifices featured by transient epithelium (e.g. iatrogenic – the scar or the stomy site) (case 8). It seems coherent that malignant tumor causing pathological immunization triggered the onset of BP. It was suggested that BP may be secondary to surgical procedures exposing sequestered antigens of colon mucosa (particularly BP180) [185,203–206]. The case is a hallmark of literature data [191–193]. As pemphigus and pemphigoid may occur as a paraneoplastic syndrome accompanying malignant tumor, it might be reasonable to form an online national registry of patients with ABD. Case 9 was included to visualize that need. Although both ABD may not contain "paraneoplastic" attribute, it is highly advisable to monitor all the patients with all ABD as group of high risk of developing malignancy [16]. There is scant data on coexistence of MMP and Hodgkin lymphoma (case 10) [207,208]. Moreover, the association between pemphigoid and non-Hodgkin lymphoma may seem to be better exemplified [19,209,210]. Nonetheless, each malignant lymphoproliferation may lead to impairment of immunological mechanisms via the change of antigen suit, cytokine production, distorted antibody production and abnormal cytokine production affecting many molecular pathways, both known and unknown. As far as case 11 is concerned, practising dermatologist, perhaps suspecting Cottini form of DH, obtained skin sample for DIF from lesion-free gluteal region (Fig. 11A). However, that area should be regarded as non-optimal for diagnosing that form of DH with DIF [211]. Luckily, BP-indicative deposits of immunoreactants were present at both lesion-free and perilesional sites. The link between malignancy and pemphigoid in case 11 may be multi-sided. Both renal and prostate cancer might be suspicious of contribution to autoaggression [23,67,71,180,212,213] and the role of radiotherapy should not be considered irrelevant. Renal cancer elicits paraneoplastic syndromes in 40% of patients, although dermatological manifestations seem to be extremely rare [70]. Cancerous lung involvement in BP (as in case 12) was previously reported [34], yet pulmonary cancer seems to be more PV-associated. The cessation of hormonal treatment seemed to trigger BP as a symptom of recurrence of prostate malignancy (case 13) [21]. BP and prostate adenocarcinoma might be interrelated by BP180 issue. It was observed, that prostatic malignant tumors may lack of hemidesmosomal structures – BP180 and less commonly BP230 [180]. Abnormal composition of detectable basement membrane antigens participating in multiple molecular pathways may disbalance mechanisms of self-tolerance consequently stimulating the pathological autoimmunity. Induction of pemphigoid by trauma (in case 14 – by hysterectomy with partial colon resection), as reported in literature [214], may seem a reasonable explanation. There is one similar report on anti-laminin-332 MMP presumably associated with endometrial carcinoma [215]. BP in case 15 may be regarded secondary to breast cancer. It may be possible, that the distortion of cell cohesion in neoplastic cells leads to exposing normally hidden antigens or new epitopes are recognized by the immunocompetent cells. There are reports mentioning overlapped breast cancer and BP [20,84] as well as reports describing the evoking of autoimmune blistering dermatosis after breast radiotherapy [216–218], that may change antigenicity of the malignant cells.

Cancer research gives molecular evidence for tumor genetic instability. Vast array of unique tumor-specific neoantigens are presented on tumor's MHC molecules. Their recognition by T-cells could induce anti-tumor immunity [219]. Antibody-assisted defense against tumor may explain the fact of spontaneous cancer remissions. The other side of the coin may be the autoimmunity caused by unspecific tumor antigens, that are displayed in many tissues being easily accessible for T-cells. Hypothetically, some ABD might be really MAABD with tumor eradicated in early phase.

7. Conclusion

The diversity of ABD results from diversity of recognizable epitopes of adhesive, desmosomal, hemidesmosomal and basement membrane antigens that interact playing complicated role in securing tissue integrity, intercellular communication and skin growth. Aberrant adhesive molecule expression via epitope spreading, bystander effect and various signaling pathways, may contribute to increased risk of developing cancer and its further prognosis. The altered expression of adhesion complex molecules is thought to be vital for carcinoma motility and invasion. The conjunction of malignancy and ABD phenomenon still remains an area of interest of researchers worldwide, as it may benefit in development of more specific diagnostic tests and precise therapeutic strategies.

Concomitance of malignancy and these serious clinical conditions may dramatically decrease the patient survivorship. The wise clinician ought to trace potential malignancy in each and every one of the patients with ABD, regardless of deceptive lack of "paraneoplastic" epithet in the currently used misleading nosology for majority of those dermatoses, as such an association between those two groups of entities, was demonstrated not to be rare. Therefore, the diagnosis of ABD should be followed not only by screening, but also monitoring/periodical checking for malignancies. Moreover, the replacement of indiscriminate immunosuppressive therapy by individualized targeted therapy should be recommended. There is burning need for awareness of such coexistence also among oncologic patients, as ADB may herald the recurrence of malignancy.

Author details

Paweł Pietkiewicz, Justyna Gornowicz-Porowska, Monika Bowszyc-Dmochowska and Marian Dmochowski

*Address all correspondence to: mkdmoch@wp.pl

Cutaneous Histopathology and Immunopathology Section, Department of Dermatology, Poznan University of Medical Sciences, Poznań, Poland

We dedicate this work to our patients suffering from malignancy concomitant with autoimmune blistering dermatosis

References

[1] Dmochowski M. Autoimmunizacyjne dermatozy pecherzowe. Poznań: Wydawnictwo Naukowe Akademii Medycznej im. Karola Marcinkowskiego; 2006.

[2] Franks AL, Slansky JE. Multiple associations between a broad spectrum of autoimmune diseases, chronic inflammatory diseases and cancer. Anticancer Research 2012;32:1119–36.

[3] Vendramini-Costa DB, Carvalho JE. Molecular Link Mechanisms between Inflammation and Cancer. Current Pharmaceutical Design 2012;18:3831–52.

[4] Gornowicz-Porowska J, Bowszyc-Dmochowska M, Dmochowski M. Autoimmunity-driven enzymatic remodeling of the dermal-epidermal junction in bullous pemphigoid and dermatitis herpetiformis. Autoimmunity 2012;45:71–80.

[5] Wolff K, Johnson R, Suurmond R. Fitzpatrick's Color Atlas & Synopsis of Clinical Dermatology. - 5th ed. United States of America: McGraw-Hill Professional; 2005.

[6] Lutkowska A, Pietkiewicz P, Szulczyńska-Gabor J, Gornowicz J, Bowszyc-Dmochowska M, Dmochowski M. Gluteal skin is not an optimal biopsy site for direct immunofluorescence in diagnostics of dermatitis herpetiformis. A report of a case of dermatitis herpetiformis Cottini. Dermatologia Kliniczna 2009;11:31–3.

[7] Nguyen VT, Ndoye A, Shultz LD, Pittelkow MR, Grando SA. Antibodies against keratinocyte antigens other than desmogleins 1 and 3 can induce pemphigus vulgaris-like lesions. Journal of Clinical Investigation 2000;106:1467–79.

[8] Langan SM, Smeeth L, Hubbard R, Fleming KM, Smith CJP, West J. Bullous pemphigoid and pemphigus vulgaris--incidence and mortality in the UK: population based cohort study. BMJ 2008;337:a180–a180.

[9] Hashimoto T, Amagai M, Garrod DR, Nishikawa T. Immunofluorescence and immunoblot studies on the reactivity of pemphigus vulgaris and pemphigus foliaceus sera with desmoglein 3 and desmoglein 1. Epithelial Cell Biology 1995;4:63–9.

[10] Dańczak-Pazdrowska A, Bowszyc-Dmochowska M, Wolnik-Trzeciak G, Dmochowski M. IgG, IgG1 and IgG4 deposits in hair follicles in relation to IgG, IgG1 and IgG4 antibodies to desmogleins in pemphigus. Dermatologia Kliniczna 2004;6:207–13.

[11] Hallaji Z, Mortazavi H, Lajevardi V, Tamizifar B, AmirZargar A, Daneshpazhooh M, Chams-Davatchi C. Serum and salivary desmoglein 1 and 3 enzyme-linked immunosorbent assay in pemphigus vulgaris: correlation with phenotype and severity. Journal of the European Academy of Dermatology and Venereology 2010;24:275–80.

[12] Frew JW, Murrell DF. Paraneoplastic pemphigus (paraneoplastic autoimmune multiorgan syndrome): clinical presentations and pathogenesis. Dermatologic Clinics 2011;29:419–425, viii.

[13] Zillikens D, Rose PA, Balding SD, Liu Z, Olague-Marchan M, Diaz LA, Giudice GJ. Tight clustering of extracellular BP180 epitopes recognized by bullous pemphigoid autoantibodies. Journal of Investigative Dermatology 1997;109:573–9.

[14] World Health Organization.WHO Media centre. Cancer Fact sheet N°297. http://www.who.int/mediacentre/factsheets/fs297/en/ (accessed 4 September 2012)

[15] GLOBOCAN 2008. IARC: Section of Cancer Information. http://globocan.iarc.fr/factsheets/populations/factsheet.asp?uno=900 (accessed 4 September 2012)

[16] Iwashita K, Matsuyama T, Akasaka E, Mizutani K, Yamamoto K, Kondoh A, Nozawa M, Yagi Y, Ikoma N, Mabuchi T, Shinagawa H, Tamiya S, Nuruki H, Ohta Y, Umezawa Y, Ozawa A. The incidence of internal malignancies in autoimmune bullous diseases. The Tokai Journal of Experimental and Clinical Medicine 2007;32:42–7.

[17] Ogawa H, Sakuma M, Morioka S, Kitamura K, Sasai Y, Imamura S, Inaba Y. The incidence of internal malignancies in pemphigus and bullous pemphigoid in Japan. Journal of Dermatological Science 1995;9:136–41.

[18] Sigurgeirsson B, Agnarsson BA, Lindelöf B. Risk of lymphoma in patients with dermatitis herpetiformis. BMJ 1994;308:13–5.

[19] Shannon JF, Mackenzie-Wood A, Wood G, Goldstein D. Cicatricial pemphigoid in non-Hodgkin's lymphoma. Internal Medicine Journal 2003;33:396–7.

[20] Gül U, Kiliç A, Demirel O, Cakmak SK, Gönül M, Oksal A. Bullous pemphigoid associated with breast carcinoma. European Journal of Dermatology 2006;16:581–2.

[21] Budzińska A, Gornowicz J, Bowszyc-Dmochowska M, Dmochowski M. [Bullous pemphigoid developed after cessation of hormonal treatment for prostate cancer.]. Dermatologia Kliniczna 2011;13:19–22.

[22] Zhu X, Zhang B. Paraneoplastic pemphigus. Journal of Dermatology 2007;34:503–11.

[23] Lindelöf B, Islam N, Eklund G, Arfors L. Pemphigoid and cancer. Archives of Dermatology 1990;126:66–8.

[24] Grainge MJ, West J, Solaymani-Dodaran M, Card TR, Logan RFA. The long-term risk of malignancy following a diagnosis of coeliac disease or dermatitis herpetiformis: a cohort study. Alimentary Pharmacology & Therapeutics 2012;35:730–9.

[25] Viljamaa M, Kaukinen K, Pukkala E, Hervonen K, Reunala T, Collin P. Malignancies and mortality in patients with coeliac disease and dermatitis herpetiformis: 30-year population-based study. Digestive and Liver Disease 2006;38:374–80.

[26] Lewis HM, Renaula TL, Garioch JJ, Leonard JN, Fry JS, Collin P, Evans D, Fry L. Protective effect of gluten-free diet against development of lymphoma in dermatitis herpetiformis. British Journal of Dermatology 1996;135:363–7.

[27] Lynfield YL, Pertschuk LP. Pemphigus vulgaris following squamous cell carcinoma of the lung. International Journal of Dermatology 1984;23:147–8.

[28] Barnadas MA, Gelpí C, Rodríguez JL, González MJ, de Moragas JM. Pemphigus vulgaris and squamous cell carcinoma of the lung. Journal of the American Academy of Dermatology 1989;21:793–5.

[29] Lam S, Stone MS, Goeken JA, Massicotte SJ, Smith AC, Folberg R, Krachmer JH. Paraneoplastic pemphigus, cicatricial conjunctivitis, and acanthosis nigricans with pachydermatoglyphy in a patient with bronchogenic squamous cell carcinoma. Ophthalmology 1992;99:108–13.

[30] Serwin AB, Bokiniec E, Chodynicka B. Pemphigus vegetans in a patient with lung cancer. Dermatology Online Journal 2005;11:13. http://dermatology.cdlib.org/111/case_reports/pemphigus/serwin.html (accessed 29 August 2012)

[31] Bastiaens MT, Zwan NV, Verschueren GL, Stoof TJ, Nieboer C. Three cases of pemphigus vegetans: induction by enalapril--association with internal malignancy. International Journal of Dermatology 1994;33:168–71.

[32] Kubota Y, Yoshino Y, Mizoguchi M. A case of herpetiform pemphigus associated with lung cancer. Journal of Dermatology 1994;21:609–11.

[33] Petropoulou H, Politis G, Panagakis P, Hatziolou E, Aroni K, Kontochristopoulos G. Immunoglobulin A pemphigus associated with immunoglobulin A gammopathy and lung cancer. Journal of Dermatology 2008;35:341–5.

[34] Takeuchi M, Okazaki A, Nakajima N, Saito Y, Nozaki M, Niibe H. [A case of lung cancer with bullous pemphigoid]. Gan No Rinsho 1986;32:529–33.

[35] Greer KE, Beacham BE, Askew FC Jr. Benign mucous membrane pemphigoid in association with internal malignancy. Cutis 1980;25:183–5.

[36] Sato Y, Endo K, Ishikawa S, Onizuka M, Mitsui K, Mitsui T. [A case of resected lung cancer associated with bullous pemphigoid]. Nihon Kyobu Geka Gakkai Zasshi 1996;44:524–8.

[37] Urano-Suehisa S, Tagami H, Yamada M, Hishiki S, Tokura Y. Bullous pemphigoid, figurate erythema and generalized pigmentation with skin thickening in a patient with adenocarcinoma of the stomach. Dermatologica 1985;171:117–21.

[38] Chamberland M. [Paraneoplastic pemphigus and adenocarcinoma of the colon]. L'unión médicale du Canada 1993;122:201–3.

[39] Koga C, Izu K, Kabashima K, Tokura Y. Pemphigus vegetans associated with gastric cancer. Journal of the European Academy of Dermatology and Venereology 2007;21:1288–9.

[40] Ashmarin II, Burov GP, Zhgun AA. [Association of pemphigus vulgaris & cancer of the stomach]. Klinicheskaia meditsina 1959;37:142–4.

[41] Lavie CJ, Thomas MA, Fondak AA. The perioperative management of the patient with pemphigus vulgaris and villous adenoma. Cutis 1984;34:180–2.

[42] Ohkawa F, Nakada K, Umezono A, Kubokawa T. [A case of oral pemphigus vulgaris involving the esophagus combined with early gastric carcinoma]. Nippon Naika Gakkai Zasshi 1987;76:1725–9.

[43] Calzavara PG, Carlino A, Coglio G. [Pemphigus and neoplasia. 2 new clinical cases and a review of the literature]. Giornale Italiano di Dermatologia e Venereologia 1989;124:25–9.

[44] Patten SF, Valenzuela R, Dijkstra JW, Bergfeld WF, Slaughter S. Unmasking the presence of circulating pemphigus antibodies in a patient with coexistent pemphigus, SLE, multiple autoantibodies, and gastric carcinoma. International Journal of Dermatology 1993;32:890–2.

[45] Gül U, Gönül M, Soylu S, Heper AO, Demiriz M. An unusual occurrence of gastric adenocarcinoma in pemphigus vulgaris. International Journal of Dermatology 2009;48:1018–20.

[46] Taniuchi K, Takata M, Matsui C, Fushida Y, Uchiyama K, Mori T, Kawara S, Yancey KB, Takehara K. Antiepiligrin (laminin 5) cicatricial pemphigoid associated with an underlying gastric carcinoma producing laminin 5. British Journal of Dermatology 1999;140:696–700.

[47] Uchiyama K, Yamamoto Y, Taniuchi K, Matsui C, Fushida Y, Shirao Y. Remission of antiepiligrin (laminin-5) cicatricial pemphigoid after excision of gastric carcinoma. Cornea 2000;19:564–6.

[48] Fujimoto W, Ishida-Yamamoto A, Hsu R, Nagao Y, Iizuka H, Yancey KB, Arata J. Anti-epiligrin cicatricial pemphigoid: a case associated with gastric carcinoma and features resembling epidermolysis bullosa acquisita. British Journal of Dermatology 1998;139:682–7.

[49] Askling J, Linet M, Gridley G, Halstensen TS, Ekström K, Ekbom A. Cancer incidence in a population-based cohort of individuals hospitalized with celiac disease or dermatitis herpetiformis. Gastroenterology 2002;123:1428–35.

[50] Murphy J, Smith J, Cosgrave P, Doyle JS. A case of dermatitis herpetiformis and chronic lymphatic leukaemia. Irish Journal of Medical Science 1982;151:50.

[51] Coricciati L. [Duhring's dermatitis herpetiformis and chronic lymphatic leukemia]. Minerva Dermatologica 1960;35:285–8.

[52] van Mook WNK, Fickers MM, Theunissen PH, van der Kley JA, Duijvestijn JA, Pas HH, Flikweert DC. Paraneoplastic pemphigus as the initial presentation of chronic lymphocytic leukemia. Annals of Oncology 2001;12:115–8.

[53] Kaplan I, Hodak E, Ackerman L, Mimouni D, Anhalt GJ, Calderon S. Neoplasms associated with paraneoplastic pemphigus: a review with emphasis on non-hematologic malignancy and oral mucosal manifestations. Oral Oncology 2004;40:553–62.

[54] Davis AK, Cole-Sinclair M, Russell P. Anaplastic large cell lymphoma presenting with paraneoplastic pemphigus. Journal of Clinical Pathology 2007;60:108–10.

[55] Seth RK, Su GW, Pflugfelder SC. Mucous membrane pemphigoid in a patient with chronic lymphocytic leukemia. Cornea 2004;23:740–3.

[56] Takahara M, Tsuji G, Ishii N, Dainichi T, Hashimoto T, Kohno K, Kamezaki K, Nagafuji K, Takeuchi S, Moroi Y, Furue M. Mucous membrane pemphigoid with antibodies to the beta(3) subunit of Laminin 332 in a patient with acute myeloblastic leukemia and graft-versus-host disease. Dermatology 2009;219:361–4.

[57] Masunaga K, Toyoda M, Kokuba H, Takahara M, Ohyama B, Hashimoto T, Furue M. Mucous membrane pemphigoid with antibodies to the β3 subunit of laminin 332. Journal of Dermatology 2011;38:1082–4.

[58] Misery L, Cambazard F, Rimokh R, Ghohestani R, Magaud JP, Gaudillere A, Perrot JL, Berard F, Claudy A, Guyotat D, Schmitt D, Vincent C. Bullous pemphigoid associated with chronic B-cell lymphatic leukaemia: the anti-230-kDa autoantibody is not synthesized by leukaemic cells. British Journal of Dermatology 1999;141:155–7.

[59] Yoshida M, Miyoshi T, Sakiyama S, Kondo K, Tangoku A. Pemphigus with thymoma improved by thymectomy: report of a case. Surgery Today 2012. [Epub ahead of print] http://www.springerlink.com/content/q51804n79416823w/fulltext.pdf (accessed 27 August 2012)

[60] Lutowiecka-Wranicz A, Sysa-Jedrzejowska A, Bartkowiak B, Waszczykowska E, Chorzelski T. [Pemphigus foliaceus preceded by pemphigoid in a patient with thymoma: coincidence or pathogenetic relationship?]. Przegląd Dermatologiczny 1987;74:460–2.

[61] Takeshita K, Amano M, Shimizu T, Oyamada Y, Abiko T, Kobayashi K, Futei Y, Amagai M, Kuramochi S, Asano K, Yamaguchi K. Thymoma with pemphigus foliaceus. Internal Medicine 2000;39:742–7.

[62] James WD. Bullous pemphigoid, myasthenia gravis, and thymoma. Archives of Dermatology 1984;120:397.

[63] Sabet HY, Davis JL, Rogers RS 3rd. Mucous membrane pemphigoid, thymoma, and myasthenia gravis. International Journal of Dermatology 2000;39:701–4.

[64] Ostlere LS, Branfoot AC, Staughton RC. Cicatricial pemphigoid and carcinoma of the pancreas. Clinical and Experimental Dermatology 1992;17:67–8.

[65] Demitsu T, Yoneda K, Iida E, Sasaki K, Umemoto N, Kakurai M, Wakatabi K, Yamada T, Ohyama B, Hashimoto T. A case of mucous membrane pemphigoid with IgG antibodies against all the alpha3, beta3 and gamma2 subunits of laminin-332 and BP180 C-terminal domain, associated with pancreatic cancer. Clinical and Experimental Dermatology 2009;34:e992–994.

[66] Matz H, Milner Y, Frusic-Zlotkin M, Brenner S. Paraneoplastic pemphigus associated with pancreatic carcinoma. Acta Dermato-Venereologica 1997;77:289–91.

[67] Van Poppel H, Aswarie H, Baert L. Bullous pemphigoid associated with renal carcinoma. British Journal of Urology 1988;61:361.

[68] Blum A, Wehner-Caroli J, Scherwitz C, Rassner G. [Bullous pemphigoid as a paraneoplastic syndrome. A case report in renal-cell carcinoma]. Hautarzt 1997;48:834–7.

[69] Rub R, Avidor Y, Messer G, Schreiber L. Bullous pemphigoid as an initial presentation of renal oncocytoma. Dermatology 1999;198:322–3.

[70] Klein T, Rotterdam S, Noldus J, Hinkel A. Bullous pemphigoid is a rare paraneoplastic syndrome in patients with renal cell carcinoma. Scandinavian Journal of Urology and Nephrology 2009;43:334–6.

[71] Saravanan K, Baer ST, Meredith A, Dyson A, von der Werth J. Benign mucous membrane pemphigoid of the upper aero-digestive tract: rare paraneoplastic syndrome presentation in renal cell carcinoma. The Journal of Laryngology & Otology 2006;120:237–9.

[72] Aessopos A, Grapsa A, Farmakis D, Sideris P, Politou M, Paikos S, Aroni K. Oral paraneoplastic pemphigus associated with renal malignancy. Acta Dermato-Venereologica 2003;83:72–3.

[73] Bowman PH, Hogan DJ. Pemphigus foliaceus and renal cell carcinoma. Cutis 1999;63:271–4.

[74] Dahl MV, Ristow S. Bullous pemphigoid and ovarian cystadenocarcinoma. Immunologic studies. Archives of Dermatology 1978;114:903–5.

[75] Mitsuya J, Hara H, Ito K, Ishii N, Hashimoto T, Terui T. Metastatic ovarian carcinoma-associated subepidermal blistering disease with autoantibodies to both the p200 dermal antigen and the gamma 2 subunit of laminin 5 showing unusual clinical features. British Journal of Dermatology 2008;158:1354–7.

[76] Shibuya T, Komatsu S, Takahashi I, Honma M, Takahashi H, Ishida-Yamamoto A, Kamiya T, Fukuda S, Hashimoto T, Iizuka H. Mucous membrane pemphigoid accompanied by ovarian cancer: A case with autoantibodies solely against $\gamma(2)$ -subunit of laminin-332. The Journal of Dermatology 2012. [Epub ahead of print] http://onlinelibrary.wiley.com/doi/10.1111/j.1346-8138.2011.01482.x/pdf (accessed 4 September 2012)

[77] Mignogna MD, Fortuna G, Leuci S, Adamo D, Ruoppo E. Metastatic prostate cancer presenting as paraneoplastic pemphigus: a favourable clinical response to combined androgen blockade and conventional immunosuppressive therapy. British Journal of Dermatology 2009;160:468–70.

[78] Marzano AV, Tourlaki A, Cozzani E, Gianotti R, Caputo R. Pemphigus herpetiformis associated with prostate cancer. Journal of the European Academy of Dermatology and Venereology 2007;21:696–8.

[79] Ota M, Sato-Matsumura KC, Matsumura T, Tsuji Y, Ohkawara A. Pemphigus foliaceus and figurate erythema in a patient with prostate cancer. British Journal of Dermatology 2000;142:816–8.

[80] Young AL, Bailey EE, Colaço SM, Engler DE, Grossman ME. Anti-laminin-332 mucous membrane pemphigoid associated with recurrent metastatic prostate carcinoma: hypothesis for a paraneoplastic phenomenon. European Journal of Dermatology 2011;21:401–4.

[81] Knoell KA, Patterson JW, Gampper TJ, Hendrix JD Jr. Localized bullous pemphigoid following radiotherapy for breast carcinoma. Archives of Dermatology 1998;134:514–5.

[82] Iuliano L, Micheletta F, Natoli S. Bullous pemphigoid: an unusual and insidious presentation of breast cancer. Clinical Oncology 2003;15:505.

[83] Cabrera-Rodríguez JJ, Muñoz-García JL, Quirós Rivero J, Ropero Carmona F, Ríos Kavadoy Y. Radio-induced bullous pemphigoid. Clinical and Translational Oncology 2010;12:66–8.

[84] Isohashi F, Konishi K, Umegaki N, Tanei T, Koizumi M, Yoshioka Y. A case of bullous pemphigoid exacerbated by irradiation after breast conservative radiotherapy. Japanese Journal of Clinical Oncology 2011;41:811–3.

[85] Olsha O, Lijoretzky G, Grenader T. Bullous pemphigoid following adjuvant radiotherapy for breast cancer. Breast Journal 2011;17:204–5.

[86] Shirahama S, Furukawa F, Takigawa M. Recurrent pemphigus vulgaris limited to the surgical area after mastectomy. Journal of the American Academy of Dermatology 1998;39:352–5.

[87] Jacobs R, Eng AM, Solomon LM. Carcinoma of the breast, pemphigus vulgaris and gyrate erythema. International Journal of Dermatology 1978;17:221–4.

[88] Guerder S, Viret C, Luche H, Ardouin L, Malissen B. Differential processing of self-antigens by subsets of thymic stromal cells. Current Opinion in Immunology 2012;24:99–104.

[89] Anderson MS, Su MA. Aire and T cell development. Current Opinion in Immunology 2011;23:198–206.

[90] Maverakis E, Goodarzi H, Wehrli LN, Ono Y, Garcia MS. The etiology of paraneoplastic autoimmunity. Clinical Reviews in Allergy and Immunology 2012;42:135–44.

[91] Nikolskaia OV, Nousari CH, Anhalt GJ. Paraneoplastic pemphigus in association with Castleman's disease. British Journal of Dermatology 2003;149:1143–51.

[92] Mimouni D, Anhalt GJ, Lazarova Z, Aho S, Kazerounian S, Kouba DJ, Mascaro JM Jr, Nousari HC. Paraneoplastic pemphigus in children and adolescents. British Journal of Dermatology 2002;147:725–32.

[93] Kim WY, Kim H, Jeon YK, Kim C-W. Follicular dendritic cell sarcoma with immature T-cell proliferation. Human Pathology 2010;41:129–33.

[94] Harding FA, McArthur JG, Gross JA, Raulet DH, Allison JP. CD28-mediated signalling co-stimulates murine T cells and prevents induction of anergy in T-cell clones. Nature 1992;356:607–9.

[95] Rau FC, Dieter J, Luo Z, Priest SO, Baumgarth N. B7-1/2 (CD80/CD86) direct signaling to B cells enhances IgG secretion. The Journal of Immunology 2009;183:7661–71.

[96] Thompson ED, Enriquez HL, Fu Y-X, Engelhard VH. Tumor masses support naive T cell infiltration, activation, and differentiation into effectors. The Journal of Experimental Medicine 2010;207:1791–804.

[97] Ramsay AG, Johnson AJ, Lee AM, Gorgün G, Le Dieu R, Blum W, Byrd JC, Gribben JG. Chronic lymphocytic leukemia T cells show impaired immunological synapse formation that can be reversed with an immunomodulating drug. Journal of Clinical Investigation 2008;118:2427–37.

[98] Görgün G, Holderried TAW, Zahrieh D, Neuberg D, Gribben JG. Chronic lymphocytic leukemia cells induce changes in gene expression of CD4 and CD8 T cells. Journal of Clinical Investigation 2005;115:1797–805.

[99] Tarasenko T, Dean JA, Bolland S. FcγRIIB as a modulator of autoimmune disease susceptibility. Autoimmunity 2007;40:409–17.

[100] Guilabert A, Lozano F, Iranzo P, Suárez-Casasús B, Martinez-De Pablo I, Julià M, Mascaró Jr. JM. A case of aggressive bullous pemphigoid associated with the defective functional variant of Fc gamma receptor IIb: Implications for pathogenesis? Journal of the American Academy of Dermatology 2011;65:1062–3.

[101] Clynes RA, Towers TL, Presta LG, Ravetch JV. Inhibitory Fc receptors modulate in vivo cytotoxicity against tumor targets. Nature Medicine 2000;6:443–6.

[102] Shan D, Ledbetter JA, Press OW. Apoptosis of malignant human B cells by ligation of CD20 with monoclonal antibodies. Blood 1998;91:1644–52.

[103] Ahmed AR, Park MS, Tiwari JL, Terasaki PI. Association of DR4 with pemphigus. Experimental and Clinical Immunogenetics 1987;4:8–16.

[104] Sinha AA, Brautbar C, Szafer F, Friedmann A, Tzfoni E, Todd JA, Steinman L, McDevitt HO. A newly characterized HLA DQ beta allele associated with pemphigus vulgaris. Science 1988;239:1026–9.

[105] Riechers R, Grötzinger J, Hertl M. HLA class II restriction of autoreactive T cell responses in pemphigus vulgaris: review of the literature and potential applications for the development of a specific immunotherapy. Autoimmunity 1999;30:183–96.

[106] Tron F, Gilbert D, Mouquet H, Joly P, Drouot L, Makni S, Masmoudi H, Charron D, Zitouni M, Loiseau P, Ben Ayed M. Genetic factors in pemphigus. J. Autoimmun. 2005;24:319–28.

[107] Gazit E, Loewenthal R. The immunogenetics of pemphigus vulgaris. Autoimmunity Reviews 2005;4:16–20.

[108] Lee E, Lendas KA, Chow S, Pirani Y, Gordon D, Dionisio R, Nguyen D, Spizuoco A, Fotino M, Zhang Y, Sinha AA. Disease relevant HLA class II alleles isolated by genotypic, haplotypic, and sequence analysis in North American Caucasians with pemphigus vulgaris. Human Immunology 2006;67:125–39.

[109] Shams S, Amirzargar AA, Yousefi M, Rezaei N, Solgi G, Khosravi F, Ansaripour B, Moradi B, Nikbin B. HLA class II (DRB, DQA1 and DQB1) allele and haplotype frequencies in the patients with pemphigus vulgaris. Journal of Clinical Immunology 2009;29:175–9.

[110] Hertl M, Eming R, Veldman C. T cell control in autoimmune bullous skin disorders. Journal of Clinical Investigation 2006;116:1159–66.

[111] Drouet M, Delpuget-Bertin N, Vaillant L, Chauchaix S, Boulanger MD, Bonnetblanc JM, Bernard P. HLA-DRB1 and HLA-DQB1 genes in susceptibility and resistance to cicatricial pemphigoid in French Caucasians. European Journal of Dermatology 1998;8:330–3.

[112] Carrozzo M, Fasano ME, Broccoletti R, Carbone M, Cozzani E, Rendine S, Roggero S, Parodi A, Gandolfo S. HLA-DQB1 alleles in Italian patients with mucous membrane pemphigoid predominantly affecting the oral cavity. British Journal of Dermatology 2001;145:805–8.

[113] Chen Y, Hu J, Liu C, Yang L, Qi Y, Li W, Yin L, Li H, Jiang J, Liang W, Li F. [Correlation between HLA-DRB1*0901 and 1501, HLA-DQB1*0301 and 0602 alleles and esophageal squamous cell carcinoma of Kazakh in Xinjiang, China]. Zhonghua Bing Li Xue Za Zhi 2009;38:816–9.

[114] Mostafa MI, Zarouk WA, El-Kamah GY. Class II alleles HLA-DQB1* 0301 among a seven-membered Egyptian family of a child with oral pemphigoid. Bratislavské lekárske listy 2011;112:591–4.

[115] Wu M-S, Hsieh R-P, Huang S-P, Chang Y-T, Lin M-T, Chang M-C, Shun C-T, Sheu J-C, Lin J-T. Association of HLA-DQB1*0301 and HLA-DQB1*0602 with different subtypes of gastric cancer in Taiwan. Japanese Journal of Cancer Research 2002;93:404–10.

[116] Lie AK, Skarsvåg S, Haugen OA, Skjeldestad FE, Olsen AO, Skovlund E, Rønningen KS. Association between the HLA DQB1*0301 gene and human papillomavirus infec-

tion in high-grade cervical intraepithelial neoplasia. International Journal of Gynecological Pathology 1999;18:206–10.

[117] Setterfield J, Theron J, Vaughan RW, Welsh KI, Mallon E, Wojnarowska F, Challacombe SJ, Black MM. Mucous membrane pemphigoid: HLA-DQB1*0301 is associated with all clinical sites of involvement and may be linked to antibasement membrane IgG production. British Journal of Dermatology 2001;145:406–14.

[118] Rico MJ, Benning C, Weingart ES, Streilein RD, Hall RP 3rd. Characterization of skin cytokines in bullous pemphigoid and pemphigus vulgaris. British Journal of Dermatology 1999;140:1079–86.

[119] Satyam A, Khandpur S, Sharma VK, Sharma A. Involvement of T(H)1/T(H)2 cytokines in the pathogenesis of autoimmune skin disease-Pemphigus vulgaris. Immunological Investigations 2009;38:498–509.

[120] D'Auria L, Cordiali Fei P, Ameglio F. Cytokines and bullous pemphigoid. European Cytokine Network 1999;10:123–34.

[121] Lee YS, Choi I, Ning Y, Kim NY, Khatchadourian V, Yang D, Chung HK, Choi D, LaBonte MJ, Ladner RD, Nagulapalli Venkata KC, Rosenberg DO, Petasis NA, Lenz H-J, Hong Y-K. Interleukin-8 and its receptor CXCR2 in the tumour microenvironment promote colon cancer growth, progression and metastasis. British Journal of Cancer 2012;106:1833–41.

[122] Kuai W-X, Wang Q, Yang X-Z, Zhao Y, Yu R, Tang X-J. Interleukin-8 associates with adhesion, migration, invasion and chemosensitivity of human gastric cancer cells. World Journal of Gastroenterology 2012;18:979–85.

[123] Hahne M, Kataoka T, Schröter M, Hofmann K, Irmler M, Bodmer JL, Schneider P, Bornand T, Holler N, French LE, Sordat B, Rimoldi D, Tschopp J. APRIL, a new ligand of the tumor necrosis factor family, stimulates tumor cell growth. The Journal of Experimental Medicine 1998;188:1185–90.

[124] Rennert P, Schneider P, Cachero TG, Thompson J, Trabach L, Hertig S, Holler N, Qian F, Mullen C, Strauch K, Browning JL, Ambrose C, Tschopp J. A soluble form of B cell maturation antigen, a receptor for the tumor necrosis factor family member APRIL, inhibits tumor cell growth. The Journal of Experimental Medicine 2000;192:1677–84.

[125] Rickert RC, Jellusova J, Miletic AV. Signaling by the tumor necrosis factor receptor superfamily in B-cell biology and disease. Immunological Reviews 2011;244:115–33.

[126] Asashima N, Fujimoto M, Watanabe R, Nakashima H, Yazawa N, Okochi H, Tamaki K. Serum levels of BAFF are increased in bullous pemphigoid but not in pemphigus vulgaris. British Journal of Dermatology 2006;155:330–6.

[127] Daneshpazhooh M, Chams-Davatchi C, Payandemehr P, Nassiri S, Valikhani M, Safai-Naraghi Z. Spectrum of autoimmune bullous diseases in Iran: a 10-year review. International Journal of Dermatology 2012;51:35–41.

[128] González DA, Díaz BB, Rodríguez Pérez M del C, Hernández AG, Chico BND, de León AC. Sex hormones and autoimmunity. Immunology Letters 2010;133:6–13.

[129] Klibson SK, Severovostokova VI, Shpanskaia LS. [The hormonal profile of patients with pemphigus and bullous pemphigoid]. Vestnik Dermatologii i Venerologii 1989:37–41.

[130] Brenner S, Wohl Y. A survey of sex differences in 249 pemphigus patients and possible explanations. Skinmed 2007;6:163–5.

[131] Shapiro S. Recent epidemiological evidence relevant to the clinical management of the menopause. Climacteric 2007;10 Suppl 2:2–15.

[132] Grulich AE, Vajdic CM, Cozen W. Altered immunity as a risk factor for non-Hodgkin lymphoma. Cancer Epidemiology, Biomarkers & Prevention 2007;16:405–8.

[133] Dar SA, Das S, Bhattacharya SN, Ramachandran VG, Ahmed T, Banerjee BD, Sonthalia S, Sood V, Banerjea AC. Possible role of superantigens in inducing autoimmunity in pemphigus patients. Journal of Dermatology 2011;38:980–7.

[134] Delogu LG, Deidda S, Delitala G, Manetti R. Infectious diseases and autoimmunity. Journal of Infection in Developing Countries 2011;5:679–87.

[135] Sagi L, Baum S, Agmon-Levin N, Sherer Y, Katz BSP, Barzilai O, Ram M, Bizzaro N, SanMarco M, Trau H, Shoenfeld Y. Autoimmune bullous diseases the spectrum of infectious agent antibodies and review of the literature. Autoimmunity Reviews 2011;10:527–35.

[136] Tufano MA, Baroni A, Buommino E, Ruocco E, Lombardi ML, Ruocco V. Detection of herpesvirus DNA in peripheral blood mononuclear cells and skin lesions of patients with pemphigus by polymerase chain reaction. British Journal of Dermatology 1999;141:1033–9.

[137] Wang G-Q, Xu H, Wang Y-K, Gao X-H, Zhao Y, He C, Inoue N, Chen H-D. Higher prevalence of human herpesvirus 8 DNA sequence and specific IgG antibodies in patients with pemphigus in China. Journal of the American Academy of Dermatology 2005;52:460–7.

[138] Jang HS, Oh CK, Lim JY, Jun ES, Kim YS, Kwon KS. Detection of human herpesvirus 8 DNA in pemphigus and chronic blistering skin diseases. Journal of Korean Medical Science 2000;15:442–8.

[139] Berkun Y, Mimouni D, Shoenfeld Y. Pemphigus following hepatitis B vaccination--coincidence or causality? Autoimmunity 2005;38:117–9.

[140] Marfatia YS, Patel S, Makrandi S, Sharma P. Human immunodeficiency virus and pemphigus vulgaris: an interesting association. Indian Journal of Dermatology, Venereology and Leprology 2007;73:354–5.

[141] Ruocco E, Lo Schiavo A, Baroni A, Sangiuliano S, Puca RV, Brunetti G, Ruocco V. Pemphigus vulgaris after coxsackievirus infection and cephalosporin treatment: a paraviral eruption? Dermatology 2008;216:317–9.

[142] Blazsek A, Sillo P, Ishii N, Gergely P Jr, Poor G, Preisz K, Hashimoto T, Medvecz M, Kárpáti S. Searching for foreign antigens as possible triggering factors of autoimmunity: Torque Teno virus DNA prevalence is elevated in sera of patients with bullous pemphigoid. Experimental Dermatology 2008;17:446–54.

[143] Lin S-S, Wang K-H, Yeh S-W, Chen WY, Tsai T-H. Simultaneous occurrence of pemphigus foliaceus and bullous pemphigoid with concomitant herpesvirus infection. Clinical and Experimental Dermatology 2009;34:537–9.

[144] Hoffman LJ, Bunker CH, Pellett PE, Trump DL, Patrick AL, Dollard SC, Keenan HA, Jenkins FJ. Elevated seroprevalence of human herpesvirus 8 among men with prostate cancer. Journal of Infectious Diseases 2004;189:15–20.

[145] Korodi Z, Wang X, Tedeschi R, Knekt P, Dillner J. No serological evidence of association between prostate cancer and infection with herpes simplex virus type 2 or human herpesvirus type 8: a nested case-control study. Journal of Infectious Diseases 2005;191:2008–11.

[146] Sutcliffe S, Giovannucci E, Gaydos CA, Viscidi RP, Jenkins FJ, Zenilman JM, Jacobson LP, De Marzo AM, Willett WC, Platz EA. Plasma antibodies against Chlamydia trachomatis, human papillomavirus, and human herpesvirus type 8 in relation to prostate cancer: a prospective study. Cancer Epidemiology, Biomarkers & Prevention 2007;16:1573–80.

[147] Lin Y, Mao Q, Zheng X, Yang K, Chen H, Zhou C, Xie L. Human papillomavirus 16 or 18 infection and prostate cancer risk: a meta-analysis. Irish Journal of Medical Science 2011;180:497–503.

[148] Hrbacek J, Urban M, Hamsikova E, Tachezy R, Eis V, Brabec M, Heracek J. Serum antibodies against genitourinary infectious agents in prostate cancer and benign prostate hyperplasia patients: a case-control study. BMC Cancer 2011;11:53.

[149] Klochkova TG, Evtushenko VI. [Role of human cytomegalovirus in the pathogenesis, growth and aggressiveness of prostate cancer]. Voprosy Onkologii 2012;58:33–40.

[150] Siguier M, Sellier P, Bergmann J-F. BK-virus infections: a literature review. Médecine et Maladies Infectieuses 2012;42:181–7.

[151] Groom HCT, Warren AY, Neal DE, Bishop KN. No evidence for infection of UK prostate cancer patients with XMRV, BK virus, Trichomonas vaginalis or human papilloma viruses. PLoS ONE 2012;7:e34221.

[152] Huo Q, Zhang N, Yang Q. Epstein-Barr virus infection and sporadic breast cancer risk: a meta-analysis. PLoS ONE 2012;7:e31656.

[153] Sugi T, Hashimoto T, Hibi T, Nishikawa T. Production of human monoclonal anti-basement membrane zone (BMZ) antibodies from a patient with bullous pemphigoid (BP) by Epstein-Barr virus transformation. Analyses of the heterogeneity of anti-BMZ antibodies in BP sera using them. Journal of Clinical Investigation 1989;84:1050–5.

[154] Pender MP. CD8+ T-Cell Deficiency, Epstein-Barr Virus Infection, Vitamin D Deficiency, and Steps to Autoimmunity: A Unifying Hypothesis. Autoimmune Diseases 2012;2012:189096.

[155] Evangelista F, Dasher DA, Diaz LA, Prisayanh PS, Li N. E-cadherin is an additional immunological target for pemphigus autoantibodies. Journal of Investigative Dermatology 2008;128:1710–8.

[156] Disis ML, Goodell V, Schiffman K, Knutson KL. Humoral epitope-spreading following immunization with a HER-2/neu peptide based vaccine in cancer patients. Journal of Clinical Immunology 2004;24:571–8.

[157] Fujinami RS, von Herrath MG, Christen U, Whitton JL. Molecular mimicry, bystander activation, or viral persistence: infections and autoimmune disease. Clinical Microbiology Reviews 2006;19:80–94.

[158] Lehmann PV, Forsthuber T, Miller A, Sercarz EE. Spreading of T-cell autoimmunity to cryptic determinants of an autoantigen. Nature 1992;358:155–7.

[159] Cooper GM. Oncogenes. 2nd ed. Boston: Jones and Bartlett Publishers;1995.

[160] Sitaru C. Autoimmune blistering diseases associated with neoplasia. Symposium of The Romanian Society of Dermatopathology, 29-31 October 2009, Timisoara, Romania. http://www.srdpat.ro/symposiums/second/summaries (accessed 2 September 2012)

[161] Beaudry VG, Jiang D, Dusek RL, Park EJ, Knezevich S, Ridd K, Vogel H, Bastian BC, Attardi LD. Loss of the p53/p63 Regulated Desmosomal Protein Perp Promotes Tumorigenesis. PLoS Genetics 2010;6.

[162] Yashiro M, Nishioka N, Hirakawa K. Decreased expression of the adhesion molecule desmoglein-2 is associated with diffuse-type gastric carcinoma. European Journal of Cancer 2006;42:2397–403.

[163] Chen Y-J, Chang JT, Lee L, Wang H-M, Liao C-T, Chiu C-C, Chen P-J, Cheng A-J. DSG3 is overexpressed in head neck cancer and is a potential molecular target for inhibition of oncogenesis. Oncogene 2007;26:467–76.

[164] Cui T, Chen Y, Yang L, Knösel T, Zöller K, Huber O, Petersen I. DSC3 expression is regulated by p53, and methylation of DSC3 DNA is a prognostic marker in human colorectal cancer. British Journal of Cancer 2011;104:1013–9.

[165] Attardi LD, Reczek EE, Cosmas C, Demicco EG, McCurrach ME, Lowe SW, Jacks T. PERP, an apoptosis-associated target of p53, is a novel member of the PMP-22/gas3 family. Genes & Development 2000;14:704–18.

[166] Grando SA. Pemphigus autoimmunity: hypotheses and realities. Autoimmunity 2012;45:7–35.

[167] Ihrie RA, Attardi LD. A new Perp in the lineup: linking p63 and desmosomal adhesion. Cell Cycle 2005;4:873–6.

[168] Ihrie RA, Marques MR, Nguyen BT, Horner JS, Papazoglu C, Bronson RT, Mills AA, Attardi LD. Perp is a p63-regulated gene essential for epithelial integrity. Cell 2005;120:843–56.

[169] Klus GT, Rokaeus N, Bittner ML, Chen Y, Korz DM, Sukumar S, Schick A, Szallasi Z. Down-regulation of the desmosomal cadherin desmocollin 3 in human breast cancer. International Journal of Oncology 2001;19:169–74.

[170] Gornowicz-Porowska J, Bowszyc-Dmochowska M, Seraszek-Jaros A, Kaczmarek E, Dmochowski M. Loss of correlation between intensities of desmoglein 2 and desmoglein 3 expression in basal cell carcinomas. Acta Dermatovenerologica Croatica 2011;19:150–5.

[171] Tsang SM, Liu L, Teh M-T, Wheeler A, Grose R, Hart IR, Garrod DR, Fortune F, Wan H. Desmoglein 3, via an interaction with E-cadherin, is associated with activation of Src. PLoS ONE 2010;5:e14211.

[172] Hoshino R, Chatani Y, Yamori T, Tsuruo T, Oka H, Yoshida O, Shimada Y, Ari-i S, Wada H, Fujimoto J, Kohno M. Constitutive activation of the 41-/43-kDa mitogen-activated protein kinase signaling pathway in human tumors. Oncogene 1999;18:813–22.

[173] Teh M-T, Parkinson EK, Thurlow JK, Liu F, Fortune F, Wan H. A molecular study of desmosomes identifies a desmoglein isoform switch in head and neck squamous cell carcinoma. Journal of Oral Pathology & Medicine 2011;40:67–76.

[174] Khan K, Hardy R, Haq A, Ogunbiyi O, Morton D, Chidgey M. Desmocollin switching in colorectal cancer. British Journal of Cancer 2006;95:1367–70.

[175] Parikka M, Kainulainen T, Tasanen K, Väänänen A, Bruckner-Tuderman L, Salo T. Alterations of collagen XVII expression during transformation of oral epithelium to dysplasia and carcinoma. Journal of Histochemistry & Cytochemistry 2003;51:921–9.

[176] Lo AK, Yuen PW, Liu Y, Wang XH, Cheung AL, Wong YC, Tsao SW. Downregulation of hemidesmosomal proteins in nasopharyngeal carcinoma cells. Cancer Letters 2001;163:117–23.

[177] Yamada T, Endo R, Tsukagoshi K, Fujita S, Honda K, Kinoshita M, Hasebe T, Hirohashi S. Aberrant expression of a hemidesmosomal protein, bullous pemphigoid an-

tigen 2, in human squamous cell carcinoma. Laboratory Investigation 1996;75:589–600.

[178] Parikka M, Kainulainen T, Tasanen K, Bruckner-Tuderman L, Salo T. Altered expression of collagen XVII in ameloblastomas and basal cell carcinomas. Journal of Oral Pathology & Medicine 2001;30:589–95.

[179] Bergstraesser LM, Srinivasan G, Jones JC, Stahl S, Weitzman SA. Expression of hemidesmosomes and component proteins is lost by invasive breast cancer cells. American Journal of Pathology 1995;147:1823–39.

[180] Nagle RB, Hao J, Knox JD, Dalkin BL, Clark V, Cress AE. Expression of hemidesmosomal and extracellular matrix proteins by normal and malignant human prostate tissue. American Journal of Pathology 1995;146:1498–507.

[181] Herold-Mende C, Kartenbeck J, Tomakidi P, Bosch FX. Metastatic growth of squamous cell carcinomas is correlated with upregulation and redistribution of hemidesmosomal components. Cell and Tissue Research 2001;306:399–408.

[182] Blumberg PM. In vitro studies on the mode of action of the phorbol esters, potent tumor promoters: part 1. Critical Reviews in Toxicology 1980;8:153–97.

[183] Olsen J, Lefebvre O, Fritsch C, Troelsen JT, Orian-Rousseau V, Kedinger M, Simon-Assmann P. Involvement of activator protein 1 complexes in the epithelium-specific activation of the laminin gamma2-chain gene promoter by hepatocyte growth factor (scatter factor). Biochemical Journal 2000;347:407–17.

[184] Fairley JA, Heintz PW, Neuburg M, Diaz LA, Giudice GJ. Expression pattern of the bullous pemphigoid-180 antigen in normal and neoplastic epithelia. British Journal of Dermatology 1995;133:385–91.

[185] Yanagi T, Kato N, Yamane N, Osawa R. Bullous pemphigoid associated with dermatomyositis and colon carcinoma. Clinical and Experimental Dermatology 2007;32:291–4.

[186] Stelkovics E, Korom I, Marczinovits I, Molnar J, Rasky K, Raso E, Ficsor L, Molnar B, Kopper L, Krenacs T. Collagen XVII/BP180 protein expression in squamous cell carcinoma of the skin detected with novel monoclonal antibodies in archived tissues using tissue microarrays and digital microscopy. Applied Immunohistochemistry and Molecular Morphology 2008;16:433–41.

[187] Kariya Y, Kariya Y, Gu J. Roles of laminin-332 and alpha6beta4 integrin in tumor progression. Mini-Reviews in Medicinal Chemistry 2009;9:1284–91.

[188] Marinkovich MP. Tumour microenvironment: laminin 332 in squamous-cell carcinoma. Nature Reviews Cancer 2007;7:370–80.

[189] Chruśliński A, Niśkiewicz I, Puchała A, Zajkowska M, Budzińska A, Bowszyc-Dmochowska M, Stryczyńska G, Adamiak E, Bajon T, Bręborowicz J, Gornowicz J, Dmo-

chowski M. [Mucocutaneous pemphigus vulgaris in a patient with oral squamous cell carcinoma treated with radiotherapy]. Dermatologia Kliniczna 2009;11:37–41.

[190] [190]Dmochowski M. [Body orifices and mucous membranes in pemphigus vulgaris]. Dermatologia Kliniczna 2007;9:124–31.

[191] Dmochowski M, Fuksiewicz W, Turczuk-Bierła I, Bowszyc-Dmochowska M. A case of trauma-induced and paraneoplastic bullous pemphigoid. Dermatologia Kliniczna 2008;10:45–6.

[192] Cecchi R, Paoli S, Giomi A. Peristomal bullous pemphigoid. Journal of the European Academy of Dermatology and Venereology 2004;18:515–6.

[193] Vande Maele DM, Reilly JC. Bullous pemphigoid at colostomy site: report of a case. Diseases of the Colon & Rectum 1997;40:370–1.

[194] Chapireau D, Adlam D, Cameron M, Thompson M. Paraneoplastic syndromes in patients with primary oral cancers: a systematic review. British Journal of Oral and Maxillofacial Surgery 2010;48:338–44.

[195] Palleschi GM, Giomi B. Herpetiformis pemphigus and lung carcinoma: a case of paraneoplastic pemphigus. Acta Dermato-Venereologica 2002;82:304–5.

[196] Carr NJ, Finch J, Ilesley IC, Chandrakumaran K, Mohamed F, Mirnezami A, Cecil T, Moran B. Pathology and prognosis in pseudomyxoma peritonei: a review of 274 cases. Journal of Clinical Pathology 2012. [Epub ahead of print] http://jcp.bmj.com/content/early/2012/06/19/jclinpath-2012-200843.full.pdf (accesed 2 September 2012)

[197] Semino-Mora C, Liu H, McAvoy T, Nieroda C, Studeman K, Sardi A, Dubois A. Pseudomyxoma peritonei: is disease progression related to microbial agents? A study of bacteria, MUC2 AND MUC5AC expression in disseminated peritoneal adenomucinosis and peritoneal mucinous carcinomatosis. Annals of Surgical Oncology 2008;15:1414–23.

[198] Gatalica Z, Foster JM, Loggie BW. Low grade peritoneal mucinous carcinomatosis associated with human papilloma virus infection: case report. Croatian Medical Journal 2008;49:669–73.

[199] Pavai S, Yap SF. The clinical significance of elevated levels of serum CA 19-9. Medical Journal of Malaysia 2003;58:667–72.

[200] Pietkiewicz P, Gornowicz-Porowska J, Bowszyc-Dmochowska M, Dmochowski M. The chancre of pemphigus on the scalp as the first symptom of mucosal-dominant pemphigus vulgaris in a elderly man taking ramipril. Dermatologia Kliniczna 2011;13:235–8.

[201] Inaoki M, Kaji K, Furuse S, Fujimoto A, Komatsu N, Takata M, Takehara K. Pemphigus foliaceus developing after metastasis of cutaneous squamous cell carcinoma to

regional lymph nodes. Journal of the American Academy of Dermatology 2001;45:767–70.

[202] Krunic AL, Garrod DR, Madani S, Buchanan MD, Clark RE. Immunohistochemical staining for desmogleins 1 and 2 in keratinocytic neoplasms with squamous phenotype: actinic keratosis, keratoacanthoma and squamous cell carcinoma of the skin. British Journal of Cancer 1998;77:1275–9.

[203] Nishimura E, Matsunaga M, Yoshida T, Shirota K, Higa K. [Recurrence of bullous pemphigoid after surgery: report of a case]. The Japanese Journal of Anesthesiology 2001;50:416–8.

[204] Neville JA, Yosipovitch G. Flare of bullous pemphigoid in surgically treated skin. Cutis 2005;75:169–70.

[205] Aho S, Uitto J. 180-kD bullous pemphigoid antigen/type XVII collagen: tissue-specific expression and molecular interactions with keratin 18. Journal of Cellular Biochemistry 1999;72:356–67.

[206] Binet O, Brunetiere RA, Rabary G, Garelly EB, Gallan A, Villet R. Immunologic studies of bullous pemphigoid associated with adenocarcinoma of the colon. New England Journal of Medicine 1983;308:460–1.

[207] Egan CA, Florell SR, Zone JJ. Localized bullous pemphigoid in a patient with B-cell lymphoma. Southern Medical Journal 1999;92:1220–2.

[208] Dega H, Laporte JL, Joly P, Gabarre J, Andre C, Delpech A, Frances C, Chosidow O. Paraneoplastic pemphigus associated with Hodgkin's disease. British Journal of Dermatology 1998;138:196–8.

[209] Parra CA, López González G, Pizzi de Parra N. [Bullous pemphigoid and lymphoblastic lymphoma]. Medicina Cutánea Ibero-Latino-Americana 1979;7:51–4.

[210] Kreutzer B, Stübiger N, Thiel HJ, Zierhut M. Oculomucocutaneous changes as paraneoplastic syndromes. German Journal of Ophthalmology 1996;5:176–81.

[211] Lutkowska A, Pietkiewicz P, Szulczyńska-Gabor J, Gornowicz J, Bowszyc-Dmochowska M, Dmochowski M. [Gluteal skin is not an optimal biopsy site for direct immunofluorescence in diagnostics of dermatitis herpetiformis. A report of a case of dermatitis herpetiformis Cottini]. Dermatologia Kliniczna 2009;11:31-33.

[212] Jedlickova H, Hlubinka M, Pavlik T, Semradova V, Budinska E, Vlasin Z. Bullous pemphigoid and internal diseases - A case-control study. European Journal of Dermatology 2010;20:96–101.

[213] Blum A, Wehner-Caroli J, Scherwitz C, Rassner G. [Bullous pemphigoid as a paraneoplastic syndrome. A case report in renal-cell carcinoma]. Hautarzt 1997;48:834–7.

[214] Korfitis C, Gregoriou S, Georgala S, Christofidou E, Danopoulou I. Trauma-induced bullous pemphigoid. Indian Journal of Dermatology, Venereology and Leprology 2009;75:617.

[215] Lenz P, Hsu R, Yee C, Yancey K, Volc-Platzer B, Stingl G, Kirnbauer R. [Cicatricial pemphigoid with autoantibodies to laminin 5 (epiligrin) in a patient with metastatic endometrial carcinoma]. Hautarzt 1998;49:31–5.

[216] Mul VEM, van Geest AJ, Pijls-Johannesma MCG, Theys J, Verschueren TAM, Jager JJ, Lambin P, Baumert BG. Radiation-induced bullous pemphigoid: a systematic review of an unusual radiation side effect. Radiotherapy and Oncology 2007;82:5–9.

[217] Clayton AS, Angeloni V. Bullous pemphigoid in a previously irradiated site. Cutis 1998;61:73–6.

[218] Ohata C, Shirabe H, Takagi K, Kawatsu T, Hashimoto T. Localized bullous pemphigoid after radiation therapy: two cases. Acta Dermato-Venereologica 1997;77:157.

[219] Pardoll DM. Inducing autoimmune disease to treat cancer. Proceedings of the National Academy of Sciences 1999;96:5340-2.

[220] Gornowicz-Porowska J, Pietkiewicz P, Bowszyc-Dmochowska M, Dmochowski M. The BP180 IgG ELISA is superior to the BP230 IgG ELISA for diagnosing IgG-mediated subepidermal autoimmune blistering dermatoses. Dermatologia Kliniczna 2012;14:111-6.

Chapter 7

Skin Cancer Prevention Strategies

Lisa Passantino, Max Costa and Mary Matsui

Additional information is available at the end of the chapter

http://dx.doi.org/10.5772/55241

1. Introduction

Ultraviolet radiation (UVR) has been identified as the primary etiologic agent for the induction and promotion of most skin cancers. The first associations between solar UVR and skin cancer were acknowledged by the scientific community in 1927. Since then, increasing evidence for the role of UVR in the causation of skin cancer has resulted in the listing of solar and artificial UVR as a human carcinogen by the International Agency for Research on Cancer (IARC) in 1992. Broad spectrum (UVA and UVB) UVR was categorized as a human carcinogen by the National Toxicology Program in 2005. UVR from the sun causes approximately 90% of malignant melanomas and non-melanoma (basal cell carcinoma [BCC] and squamous cell carcinoma [SCC]) skin cancers [1]. The non-melanoma skin cancers make up one third of all cancers around the world [2]. According to the National Cancer Institute, in the United States melanoma has one of the fastest increasing incidence rates. It is estimated that more than two million new cases of skin cancer will be diagnosed in 2012 [3-5]. Prevention of skin cancer is possible since UVR is known to be the central causative agent. National educational programs have emerged globally to deliver the message that unprotected sun exposure increases the risk for developing skin cancer, and present multiple behaviors that when followed together reduce the risk of photocarcinogenesis.

The goal of this chapter is to present a variety of skin cancer prevention strategies in the context of existing scientific knowledge on photocarcinogenesis. The connection between UVR exposure and skin cancer has been shown in numerous epidemiological, *in-vivo*, and *in-vitro* studies. Health professionals and government agencies have been communicating the dangers of UV exposure and the benefits of adopting primary and secondary prevention practices to lessen skin cancer incidence and mortality [1, 6]. Primary prevention strategies to protect against skin cancer are to wear broad spectrum sunscreen, seek shade, avoid the outdoors during peak daytime hours, and to wear protective clothing. Intentional UVR exposure for the purpose of tanning (indoor or outdoor) or stimulation of vitamin D synthesis is strongly discouraged. There is scientific evidence that indicates oral and topical supplementation with antioxidants, vitamins, and phytochemicals is beneficial for chemoprevention. Secondary prevention for skin cancer is performing periodic examinations of the skin for suspicious growths, and having dangerous-looking growths excised by a dermatologist. Practicing a combination of these skin cancer prevention strategies will reduce the risk of skin cancer.

2. Photocarcinogenesis

Solar UVR is composed of UVA (320-400 nm), UVB (290-320 nm), and UVC (200-290 nm). The atmospheric ozone layer inhibits all UVC and some UVB from reaching the surface of the Earth. The composition of UVR that reaches humans is approximately 95% UVA and 5% UVB, depending on factors such as cloud coverage, weather, thickness of the ozone layer, and latitude. UVA can penetrate deep into the dermis, while most UVB is absorbed by the stratum corneum in the epidermis but some passes into the upper dermis [7]. Human skin has evolved protective mechanisms against solar UVR. Melanocytes produce melanin that absorbs and scatters light in the lower epidermis [8]. The stratum corneum scatters UV light, and stratum corneum, spinosum, and basale can absorb UV light. Endogenously produced antioxidants and DNA repair enzymes protect skin cells from the damaging effects of UVR [9, 10].

Irradiation of the skin with UV damages the tissue and cellular components, and contributes to skin aging and carcinogenesis. The characteristic adverse effects of UVB include sunburn, inflammation, immunosuppression, erythema, and DNA damage. UVA exposure is primarily associated with the generation of reactive oxygen species (ROS), some oxidative DNA damage, cell membrane oxidation, and can result in immunosuppression. UVA indirectly causes oxidative DNA damage through the generation of ROS. The oxidation of guanine bases to 8-hydroxy-2'deoxyguanine (8-OH-dG) is primarily associated with UVA irradiation. UVB can induce oxidative stress indirectly through the activation of the inflammatory cells. Signature mutagenic DNA lesions caused by UVB consistently found in skin cancers are cyclobutane pryimidine dimers (CPD), pyrimidine-(6-4)-pyrimidine photoproducts, and C → T transitions [6, 7, 11-16]. Signature UVB mutations, CPDs and G:C → A:T transitions, have been found to localize in the superficial epithelial layers of human SCC samples, while signature UVA mutations, 8-OH-dG and A:T → C:G transversions, localized in the basal layers [15]. This distribution of DNA lesions is consistent with knowledge that UVA penetration into the skin is deeper than UVB penetration. Signature gene mutations found in skin cancers are those of tumor protein 53 (p53) tumor suppressor gene and proto-oncogene B-raf. Mutations to p53 are particularly detrimental because p53 plays a central role in pausing the cell cycle to allow time for DNA repair [2, 13]. UVR exposure can induce signal transduction pathways, such as mitogen-activated protein kinase (MAPK) and activation of transcription factor AP-1 that regulate cell growth, differentiation, apoptosis, and production of pro-inflammatory cytokines [17].

Inappropriate cell proliferation and survival contributes to carcinogenesis. Severely damaged DNA that cannot be repaired triggers skin cells to undergo apoptosis. Cells that survive the damage could carry mutations if the repair was not carried out perfectly [18]. There is a greater tendency for damaged keratinocytes to undergo apoptosis than damaged melanocytes, possibly to preserve melanin-producing cells for photoprotection [19]. In addition to genotoxic effects, UVB exposure increases cell proliferation as is observed in animal models where hyperproliferation of the epidermis and inflammation are the result of prostaglandin and epidermal growth factor receptor activation by UVB [9].

UV exposure causes immunosuppression that promotes the development of skin cancer because the immune system is less likely to detect and eliminate cancer cells. UVA and UVB separately can suppress cutaneous immune responses in humans, and the magnitude of immunosuppression is greater when they are combined [20]. UVR induces physical alterations to cell surface proteins in the epidermis. These structural changes create neoantigens that would be attacked by the immune system. It is believed that the human adaptive immune system has evolved such that recognition of antigens is suppressed by UVR, thus reducing the risk of auto-sensitization. Langerhans cells, the antigen presenting cells of the skin, migrate out of the epidermis to local lymph nodes for several days after UV exposure [18]. The Langerhans cells activate T helper type 2 cells, which suppress immune reactions by releasing immunosuppressive cytokines [13, 21]. The downside to this mechanism is that cancer detection capabilities are suppressed in addition to autoimmune reactions [18].

UVR is considered to be a complete carcinogen since it can induce tumor formation by itself, and both UVA and UVB contribute to skin carcinogenesis. Since UVB is a more potent and direct inducer of DNA damage than UVA, it is thought to play more of a role in the initiation stage of tumorigenesis while the effects of UVA are thought to promote the development of the tumor [7]. UVR can be coupled with other chemical carcinogens to promote tumor development. The combination of solar UV and sodium arsenite causes SCC in mice, but sodium arsenite alone cannot cause SCC. This is an example of how UVR can act as a cocarcinogen [22].

3. Susceptibility factors for UV-induced skin damage and cancer

Relative endogenous protection capacity against UVR is a major factor in determining susceptibility to skin cancer. Individual differences in skin pigmentation, DNA repair, endogenous antioxidant levels, and impact the biological response to UVR [17]. The Fitzpatrick skin type (FST) was created in the 1970s as a method to classify people by the intensity of their erythema response to UVR. It can be used to predict response and susceptibility to skin cancer since lighter-skinned individuals with low FST tend to be more sensitive to UVR than darker-skinned individuals with high FST. There are six FSTs, with FST I being the most sensitive to sunlight and FST VI being the least sensitive. People that are FST I have white skin, may have freckles, blue or green-colored eyes, and red hair. People that are FST VI have black skin and hair, dark-brown eyes, and rarely experience sunburn [8]. Constitutive skin color should not be confused with FST because FST is based on the biological response not ethnicity [23]. It is no coincidence that the highest incidence rates of non-melanoma skin cancer are found in regions with light-skinned populations such as Australia, Switzerland, and Ireland [2], and that the highest registered incidence of melanoma is found in Australia (Geller et.al, 2012). There is a 20 times greater incidence of malignant melanoma in Caucasians than in African-Americans in the United States [19]. One reason for this difference is that darkly pigmented skin responds to UVR differently than light pigmented skin. In African-Americans, DNA damage is not prominent below the epidermis, and damaged skin cells are more likely to undergo apoptosis. It is believed that the melanin in more highly pigmented individuals provides a higher level of protection than in light skinned individuals. By absorbing UV light, melanin is protective, but it is not enough to give 100% protection, so more highly pigmented people are still prone to UV-induced skin damage and can still get skin cancer [23].

The effects of UV damage on the skin are cumulative. The total number of severe sunburn incidences and lifetime dose of UVR are important factors to consider when determining skin cancer susceptibility. Outdoor workers have a greater risk of developing SCC than indoor workers because their skin experiences chronic irradiation with solar UV. Spending long periods of time outdoors for recreational purposes is associated with increased risk of melanoma [17]. Major risk factors for developing melanoma are the number of nevi and number sunburns experienced during childhood and adolescence [6, 17].

4. Photoprotective behaviors

Acute UVR exposure has deleterious effects on the skin, and contributes to the cumulative effects of lifetime UV exposure. Cellular damage and DNA mutations caused by UVR, if not repaired, can accumulate in the skin and contribute to skin aging and increase skin cancer risk. Melanomas typically develop in areas of the skin that are occasionally exposed to sunlight, while non-melanomas tend to develop in areas of the skin that are frequently exposed to sunlight [19]. Therefore, it is important to protect all areas of skin from UVR by practicing a combination of photoprotective behaviors. The most common form of sun protection that comes to mind is sunscreen, but it is not the only method. Comprehensive sun protection programs endorsed by healthcare professionals include the use of broad spectrum sunscreen, wearing protective clothing, staying in the shade and limiting sun exposure especially at times of peak intensity (10am-2pm), and avoiding indoor tanning devices [8, 9, 24]. Sand, water, and snow reflect UV rays, so protective measures should be taken seriously when in these environments[19]. These core photoprotective methods should be followed by all people regardless of skin color and FST, and especially followed by susceptible populations. However, only 60.6% of adults surveyed in the United States in 2010 reported that they usually or always follow at least one photoprotective behavior when spending time outdoors [25].

Wearing protective clothing means that the clothing should be a physical barrier to sunlight, and should cover as much of the body as possible. Protective clothing includes wearing long pants or a long skirt, and long sleeves. Hats that shade the face, neck and ears are part of protective clothing. Most men wear a baseball cap for protection, but these caps do not shade the face, neck, and ears as well as a wide-brimmed hat that offers more coverage

[25]. Sunglasses also fall under protective clothing as they protect the eyes and areas around the eyes from UVR and reduce the risk of developing ocular melanoma. The best protection against solar UVR would be obtained by through a combination of protective clothing and sunscreen [26].

Consumers are advised to select sunscreens that offer broad spectrum (UVA and UVB) protection with a sun protective factor (SPF) of 15 or greater by the United States Food and Drug Administration (FDA) [1]. Sunscreens are applied directly onto the skin and they reduce UVR penetration by reflection or absorption [9]. Broad spectrum sunscreens can protect against UV-induced erythema and immunosuppression [21]. Sunscreen use is a method of chemoprevention, meaning it can suppress or prevent the progression of premalignant skin lesions into cancer [19]. Sunscreen with SPF of 15 or greater reduces skin cancer risk, and prevents both melanoma and non-melanoma skin cancers [24]. The amount of protection is related to the SPF level and the amount of sunscreen applied. Lower SPF sunscreens are less effective, especially when applied inadequately, than higher SPF sunscreens [27].

Consistent daily application of sunscreen is especially recommended for individuals who are more susceptible to developing melanoma [19]. Consistent long-term daily application of broad spectrum sunscreen to the head and arms was shown to decrease the incidence of malignant melanoma compared to discretionary sunscreen use in a randomized controlled prospective study of Australians [28]. Fewer melanocytic nevi develop on Caucasian children who routinely used SPF 30 broad spectrum sunscreen when going outdoors for more than 30 minutes than children who do not use sunscreen [29]. Sunscreen itself is safe and does not increase the risk of skin cancer. Meta-analysis of 11 case-control studies did not find an association between sunscreen use and increased risk of developing melanoma [30]. Some studies have reported an association between topical sunscreen use and melanoma, but this relationship is probably connected to inappropriate and compensatory use of sunscreen.

The compensation hypothesis is that people tend to wear less protective clothing and/or prolong the amount of time spent in the sun when they use higher SPF sunscreens. This compensatory behavior actually defeats the purpose of using sunscreen, and it increases risk of skin cancer because the risk of sunburn is increased [1, 17, 24]. In an observational study of European sunbathers, it was found that the duration of time spent sunbathing was up to 25% longer for those who used SPF 30 than those who used SPF 10 [31]. Sunscreen is meant to be used as an adjunct to other methods of photoprotection and not to extend the amount of intentional sun exposure time. Consumers generally have a false sense of security when wearing high SPF sunscreens, especially those of SPF of 50 and greater, and they often forgo other methods of photoprotection, such as wearing protective clothing. Interestingly, the consumers who wear sunscreen and spend more time sunbathing are generally those who are more sensitive to UVR. This likely explains why the incidence of melanoma continues to increase despite more people wearing sunscreen [26].

Another behavior that compromises the effectiveness of sunscreen is inadequate sunscreen application thickness. Sunscreen accumulates in fissures on the skin, so it is necessary to apply enough product to fill in the fissures and to fully cover epidermal ridges [32]. Most consumers apply sunscreen below the standard thickness used for the international SPF test, which is 2 mg/cm^2 [1]. Consumers apply between 0.5 and 1.2 mg/cm^2 sunscreen and consequently do not receive the expected amount of sun protection. The actual SPF of the sunscreen can be decreased by 20-50% compared to the rated SPF when it is applied improperly [19, 27, 32]. The reduction of actual SPF as a function of application thickness was recently demonstrated during a study in which Chinese women applied SPF 4,15, 30, or 55 sunscreen at 0.5, 1, 1.5, or 2 mg/cm^2. The actual SPF was calculated for each individual after exposure to solar simulated UVR. It was determined that at the standard application thickness of 2 mg/cm^2 the observed SPF was similar to the rated SPF. However, as application thickness decreased there was an observed linear decrease in actual SPF for SPF 4 and 15 sunscreens, and an exponential decrease in the actual SPF for the SPF 30 and 55 sunscreens [27]. Inadequate application of lower SPF sunscreens may put consumers at greater risk of sunburn and skin cancer than inadequate application of higher SPF sunscreens.

To compensate for inadequate application thickness, the American Academy of Dermatology recommends using a minimum of SPF 30 sunscreen, which is higher than the FDA's recommendation of 15. High SPF sunscreen should especially be used when going outdoors on days when the UV index is predicted to be high and there is greater risk of overexposure. Spending even 45 minutes outdoors unprotected on a day of moderate UV index value can cause skin damage [33]. One application of sunscreen may not be enough if an individual stays outdoors for long periods of time and/or is involved in activities that cause the skin to perspire or get wet.

Proper use of sunscreen includes reapplication every two hours, and more frequently when sweating, swimming, or towel drying [24]. It is important to reapply sunscreen because the active components may become unstable and lose activity during exposure to sunlight [27]. The FDA does not currently require a photostability test for sunscreens [1]. The duration of water resistance is limited, so water resistant sunscreens need to be reapplied frequently when swimming or sweating [24]. It is required by USFDA monograph that the duration of water resistance (40 or 80 minutes) be indicated on the label to instruct consumers about when they should reapply the sunscreen [1]. Spray on sunscreen is thought to be less effective than traditional sunscreens because it is not rubbed directly onto the skin. The FDA is currently investigating the effectiveness of spray on sunscreens, and is performing inhalation safety testing as well [24].

Indoor tanning is a popular alternative to natural tanning because it can be done at any time of the year, but it is actually very dangerous because the skin is intentionally exposed to intense UVR repeatedly over short periods of time. Tanning bulbs emit predominantly UVA, which is known to cause high levels of oxidative stress in the skin and contribute to greater risk of melanoma [26]. They also emit a small amount of UVB that primarily damages the DNA in skin cells during indoor tanning sessions. Artificial UVR from indoor tanning equipment is considered to be carcinogenic along with solar UVR, yet approximately 28 million people expose themselves to it annually in the United States [34].The likelihood of developing SCC is 2.5 times greater for people who use tanning beds, and the likelihood of developing BCC is 1.5 times greater [35]. Individuals who have ever used tanning beds have a 15% greater risk of developing melanoma than individuals who have never been in a tanning bed [19]. The age at which people start using indoor tanning technologies is a risk factor for developing skin cancer as well. The lifetime risk of developing melanoma is 75% higher in people who first use indoor tanning beds before the age of 35 [35]. Younger people have a greater tendency to use indoor tanning devices, possibly because of the social perception that having a tan is attractive. More people between the ages of 18-24 used indoor tanning devices than people over the age of 25 in 2010. In both age groups, females exposed themselves to artificial UVR to obtain a tan more than males did. Most of these adults were non-Hispanic whites [25]. The high skin cancer risk associated with indoor tanning coupled with the addictiveness of the behavior has caused many states in the U.S. to pass laws restricting the use of indoor tanning devices by minors in 2012 [19].

Consumers should be aware of their skin's reaction to sunlight when they are outdoors, and take appropriate action when noticing adverse reactions to sun exposure. Regardless of sunscreen application and whether sun exposure is intentional or unintentional, if the skin becomes red (indicative of cellular damage) and uncomfortable at any time it is prudent to immediately find shade and put on protective clothing [26]. Parents should be vigilant of signs of redness in their childrens' skin as well. Infants and children should be kept in the shade out of direct sunlight [2]. Self-examination of skin for suspicious growths and nevi is also recommended for early detection of skin cancer [2, 17].

5. Chemoprevention with topical and dietary antioxidants, phytochemicals, and vitamin supplementation

Chemoprevention is the use of natural or synthetic agents to prevent or reverse the development of cancer [21]. Sunscreen use is considered a form of chemoprevention because it contains compounds, such as avobenzone and octyl salicylate, that inhibit UVR from damaging the skin. Supplementation of sunscreens with various phytochemicals and antioxidants has been shown to improve the function of sunscreens in preventing photodamage [13]. Oral intake of certain vitamins, antioxidants, and plant extracts can provide systemic protection as well.

A diet rich in fruits and vegetables has generally been associated with lowering the risk of a variety of diseases and cancers, including skin cancer. Regular consumption of fruits and vegetables was associated with a decreased risk of SCC in a dietary study of 1360 adults in Nambour, Australia. In this study it was also found that a diet high in meat and fat was positively associated with the development of SCC but not BCC [36]. Fruits and vegetables contain bioactive phytochemicals, such as flavonoids, polyphenols and carotenoids. These compounds can boost antioxidant and immune system defenses in the body, including in the skin [37]. Carotenoids and flavonoids naturally protect plants from solar UVR, and consumption of these phytochemicals can provide systemic photoprotection for humans [8]. Polyphenols from tea have been shown to protect against UVB-induced contact sensitization, inflammation, carcinogen-induced cancer of the skin, lung, and esophagus in rodent models [37].

Photooxidative damage occurs when the antioxidant defense mechanisms of the skin are overwhelmed by UV-induced ROS, particularly from UVA. ROS that contribute to photocarcinogenesis and photoaging include singlet oxygen, superoxide radical anion, hydroxyl radical, perhydroxyl radical, and hydrogen peroxide [10, 13, 37-39]. Endogenous antioxidants that scavenge for ROS include superoxide dismutase, glutathione peroxidase, ascorbate, alpha-lipoic acid, and catalase [16]. Excessive ROS generated during UV exposure depletes endogenous antioxidants, and causes a state of oxidative stress in cells that can damage cellular proteins, lipids, DNA, trigger apoptosis, and contribute to photocarcinogenesis [14]. Incorporating antioxidants into sunscreens can ameliorate UV-induced tissue damage and promote DNA repair [13].

Human studies with antioxidant supplementation to sunscreens have been successful at demonstrating the benefits of including antioxidants in the formulation. In a human study, the combination of a several antioxidants, including ascorbyl phosphate, tocopherol acetate, *Echinacea pallida* extract, chamomile extract, and caffeine, with sunscreen best protected the skin compared to sunscreen alone after repetitive irradiation with solar simulated UVR [40]. A significant inhibition of UVR-induced melanin synthesis was observed in the presence of antioxidants alone. There was a synergy between the antioxidants and broad spectrum sunscreen, making the combination more protective than either the antioxidants or sunscreen alone. The antioxidant alone was able to prevent hyperproliferation and thickening of the epidermis that is a typical biological response to chronic UVR exposure. UV-induction of cytokeratin 16 and MMP9 was also suppressed by antioxidant cocktail and sunscreen combination [40]. In another study using a similar combination of antioxidants, sunscreen with antioxidants or sunscreen alone were equally able to protect against immunosuppression as measured by immunohistochemical staining for Langerhans cells. Less induction of tissue remodeling protein MMP1 was observed with the sunscreen plus antioxidant formulation [13]. Taken together, this data demonstrates additive or synergistic effects of antioxidants for photoprotection.

5.1. Green tea

Tea (*Camellia sinensis*) drinking has been associated with health in many cultures. Green tea consumption has been associated with reduced cancer risk, including SCC [17]. It has been demonstrated in mouse skin tumor models that green tea inhibits photocarcinogenesis [37]. Epigallocatechin-3-gallate (EGCG) makes up approximately 40% of all the polyphenols found in green tea, and it is believed to be the main polyphenol responsible for the beneficial health effects of green tea [12, 37]. White and black teas also have protective effects. Theaflavins, the polyphenols found in black tea, can inhibit the UVB-induced activation of cell signaling through AP-1, MAPK, and extracellular matrix receptor-activated kinase [17]. Topical application of white or green teas have been shown to protect against the loss of Langerhans cells after solar simulated UVR exposure in both human subjects and in an *ex vivo* skin explant model [21]. In another human study, EGCG inhibited UVB-induced erythema and inflammation. Fewer leukocytes infiltrated the skin when EGCG was applied prior to irradiation with UVB, and less prostanoids were synthesized [37]. In addition to being able to suppress the

http://dx.doi.org/10.5772/55241

inflammatory and immunosuppressive effects of UVB, topical application of green or white tea has been shown to completely prevent the formation of 8-OH-dG adducts in human skin [21]. The reduction of DNA damage, aberrant cell signaling, inflammation, and immunosuppression are mechanisms exhibited by teas and tea extracts that contribute to their anti-cancer properties.

The amount of pre-treatment time and concentration of green tea polyphenols required to obtain optimal protection on human skin was elucidated in a study by Elmets et.al. In this study, skin on the back of six human subjects was pre-treated for 30 minutes with 0.25-10% solutions of green tea polyphenols. The skin was then irradiated with a solar simulator at twice the individual's minimal erythema dose (MED). At 24, 48, and 72 hours post-exposure erythema was quantified with a chromameter and biopsies were taken from the exposed sites. Erythema was found to be reduced in a dose-dependent manner at all time points and with all doses of green tea polyphenol that were used (figure 1). Pre-treatment with the polyphenols was noted to work best when applied immediately before exposure as opposed to several hours before exposure. Analysis of the biopsies revealed a 66% reduction in the number of sunburn cells, significantly less Langerhans cell migration at 4 days post-exposure, and a 55% reduction in DNA lesions. Subjects were also irradiated with 135 J/cm^2 UVA only, and pre-treatment with 5% green tea polyphenols significantly protected against UVA-induced erythema in that experiment [9]. The results of this study indicate that the use of green tea polyphenols is most effective at protecting the skin from UVR when used at a concentration of 0.25% or greater, with the greatest protection observed when applying a 10% solution 30 minutes before irradiation. Adding green tea polyphenols to sunscreens could enhance broad spectrum protection since they have been demonstrated to reduce UVA-induced erythema.

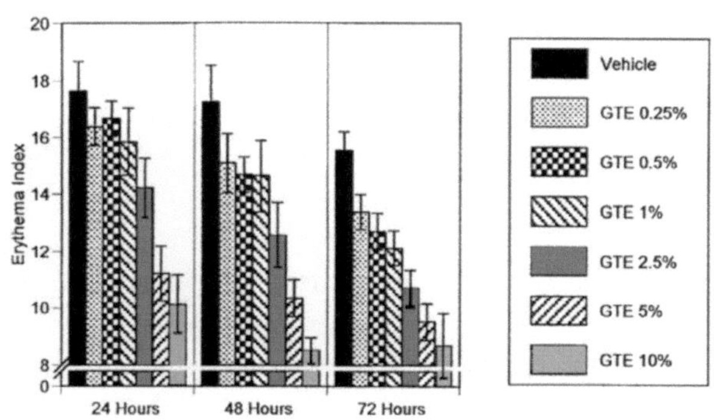

Figure 1. Effect of green tea polyphenols (GTP) on the erythema response evoked by 2-MED solar simulated radiation. Data represent the mean ± standard error of the mean erythema index at 24, 48, and 72 hours after irradiation with a solar simulator. Measurements were made with a chromameter on 6 volunteers. Areas of skin were pretreated with indicated concentration of an extract of green tea (GTE) 30 minutes before UV exposure. Reprinted from Cutaneous photoprotection from ultraviolet injury by green tea polyphenols, Journal of the American Academy of Dermatology, 44(3):425-32, Elmets CA, Singh D, Tubesing K, Matsui M, Katiyar S, Mukhtar H, (2001) with permission from Elsevier.

In a parallel experiment, Elmets et.al tested separate green tea polyphenols for ability to inhibit erythema on human subjects irradiated with solar simulated UVR. The polyphenols tested were 5% solutions of EGCG, epicatechin (EC), epigallocatechin (EGC), or epicatechin-3-gallate (ECG). EC and EGC were not effective at inhibiting erythema, but EGCG and ECG were. The authors were intrigued by this finding because EGCG and ECG both contain a galloyl group at the 3 position, and this common structure between them could be the source of their effectiveness compared to the other polyphenols that were tested [9]. These results confirmed that EGCG is one of the polyphenols that contributes the most to the photoprotective effects of green tea.

5.2. Resveratrol

Resveratrol is a chemopreventive phytochemical found in grape skin and seeds, red wine, peanuts, and fruits. Topical application of resveratrol in hairless mice has been shown to reduce signs of oxidative stress and inflammation induced by UVB exposure [12]. Daily topical application of resveratrol in humans prior to irradiation with solar simulated UVR for four consecutive days provided significant protection against erythema, melanin synthesis, tanning, and sunburn cell formation compared to unprotected skin [10].

5.3. Pomegranate

Pomegranate is known for its strong anti-inflammatory, antioxidant, anti-proliferative, and anti-tumorigenic properties. Anthocyanidins and hydrolysable tannins are polyphenols found in pomegranate. In an animal study, hairless mice were irradiated with 180 mJ/cm^2 UVB after consuming 0.2% (wt/vol) pomegranate extract for two weeks. Analysis of skin biopsies taken from the mice revealed that pomegranate consumption resulted in the inhibition of UVB-induced skin edema, cell proliferation, infiltration of leukocytes, NFκB activation, COX-2 expression, CPDs, 8-OH-dG, and generation of hydrogen peroxide and lipid peroxidation [11]. These results suggest that regular consumption of pomegranate could provide systemic protection from UVB.

5.4. Lycopene

Lycopene is a carotenoid found in tomatoes, red bell peppers, watermelon and other red-colored fruits and vegetables. Lycopene consumption is believed to aid in the prevention of cardiovascular disease, diabetes, and cancer because of its strong antioxidant property. The bioavailability of lycopene is greater in cooked and processed foods than from fresh fruits. It has been recognized as one of the most powerful quenchers of singlet oxygen of all the carotenoids [41]. Dietary intake of lycopene or foods rich in lycopene can provide systemic photoprotection. Daily consumption of 55 grams of tomato paste with olive oil for 12 weeks protected individuals from solar simulated UVR-induced mitochondrial DNA damage compared to individuals who ate olive oil alone. Less induction of matrix metalloproteinases was also found, and the skin of the group that ate tomato paste tended to have a higher MED than the group that did not [41]. In another human study, individuals that consumed lycopene for 10-12 weeks developed about 40% less erythema than those that did not [8].

http://dx.doi.org/10.5772/55241

5.5. Chocolate

Fresh cocoa beans contain high levels of polyphenols that are potent antioxidants. Most commercially available chocolate does not contain high antioxidants because conventional chocolate making diminishes antioxidant capacity. Chocolate that is specially prepared to retain high amounts of active flavanols can increase the MED in human subjects who ate it every day for 12 weeks compared to subjects who ate conventional chocolate [42].

5.6. Beta-carotene

β-carotene is a fat soluble antioxidant carotenoid found in many plants, and gives orange color to many fruits and vegetables, such as carrots and yams. It is a precursor to vitamin A, also known as provitamin A [43]. The effectiveness of β-carotene as a systemic photoprotectant in humans is dependent upon the dose and the duration of consumption before irradiation with UVR. Reports suggest that in order for β-carotene pre-treatment to be effective it should be consumed at a dose of 20 mg per day for at least 10 weeks, and moderate intake is insufficient to achieve photoprotection [8]. Meta-analysis of seven human studies on sunburn protection and β-carotene arrived at the same conclusion, and added that the mean photoprotection provided by β-carotene increases for each month beyond 10 weeks of consistent consumption, and β-carotene can provide system photoprotection with a maximal SFP of 4. [43].

While dietary supplementation with β-carotene protects against sunburn, it is not effective for preventing skin cancer when used alone. A data review of randomized control studies did not find a positive association between oral β-carotene supplementation and the prevention of melanoma or non-melanoma [44]. β-carotene supplementation could be used in combination with other photoprotective methods to reduce sunburn. However, dietary supplementation with β-carotene should be done with caution because at high levels it can create a prooxidative state that is damaging to the body. Consuming high amounts of β-carotene is not suggested for smokers, as it has been shown to increase lung cancer risk [44].

5.7. Vitamin C and Vitamin E

Vitamin C (ascorbic acid) and vitamin E (α-tocopherol) are photoprotective antioxidants that can be combined with other antioxidants like β-carotene or added into sunscreen to protect the skin from UVR. Vitamin E is a potent inhibitor of lipid peroxidation, and it is typically found in plant derived oils. Vitamin C has functions as a reducing agent and is an essential vitamin for humans. Vitamins C and E have a synergistic relationship; vitamin C can regenerate oxidized vitamin E at the cell membrane [38, 39]. Oral administration of 200mg/day vitamin C and 1000IU/day of vitamin E for eight days in humans reduces sensitivity to solar simulated UVR as observed by higher MED in subjects [38]. The combination of vitamin E with β-carotene has been shown to suppress UVR-induced erythema better than β-carotene alone when administered orally for 12 weeks [39]. Topical application of vitamin E onto hairless mice prior to irradiation with solar simulated UV has been reported to prevent immunosuppression [16].

5.8. Polypodium leucotomos

An organic extract of the tropical South American fern *Polypodium leucotomos*, given the commercial name "Fernblock", can be used orally or topically to protect the skin from solar UVR. This extract protects against the genotoxic effects of UVB by preventing the formation of CPDs, 8-OH-dG, and mitochondrial DNA damage. It induces the p53 tumor suppressor protein. The extract prevents UVR-induced inflammation through the inhibition of pro-inflammatory molecules (tumor necrosis factor alpha and nitric oxide synthase), COX-2, apoptosis of keratinocytes and fibroblasts, and general reduction of erythema and sunburn. One component of Fernblock, caffeic acid, prevents oxidative stress by inhibiting the formation of peroxide and nitric oxide upon exposure to UVR. Fernblock also prevents the immunosuppressive effects of UVR by suppressing the migration of Langerhans cells and activation of T helper type 2 cells. Remodeling of the dermal extracellular matrix by matrix metalloproteinase 3 is inhibited by the extract, and both collagen and elastin proteins are up regulated indicating that the extract may also fight photoaging. Topical application of the extract on hairless mice was reported to block UVB-induced skin tumor formation. All of these positive protective effects make Fernblock a potentially powerful photocarcinogenesis protective agent [14].

6. Vitamin D

Vitamin D is important for bone health, intestinal uptake of calcium and phosphate, and regulation of calcium and phosphate levels in the blood [2, 4]. Vitamin D is associated with the prevention of autoimmune disease, cardiovascular disease, and believed to have anti-inflammatory and anti-proliferative effects [45, 46]. The current recommended daily allowance for vitamin D is 400 IU for infants under 1 year old, 600 IU for persons 1-70 years old, and 800 IU for persons older than 70 years [47]. People who have vitamin D insufficiency are recommended to take 1,000 IU of vitamin D daily [48].

Lack of vitamin D results in poor enteral absorption of calcium that causes decreased blood levels of ionized calcium. This decrease promotes the breakdown of bone by osteoclasts to release calcium. By this mechanism, vitamin D insufficiency in adults can lead to osteoporosis. Childhood vitamin D deficiency causes Rickets disease. During the late 1800s to early 1900s Rickets disease afflicted more than 80% of North American and European children who lived in industrialized cities. After it was learned that a deficiency in vitamin D was to blame for the bone deformities caused by this disease, increasing exposure to sunlight and fortification of milk with vitamin D in the 1930s helped to reduce the incidence of Rickets in the United States [46, 47]. In addition to dietary sources, vitamin D can be obtained by cutaneous synthesis upon exposure to sunlight (figure 2). Upon irradiation with UVB, 7-dehydrocholsterol (provitamin D) in the skin is converted into pre-cholecalciferol (previtamin D_3). Pre-cholecalciferol undergoes a spontaneous isomerization into cholecalciferol (vitamin D_3). Vitamin D-binding protein (DBP) transports vitamin D_3 to the liver where it is hydroxylated by cytochrome p450 27A1 into 25-hydroxyvitamin D (25(OH)D_3) [2]. Further hydroxylation in the kidney or at the

http://dx.doi.org/10.5772/55241

skin modifies the vitamin into its active form called calcitriol ($25(OH)_2D_3$) [49]. Calcitriol binds to the nuclear vitamin D receptor (VDR), which then forms a heterodimer with the retinoid-X receptor and becomes a transcription factor that regulates the expression of cell cycle, cell proliferation, and apoptosis genes [2].

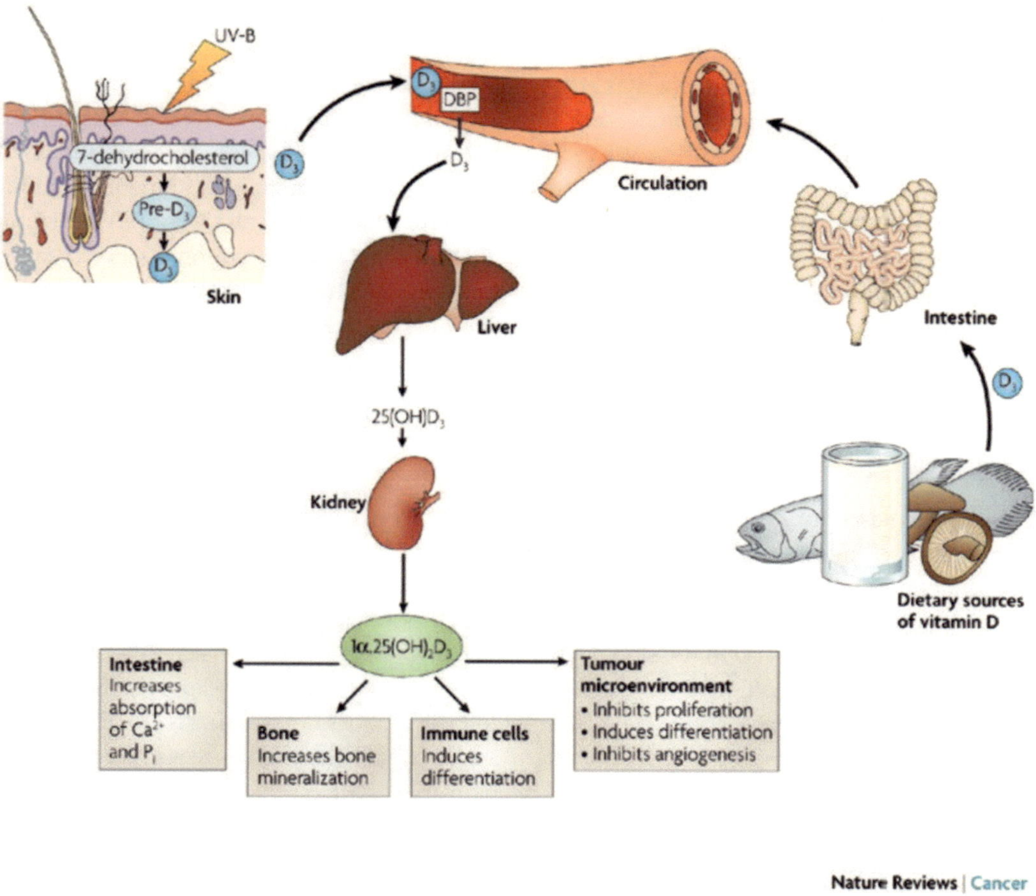

Figure 2. Vitamin D synthesis and biological effects. Reprinted by permission of Macmillan Publishers Ltd: Nature Reviews Cancer, Deeb KK, Trump DL, Johnson CS, Vitamin D signaling pathways in cancer: potential for anticancer therapeutics, 07(9):648-700 (2007).

There is contradictory evidence about whether vitamin D protects against cancer. A study conducted by the National Institutes of Health did not find a correlation between vitamin D levels and internal cancers [49]. Other studies have found that vitamin D can reduce the risk of internal cancers, particularly prostate and colorectal cancer [48]. It was reported in an observational study that individuals with the lowest serum levels of $25(OH)D_3$ had a 26% higher mortality rate when compared to those with higher vitamin D levels [45]. It is hypothesized that high blood levels of $25(OH)D_3$ result in higher levels of calcitriol that regulates cell proliferation. A number of cells in the body, including breast, colon, and skin, have the enzymes required to make calcitriol. It is suggested that when vitamin D levels are high local production of calcitriol keeps cell proliferation in check and reduces risk of carcinogenesis [46]. Thus, it is speculated that vitamin D production in the skin is protective and sunscreen use diminishes protection by inhibiting vitamin D synthesis.

There is almost no evidence supporting the idea that the vitamin D deficiency epidemic is correlated to the overuse of sunscreen [48]. Sunscreen use may diminish photosynthesis of vitamin D, but it is not necessary or recommended to obtain vitamin D from intentional sun exposure. To maximize cutaneous synthesis of vitamin D, individuals would have to expose themselves to sunlight for the amount of time required to achieve one third of their MED, meaning the skin would incur damage to make vitamin D. Incidental sun exposure for 10-20 minutes on skin protected with SPF 15 or greater sunscreen could maximize cutaneous vitamin D synthesis while protecting the skin because sunscreen does not block all UV [48]. While some people find the idea of synthesizing their own vitamin D through intentional sun exposure holistic and appealing, the better option is to continue protecting skin from solar UVR with sunscreen and protective clothing, and to obtain vitamin D from dietary sources and incidental protected sun exposure. A variety of foods including milk, bread, cereal, yogurt, and multi-vitamins are fortified with vitamin D in the United States and are good alternatives to intentional exposure to sunlight. The use of indoor tanning beds to increase vitamin D levels is not advised [4, 48, 50].

Populations susceptible to vitamin D deficiency are the eldery, people with darkly pigmented skin, breastfed infants, and obese people. The suggestion that elderly and darkly pigmented populations intentionally expose themselves to UVR is not a good solution because these susceptible populations generally have poor cutaneous vitamin D synthesis. The ability to photosynthesize vitamin D in the skin decreases with age because there is less 7-dehydrocholesterol in the skin. People with darkly pigmented skin have increased melanin in the epidermis that inhibits cutaneous vitamin D synthesis [2, 46, 48]. It does not make sense for the elderly or people with darkly pigmented skin to intentionally expose themselves to sunlight to make vitamin D since the process is inefficient in their skin. Rather, they should take dietary supplements and incorporate foods fortified with vitamin D. Obesity is also a risk factor for deficiency of vitamin D. Vitamin D_3 is stored deep in the body fat of obese individuals and is not readily bioavailable to them during winter months, so they can only mobilize about half the amount of vitamin D_3 as persons with healthy weights [46]. Human breast milk contains less than 78 IU vitamin D per liter so it is recommended that infants also receive vitamin D supplementation [47]. Infants should not be exposed to solar UV to increase vitamin D synthesis [2]. Dietary supplementation with vitamin D is the best option for all people, especially those with reduced ability to synthesize and maintain vitamin D levels in their body.

7. Sun protection education

Social perceptions and miscommunications about the dangers of UVR exposure contribute to the continued incidence of sunburns and skin cancer. The message that sun safety should be practiced daily is not widely followed, as evident by the fact that people are more likely to follow skin protection methods while on vacation or at the beach than when participating in other outdoor recreational activities [19]. Intentional unprotected sun exposure for cosmetic purposes is prominent in young adults because of the perception that tanned skin is more attractive [48]. About 50% of people in the U.S. between the ages of 18 and 24 years old report having a sunburn in the last year, compared to about 35% of people over the age of 25 who reported having a sunburn in the last year [25]. This is coincides with the tendency for young people to expose themselves to solar and artificial UVR for tanning. Over one million people go to tanning salons on an average day in the United States [34], and most are under the age of 25 [25]. This risky behavior may contribute to melanoma being the second most common cancer in young adults between the ages of 15 and 29 years old [4]. In 2004, it was found that 69% of youths between the ages of 11 and 18 reported in a cross-sectional study survey that they had been sunburned that summer [19]. Summertime sunburns should not be taken lightly or treated as a normal occurrence. The risk of developing melanoma more than doubles for individuals who report having five or more severe sunburns during adolescence [19]. A study by the University of Miami on sun protection behavior in high school students found that white-Hispanics were not likely to use sunscreens, more than twice as likely to go tanning, and generally did not believe that they had a risk of getting skin cancer compared to white non-Hispanics [23]. This is an example of the need to educate young adults and teenagers who are unaware of the health risks associated with sun exposure.

Physicians play in important role in educating patients about sun protection. Primary care physicians should actively promote broad spectrum sunscreen use, and review proper application techniques with patients to reduce sunburn. They should educate patients about the use of sunscreen as an adjunct to the other sun protection methods, and warn patients not to use sunscreen as a tool for prolonging sun exposure because that behavior increases the risk of sunburn [19, 26]. They could point patients towards many informative public education websites about sun protection and skin cancer prevention that are available from government and non-profit organizations.

Skin cancer prevention awareness is spreading with the help of government organizations, such as the National Institutes of Health and National Council on Skin Cancer. Increasing numbers of advertisements for skin cancer prevention are seen on television, heard on the radio, and posted in public places. Major awareness advocates, programs, and campaigns include the SunSmart campaign in Australia and the United Kingdom, the European Skin Cancer Foundation, the SunAWARE non-profit educational organization in the U.S., the USEPA SunWise program, American Academy of Dermatology, the Skin Cancer Foundation in the U.S., and the American Cancer Society. These groups and programs aim to educate the public about skin cancer and encourage multi-step behavioral modifications to reduce the risk of developing skin cancer. The SunAWARE organization uses AWARE as an easy acronym to help people remember the steps of sun protection (figure 3). Skin cancer incidence rates have been stabilizing when compared to the rapid increases seen before the rise in establishment of government-sponsored sun protection programs [19]. The message is starting to be heard, as evident by an overall increase in adult sunscreen use between 2005 and 2010 [25]. Sun safety awareness is encouraged by campaigns such as national "Don't Fry Day" that takes place on the Friday before Memorial Day in the U.S. and is supported by the National Council on Skin Cancer and SunWise program [5, 51].

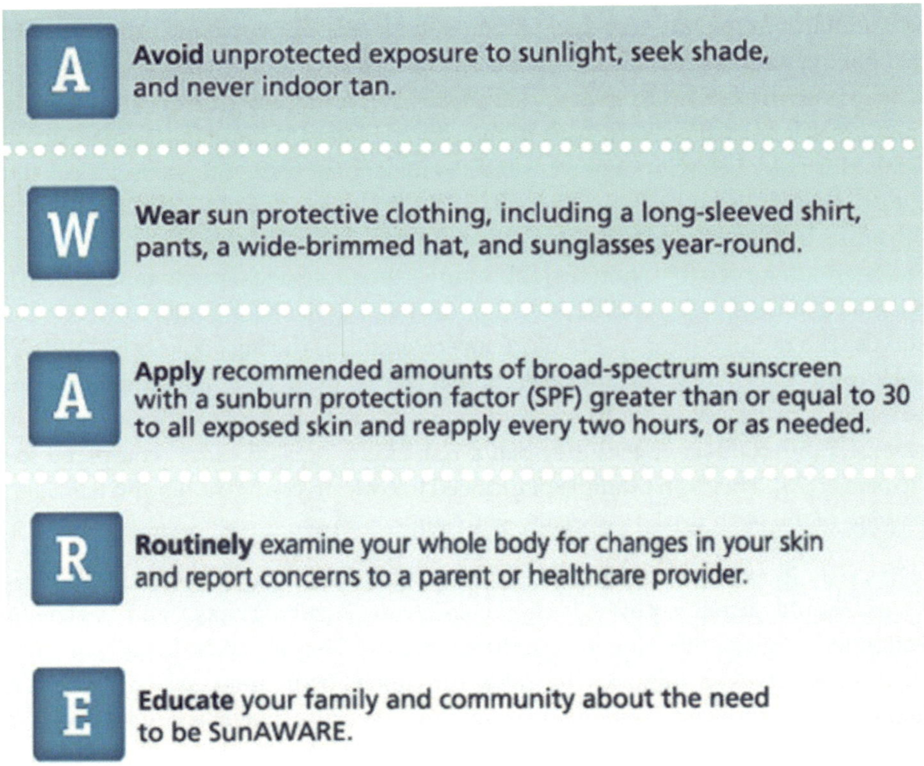

Figure 3. Sun protection advice displayed on SunAWARE website using the acronym AWARE. http://www.sunaware.org/be-sunaware/

Product labeling is another means for providing specific information on how to protect the skin. Sunscreen labels are strictly regulated by the USFDA. In the most recent law passed on sunscreen labeling in 2011, known as the "final rule", the USFDA required a new indication statement, simpler labeling, and clearer instructions for the usage of water resistant sunscreen [1]. Instead of indicating protection against UVA and/or UVB, labels are required to state "broad spectrum" to simplify the choice for consumers. The effectiveness rating of the sunscreen must be listed next to the broad spectrum phrase in the same size and style font to encourage consumers to look for broad spectrum sunscreens with a high SPF rating. To teach consumers that broad spectrum sunscreens with SPF 15 and greater are more protective when combined with other sun protection measures than sunscreens with low SPF that are not broad spectrum, the following indication statement is required on all broad spectrum SPF 15 and greater sunscreens:

"**Sun Protection Measures**. Spending time in the sun increases your risk of skin cancer and early skin aging. To decrease this risk, regularly use a sunscreen with a Broad Spectrum SPF of 15 or higher and other sun protection measures including: • limit time in the sun, especially from 10 a.m. - 2 p.m. • wear long-sleeved shirts, pants, hats, and sunglasses" [1]

Previous labeling requirements were confusing and misleading about water resistance. Sunscreens resistant to water must be called "water resistant" and not "waterproof" because there is a limit to the amount of time that they are effective on wet skin. Likewise, the term "sweatproof" is also not permitted. Previous labeling indicating that a sunscreen was "water resistant" or "very water resistant" did not clearly differentiate between the two. It is now required that the label state how much time can be spent in the water, for example "water resistant (40 minutes)" or "water resistant (80 minutes)" is very clear about the duration of protection. Emphasis on the duration of water resistance encourages re-application of the sunscreen at appropriate time intervals [1].

Screening for skin cancer is an effective means of secondary prevention. There is a good chance that skin cancer is curable when detected early enough. Simple excision of the lesion that can be performed as an outpatient procedure by a dermatologist is an effective means of removing the cancer and increasing survival [17]. Designated skin cancer screening days help to identify malignant lesions before they progress to more dangerous stages. Organized skin cancer screenings in Germany have resulted in a 50% reduction in melanoma mortality in the screened population, indicating the usefulness and success of mass skin cancer screenings [6].

8. Conclusion

It is predicted that 40-50% of Americans will have non-melanoma skin cancer at least once before the age of 65 [25]. The lifetime accumulation of skin damage contributes to the development of skin cancer. Skin damage incurred by natural and artificial UVR affects cellular proteins, cell signaling, damages DNA, suppresses the ability of the immune system to detect cancer cells, causes tissue damage, and cell death. Fortunately, melanoma and non-melanoma skin cancers can be prevented by reducing exposure to UVR through a number of behavioral practices. These practices include avoiding excess UV exposure, applying adequate amounts of broad spectrum sunscreen with SPF of 15 or greater and remembering to reapply when necessary, wearing protective clothing including hats and sunglasses, seeking shade, avoiding cosmetic tanning, acquisition of vitamin D from dietary sources rather than intentional UV exposure, and routinely checking the body for suspicious growths on the skin. Dietary intake of phytochemicals and antioxidants has been shown to provide systemic protection from erythema and is a good addition to the recommended sun protection program. Many of these photoprotective compounds are currently included in sunscreen formulations for added protection. It is strongly encouraged that all individuals regardless of ethnicity or skin type follow these sun protection measures to reduce skin cancer risk. Public education through awareness programs is critical for correcting social perceptions and teaching sun protective behaviors.

Author details

Lisa Passantino[1*], Max Costa[1] and Mary Matsui[2]

*Address all correspondence to: lisa.passantino@gmail.com

1 Nelson Institute of Environmental Medicine, New York University, New York, N.Y., USA

2 Estee Lauder Companies, Inc., Melville, N.Y., USA

References

[1] Food and Drug Administration. Labeling and Effectiveness Testing; Sunscreen Drug Products for Over-the-Counter Human Use. In: Health and Human Services, editor.: Federal Register; 2011. p. 35620-65.

[2] Barysch MJ, Hofbauer GF, Dummer R. Vitamin D, ultraviolet exposure, and skin cancer in the elderly. Gerontology. 2010;56(4):410-3. PubMed PMID: 20502035. Epub 2010/05/27. eng.

[3] National Cancer Institute. Skin Cancer 2012 [cited 2012 September 20, 2012]. Available from: http://www.cancer.gov/cancertopics/types/skin.

[4] American Academy of Dermatology. Don't seek the sun: Top reasons to get vitamin D from your diet [web page]. 2012 [april 12, 2011]. Available from: http://www.aad.org/media-resources/stats-and-facts/prevention-and-care/vitamin-d.

[5] National Council on Skin Cancer Prevention. A growing epidemic: skin cancer in America 2010 [updated September 21, 2012; cited 2012 September 21, 2012]. Available from: http://www.skincancerprevention.org/.

[6] Greinert R, Boniol M. Skin cancer--primary and secondary prevention (information campaigns and screening)--with a focus on children & sunbeds. Progress in biophysics and molecular biology. 2011 Dec;107(3):473-6. PubMed PMID: 21906618. Epub 2011/09/13. eng.

[7] Matsui MS, DeLeo VA. Longwave ultraviolet radiation and promotion of skin cancer. Cancer cells (Cold Spring Harbor, NY : 1989). 1991 Jan;3(1):8-12. PubMed PMID: 2025494. Epub 1991/01/01. eng.

[8] Stahl W, Heinrich U, Aust O, Tronnier H, Sies H. Lycopene-rich products and dietary photoprotection. Photochemical & photobiological sciences : Official journal of the European Photochemistry Association and the European Society for Photobiology. 2006 Feb;5(2):238-42. PubMed PMID: 16465309. Epub 2006/02/09. eng.

[9] Elmets CA, Singh D, Tubesing K, Matsui M, Katiyar S, Mukhtar H. Cutaneous photoprotection from ultraviolet injury by green tea polyphenols. Journal of the American

Academy of Dermatology. 2001 Mar;44(3):425-32. PubMed PMID: 11209110. Epub 2001/02/24. eng.

[10] Wu Y, Jia LL, Zheng YN, Xu XG, Luo YJ, Wang B, et al. Resveratrate protects human skin from damage due to repetitive ultraviolet irradiation. Journal of the European Academy of Dermatology and Venereology : JEADV. 2012 Jan 5. PubMed PMID: 22221158. Epub 2012/01/10. Eng.

[11] Afaq F, Khan N, Syed DN, Mukhtar H. Oral feeding of pomegranate fruit extract inhibits early biomarkers of UVB radiation-induced carcinogenesis in SKH-1 hairless mouse epidermis. Photochemistry and photobiology. 2010 Nov-Dec;86(6):1318-26. PubMed PMID: 20946358. Pubmed Central PMCID: PMC3016092. Epub 2010/10/16. eng.

[12] Afaq F, Mukhtar H. Botanical antioxidants in the prevention of photocarcinogenesis and photoaging. Experimental dermatology. 2006 Sep;15(9):678-84. PubMed PMID: 16881964. Epub 2006/08/03. eng.

[13] Matsui MS, Hsia A, Miller JD, Hanneman K, Scull H, Cooper KD, et al. Non-sunscreen photoprotection: antioxidants add value to a sunscreen. The journal of investigative dermatology Symposium proceedings / the Society for Investigative Dermatology, Inc [and] European Society for Dermatological Research. 2009 Aug; 14(1):56-9. PubMed PMID: 19675555. Epub 2009/08/14. eng.

[14] Gonzalez S, Gilaberte Y, Philips N, Juarranz A. Fernblock, a nutriceutical with photoprotective properties and potential preventive agent for skin photoaging and photoinduced skin cancers. International journal of molecular sciences. 2011;12(12): 8466-75. PubMed PMID: 22272084. Pubmed Central PMCID: PMC3257081. Epub 2012/01/25. eng.

[15] Agar NS, Halliday GM, Barnetson RS, Ananthaswamy HN, Wheeler M, Jones AM. The basal layer in human squamous tumors harbors more UVA than UVB fingerprint mutations: a role for UVA in human skin carcinogenesis. Proceedings of the National Academy of Sciences of the United States of America. 2004 Apr 6;101(14): 4954-9. PubMed PMID: 15041750. Pubmed Central PMCID: PMC387355. Epub 2004/03/26. eng.

[16] Halliday GM. Inflammation, gene mutation and photoimmunosuppression in response to UVR-induced oxidative damage contributes to photocarcinogenesis. Mutation research. 2005 Apr 1;571(1-2):107-20. PubMed PMID: 15748642. Epub 2005/03/08. eng.

[17] Harris RB, Alberts DS. Strategies for skin cancer prevention. International journal of dermatology. 2004 Apr;43(4):243-51. PubMed PMID: 15090005. Epub 2004/04/20. eng.

[18] Cooper KD, Baron ED, Matsui MS. Implications of UV-induced inflammation and immunomodulation. Cutis; cutaneous medicine for the practitioner. 2003 Sep;72(3 Suppl):11-5; discussion 6. PubMed PMID: 14533825. Epub 2003/10/10. eng.

[19] Geller AC, Swetter S. Primary prevention of melanoma UpToDate2012 [updated June 7, 2012; cited 2012 September 10, 2012]. Available from: http://www.uptodate.com/contents/primary-prevention-of-melanoma.

[20] Halliday GM, Rana S. Waveband and dose dependency of sunlight-induced immunomodulation and cellular changes. Photochemistry and photobiology. 2008 Jan-Feb; 84(1):35-46. PubMed PMID: 18173699. Epub 2008/01/05. eng.

[21] Camouse MM, Domingo DS, Swain FR, Conrad EP, Matsui MS, Maes D, et al. Topical application of green and white tea extracts provides protection from solar-simulated ultraviolet light in human skin. Experimental dermatology. 2009 Jun;18(6): 522-6. PubMed PMID: 19492999. Epub 2009/06/06. eng.

[22] Rossman TG, Uddin AN, Burns FJ. Evidence that arsenite acts as a cocarcinogen in skin cancer. Toxicology and applied pharmacology. 2004 Aug 1;198(3):394-404. PubMed PMID: 15276419. Epub 2004/07/28. eng.

[23] Domingo DS, Matsui MS. Photoprotection in Non-Caucasian Skin Based Therapies for Skin of Color. In: Baron E, editor.: Springer London; 2009. p. 111-34.

[24] Wang SQ, Lim HW. Current status of the sunscreen regulation in the United States: 2011 Food and Drug Administration's final rule on labeling and effectiveness testing. Journal of the American Academy of Dermatology. 2011 Oct;65(4):863-9. PubMed PMID: 21821312. Epub 2011/08/09. eng.

[25] National Cancer Institute. Cancer Trends Progress Report - 2011/2012 update. Bethesda, MD: NIH, 2012 August 2012. Report No.

[26] Planta MB. Sunscreen and melanoma: is our prevention message correct? Journal of the American Board of Family Medicine : JABFM. 2011 Nov-Dec;24(6):735-9. PubMed PMID: 22086817. Epub 2011/11/17. eng.

[27] Liu W, Wang X, Lai W, Yan T, Wu Y, Wan M, et al. Sunburn protection as a function of sunscreen application thickness differs between high and low SPFs. Photodermatology, photoimmunology & photomedicine. 2012 Jun;28(3):120-6. PubMed PMID: 22548392. Epub 2012/05/03. eng.

[28] Green AC, Williams GM, Logan V, Strutton GM. Reduced melanoma after regular sunscreen use: randomized trial follow-up. Journal of clinical oncology : official journal of the American Society of Clinical Oncology. 2011 Jan 20;29(3):257-63. PubMed PMID: 21135266. Epub 2010/12/08. eng.

[29] Gallagher RP, Rivers JK, Lee TK, Bajdik CD, McLean DI, Coldman AJ. Broad-spectrum sunscreen use and the development of new nevi in white children: A randomized controlled trial. JAMA : the journal of the American Medical Association. 2000 Jun 14;283(22):2955-60. PubMed PMID: 10865273. Epub 2000/06/24. eng.

[30] Huncharek M, Kupelnick B. Use of topical sunscreens and the risk of malignant melanoma: a meta-analysis of 9067 patients from 11 case-control studies. American jour-

nal of public health. 2002 Jul;92(7):1173-7. PubMed PMID: 12084704. Pubmed Central PMCID: PMC1447210. Epub 2002/06/27. eng.

[31] Autier P, Boniol M, Dore JF. Sunscreen use and increased duration of intentional sun exposure: still a burning issue. International journal of cancer Journal international du cancer. 2007 Jul 1;121(1):1-5. PubMed PMID: 17415716. Epub 2007/04/07. eng.

[32] Schalka S, dos Reis VM, Cuce LC. The influence of the amount of sunscreen applied and its sun protection factor (SPF): evaluation of two sunscreens including the same ingredients at different concentrations. Photodermatology, photoimmunology & photomedicine. 2009 Aug;25(4):175-80. PubMed PMID: 19614894. Epub 2009/07/21. eng.

[33] USEPA. UV Index 2012 [updated December 7, 2011; cited 2012 September 23, 2012]. Available from: http://www.epa.gov/sunwise/uvindex.html.

[34] American Academy of Dermatology. Indoor Tanning 2012 [cited 2012 September 24, 2012]. Available from: http://www.aad.org/media-resources/stats-and-facts/prevention-and-care/indoor-tanning.

[35] National Council on Skin Cancer Prevention. Indoor Tanning Beds 2012 [updated September 23, 2012; cited 2012 September 23, 2012]. Available from: http://www.skincancerprevention.org/skin-cancer/tanning-beds.

[36] Ibiebele TI, van der Pols JC, Hughes MC, Marks GC, Williams GM, Green AC. Dietary pattern in association with squamous cell carcinoma of the skin: a prospective study. The American journal of clinical nutrition. 2007 May;85(5):1401-8. PubMed PMID: 17490979. Epub 2007/05/11. eng.

[37] Katiyar SK, Matsui MS, Elmets CA, Mukhtar H. Polyphenolic antioxidant (-)-epigallocatechin-3-gallate from green tea reduces UVB-induced inflammatory responses and infiltration of leukocytes in human skin. Photochemistry and photobiology. 1999 Feb;69(2):148-53. PubMed PMID: 10048310. Epub 1999/02/27. eng.

[38] Eberlein-Konig B, Placzek M, Przybilla B. Protective effect against sunburn of combined systemic ascorbic acid (vitamin C) and d-alpha-tocopherol (vitamin E). Journal of the American Academy of Dermatology. 1998 Jan;38(1):45-8. PubMed PMID: 9448204. Epub 1998/02/03. eng.

[39] Stahl W, Heinrich U, Jungmann H, Sies H, Tronnier H. Carotenoids and carotenoids plus vitamin E protect against ultraviolet light-induced erythema in humans. The American journal of clinical nutrition. 2000 Mar;71(3):795-8. PubMed PMID: 10702175. Epub 2000/03/04. eng.

[40] Wu Y, Matsui MS, Chen JZ, Jin X, Shu CM, Jin GY, et al. Antioxidants add protection to a broad-spectrum sunscreen. Clinical and experimental dermatology. 2011 Mar; 36(2):178-87. PubMed PMID: 20804506. Epub 2010/09/02. eng.

[41] Rizwan M, Rodriguez-Blanco I, Harbottle A, Birch-Machin MA, Watson RE, Rhodes LE. Tomato paste rich in lycopene protects against cutaneous photodamage in hu-

mans in vivo: a randomized controlled trial. The British journal of dermatology. 2011 Jan;164(1):154-62. PubMed PMID: 20854436. Epub 2010/09/22. eng.

[42] Williams S, Tamburic S, Lally C. Eating chocolate can significantly protect the skin from UV light. Journal of cosmetic dermatology. 2009 Sep;8(3):169-73. PubMed PMID: 19735513. Epub 2009/09/09. eng.

[43] Kopcke W, Krutmann J. Protection from sunburn with beta-Carotene--a meta-analysis. Photochemistry and photobiology. 2008 Mar-Apr;84(2):284-8. PubMed PMID: 18086246. Epub 2007/12/19. eng.

[44] Druesne-Pecollo N, Latino-Martel P, Norat T, Barrandon E, Bertrais S, Galan P, et al. Beta-carotene supplementation and cancer risk: a systematic review and metaanalysis of randomized controlled trials. International journal of cancer Journal international du cancer. 2010 Jul 1;127(1):172-84. PubMed PMID: 19876916. Epub 2009/10/31. eng.

[45] Melamed ML, Michos ED, Post W, Astor B. 25-hydroxyvitamin D levels and the risk of mortality in the general population. Archives of internal medicine. 2008 Aug 11;168(15):1629-37. PubMed PMID: 18695076. Pubmed Central PMCID: PMC2677029. Epub 2008/08/13. eng.

[46] Holick MF. The vitamin D epidemic and its health consequences. The Journal of nutrition. 2005 Nov;135(11):2739S-48S. PubMed PMID: 16251641. Epub 2005/10/28. eng.

[47] National Institutes of Health Office of Dietary Supplements. Dietary supplement fact sheet: Vitamin D 2012 [cited 2012 September 27, 2012]. Available from: http://ods.od.nih.gov/factsheets/VitaminD-HealthProfessional/.

[48] Gilchrest BA. The a-B-C-ds of sensible sun protection. Skin therapy letter. 2008 Jun; 13(5):1-5. PubMed PMID: 18648712. Epub 2008/07/24. eng.

[49] Freedman DM, Looker AC, Chang SC, Graubard BI. Prospective study of serum vitamin D and cancer mortality in the United States. Journal of the National Cancer Institute. 2007 Nov 7;99(21):1594-602. PubMed PMID: 17971526. Epub 2007/11/01. eng.

[50] American Academy of Dermatology and AAD Foundation. Position Statement on Vitamin D. 2010 December 22, 2010. Report No.

[51] USEPA. Don't Fry Day 2012 [updated July 13, 2012; cited 2012 September 27, 2012]. Available from: http://www.epa.gov/sunwise/dfd.html.

Chapter 8

Photodynamic Therapy for Non-Melanoma Skin Cancer

Cintia Teles de Andrade, Natalia Mayumi Inada,
Dora Patricia Ramirez,
Vanderlei Salvador Bagnato and Cristina Kurachi

Additional information is available at the end of the chapter

http://dx.doi.org/10.5772/55242

1. Introduction

Skin cancer shows the highest incidence worldwide, among all cancer types, and is mainly classified in melanoma and non-melanoma subtypes.

Clinical evaluation through dermatoscopy is a widely performed practice, and it is a noninvasive technique that uses magnification to allow better visualization of the structures immediately below the skin surface. This examination provides morphological criteria for distinguishing various lesions types.

Histopathology is considered the gold standard for diagnosis of skin cancer and other dermal disorders. These two exams together, as well as the location and extent of the injury will determine the choice of treatment.

Treatments such as surgical excision, cryotherapy, topical application of imiquimod cream and 5-fluorouracil cream, and radiotherapy are commonly chosen based on the depth and extension of the lesions. Limitations and side-effects of the conventional therapies motivate the development of other techniques. Photodynamic therapy (PDT) is presented as an alternative treatment for basal cell carcinoma (BCC).

PDT has proven to be effective with an excellent cosmetic outcome in the treatment of superficial BCC (sBCC), and recently published guidelines state that PDT can be an effective and reliable treatment option for the treatment of thin nodular BCC (nBCC), and actinic keratosis (AK) [1]. It is a technically simple noninvasive procedure that offers patients at least equal efficacy and a high level of satisfaction and other cosmetic outcome when compared with cryotherapy and topical treatments [2].

The term *field cancerisation* or *field effect* is frequently used to describe extensive UV damage with recurrent, multiple AK, and the presence of a tissue with genetically altered cells is a risk factor for cancer development, representing an indication for topical PDT [3].

Our group has extensive experience in clinical PDT in various areas of medicine as in gynecology [4], infectious disease [5], and in particular in dermatology [6-7], and in this chapter will be discussed the advantagens and indications of the PDT for non-melanoma skin cancer and others conditions.

2. Basic principles

Photosensitized oxidations have been of interest to chemists and biologists since Raab's discovery that microorganisms are killed by light in the presence of oxygen and sensitizing dyes [1].

The mechanism of action of photosensitizers is divide in two different types and generally involves direct oxidation by hydrogen peroxide (H_2O_2), superoxide anion radical (O^2 •) and hydroxyl radical (•OH) (Type I reaction) of biological targets (membranes, proteins, and DNA), as well as oxidation mediated by singlet oxygen ($^1O_2$) that is mainly formed through energy transfer from triplet states to molecular oxygen (Type II reaction) [8-10].

The generation of Reactive Oxygen Species (ROS), in both types I or II, are dependent on the uptake of a photosensitizing dye, often a haematoporphyrin derivative, by the tumor or other abnormal target tissue, the subsequent irradiation of the tumor with visible light of an appropriate wavelength, and the presence of molecular oxygen [10]. An adequate concentration of molecular oxygen is also needed for tissue damage. If any one of these components is absent, there is no photodynamic response, and the overall effectiveness therefore requires careful planning of both tissue photosensitization and light dosimetry.

PDT response is induced by more than one cellular mechanism. A photosensitiser can directly target the tumor cells, inducing necrosis or apoptosis (Figure 1) [11]. Alternatively, tumor necrosis can be induced by damaging its vasculature [12].

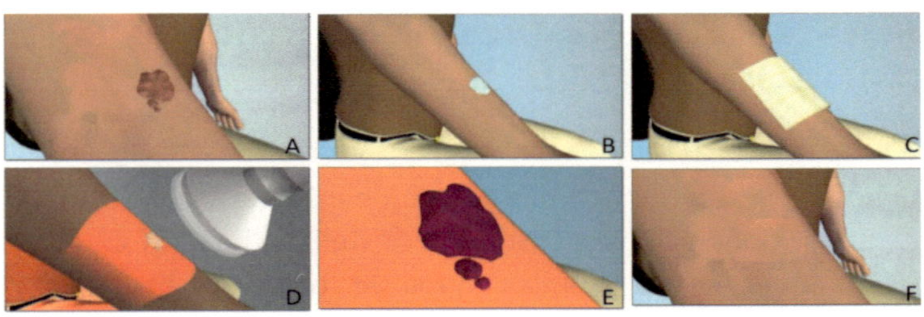

Figure 1. Treatment procedure for topical PDT. A) Skin cancer lesion; B) Cream application (MAL or ALA); C) Occlusion of the lesion; D) Illumination; E) Inflammation and tecidual necrosis; F) Curative

http://dx.doi.org/10.5772/55242

3. Photosensitizers

The photosensitizers are by definition any substance capable of making an organism, a cell or a substance photosensitive, with the photo-excitation of several types of molecules through energy transfer processes. Porphyrins, chlorines, phthalocyanines are the three main groups of studied photosensitizers (PSs). Porphyrins are the most frequently used PSs, but its systemic administration shows an important adverse factor in Dermatology. Due to the high accumulation and slow drug clearance from the skin, porphyrins lead to prolonged photosensitization of the organism after application [13]. The commercially available compounds promote a patient photosensitization that lasts for 4-6 weeks. These PDT patients must avoid sun exposure during this period, otherwise skin burns can be induced. This is the major drawback for indication of PDT in Dermatology.

The development of an ideal PDT sensitizer is still a major challenge since several characteristics must be contemplated. Main characteristics are: a) photo-excitation with red-infrared light; b) low dark toxicity; c) high stability; d) rapid clearance from the body; e) high affinity to abnormal cells (selectivity), and f) high rate of ROS production.

The main reactions observed with biological molecules are lipid peroxidation (cholesterol), cycloaddition (2 +2)-protein (reaction with tryptophan) and Diels-Alder reactions upon molecules in the genetic code (guanine). Porphyrin derivatives are indeed intersting molecules. Compounds such as porphyrins and chlorins, have the characteristics suitable for use in PDT due to the high molar extinction coefficients, high absorptivities in the region of the "therapeutic window" (600-800 nm) and with high quantum yields of singlet oxygen production.

PDT can also be performed with topical use of 5-aminolevulinic acid (5-ALA) or by its ester methyl-aminolevulinate (MAL), which are both precursors in the biosynthesis of protoporphyrin IX (PpIX), a native photosensitizing compound that accumulates in the cells. Protoporphyrin IX (PpIX) has absorption peaks at 505, 540, 580 and 630 nm.

These compounds must be stored in the form of hydrochloride (R-NH3Cl), since in its neutral form rapidly suffers degradation. Studies including a few with 5-year follow-up have shown that ALA and MAL-PDT are comparable to other modalities in the treatment of superficial lesions considering their efficacy and with equivalent or superior cosmetic outcomes [14-15]. ALA and MAL are not photosensitizers, they are precursors of endogenous PpIX (Figure 2).

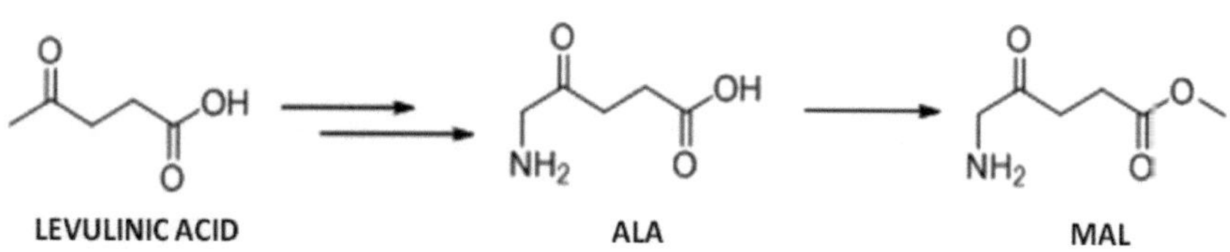

Figure 2. Molecular structures of the PpIX precursors.

The fundamental difference between ALA and its methyl ester (MAL) is the more hydrophobic character of the MAL. Thus, MAL can better penetrate through the cell membranes and more easily reaches the deepest epidermal layers. However, the biosynthesis of protoporphyrin IX production from MAL is slightly more time consuming because of the need of hydrolysis of this compound.

Chlorin is a photosensitizer indicated in the cases of PDT using *i.v.* medication. It is derived from natural or synthetic tetrapyrroles, and an important feature is their strong light absorption in the spectral region usually above 660 nm. A significant advantage of PDT using chorins is the reduced duration of cutaneous photosensitivity as compared with other photosensitizers [16].

Recently, eight new chlorins with amphiphilic properties were synthesized from PpIX. Biological studies of some of these new chlorins indicate the great potential of these compounds as photosensitizers in PDT [17].

4. Dosimetry

Distinct light sources can be used for PDT. For therapy, the tissue must be irradiated with light at appropriate wavelengths (within the absorption spectrum of porphyrins). The porphyrins exhibit a very typical absorption spectrum with the highest peak at approximately 405 nm, called the Soret-band. Other lower absorption peaks, the Q-bands, are centered at 510, 545, 580 and 630 nm. The absorption band at 630 nm is preferentially used for irradiation since light at the red spectrum results in a higher skin penetration. Lasers and incoherent light sources (lamps, light-emitting-diode – LED – lamps and, intense pulsed light – IPL) have been used. When endoscopic applications are necessary, the activating light has to be delivered through optical fibers, and laser systems are the best option for this purpose. For dermatological application, incoherent light sources are more attractive, due to the possibility of distinct emission geometries and comparable lower cost [18-20].

The therapeutic efficacy of PDT involves administration to the patient of a photosensitizer or a pro-drug, a waiting time to allow adequate concentration of the sensitizer molecules in the tumor, and irradiation of the target tissue with a proper wavelength to activate the photosensitizer generating cytotoxic products, mainly the singlet-oxygen. To trigger cell death, a minimum number of singlet-oxygen molecules have to be produced. The minimal energy dose required to achieve the irreversible tissue damage, resulting in tumor necrosis, is called the threshold dose.

The energy dose is given in Joules per centimeter square (J/cm^2), that is the amount of energy delivered to the tissue per unit area. Light intensity is measured in Watts (W) and corresponds to the energy per unit of time. One W corresponds to 1 J per 1 second. Irradiance is measured in Watts per centimeter square (W/cm^2), representing the light power delivered to the tissue surface [19, 21-22]. A simple relationship between light dose (D), irradiance (I) and time (t) is:

$$D = I.t \tag{1}$$

Energy doses delivered for the treatment of basal cell carcinoma and other dermal conditions are in the range of 40-150 J/cm^2 and with irradiances of 40-150 mW/cm^2. The PDT illumination of a BCC lesion of 2 cm of diameter, for example, may be of 8 to 20 minutes, depending on the chosen irradiation parameters.

5. Clinical results

Nonmelanoma skin cancer is the most frequent one in the world population. Currently, therapeutic options are surgical ressection, electrocoagulation, curettage, cryotherapy, immunomodulating agents, cytotoxic agents, chemotherapy, PDT, among others. PDT is a noninvasive technique with excellent cosmetic outcome, well tolerated by patients and with good healing results, when used for the initial stages of cancer lesions. Different studies show the technique effectiveness for BCC (Figure 3 and 4), presenting curative rates ranging from 52.2% to 100% [7, 23-28].

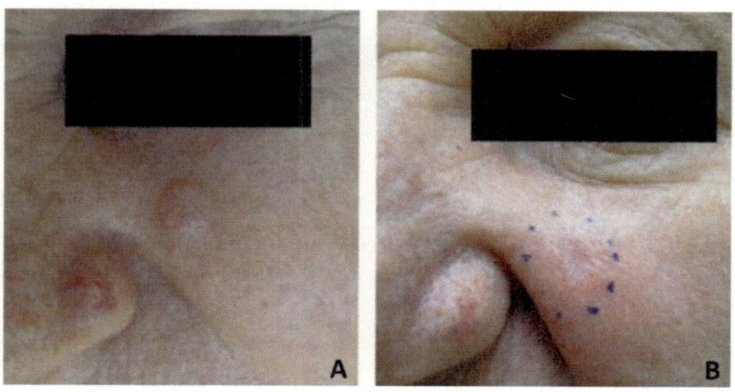

Figure 3. Nodular BCC before (A) and 30 days after (B) PDT, treated with MAL 20% in 2 sessions and dose of 100J/cm^2

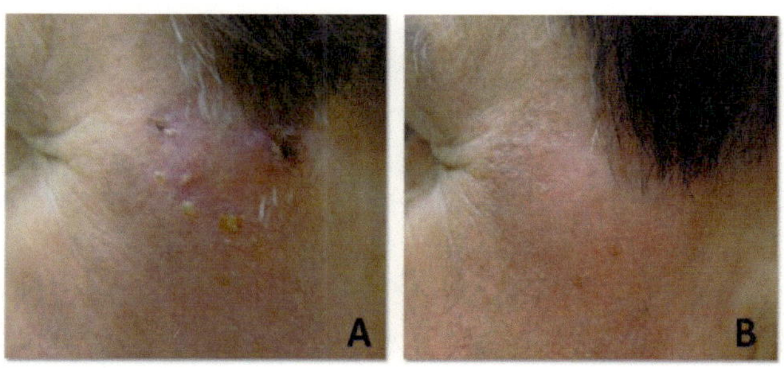

Figure 4. Superficial BCC before (A) and 30 days after (B) PDT, treated with MAL 20% in 2 sessions and dose of 100J/cm^2

Wolf et al., (1993), in their study treated 70 different lesions – superficial BCC, actinic keratosis (AK), nodular-ulcerative BCC, squamous cell carcinoma (SCC) and melanoma – using ALA cream, with dose of 30J/cm^2 for superficial BCC and AK and 100 J/cm^2-300 J/cm^2 for other lesions. Results at 12 months showed complete response for AK, 36 of 37 superficial BCC lesions showed good responses, 5 of 6 SCC, 8 cutaneous metastases of malignant melanoma were therapeutic failures and other lesions showed a partial response after treatment [23]. In the study by Calzavara (1994), which also included several lesions (AK, BCC, nodular BCC, pigmented BCC and SCC), all treated with ALA 20%, there were complete response in 100% for BCC and AK cases, decreasing to 80% in nodular lesions. Other treated lesions exhibited low curative rate when evaluated 30 days after treatment. These curative rates decreased to 86.9% in BCC and 50% in nodular BCC in the clinical follow-up done for 29 months [27]. According to the study of Souza et al., (2009), after evaluating 20 patients (showing difficulties, impediment high risk or rejection of surgical procedure) with BCC and Bowen's disease (BD) treated with ALA 20%, irradiated at wavelength of 630 nm and doses of 100 to 300 J\cm^2, showed that, after 1 session, presented curative rates of 91.2% at three months and 57.7% at sixty months [7].

Horn et al., (2003), treated 94 patients with 108 superficial, nodular and mixed BCC lesion with difficult to treatment (resulting scars from reconstructive surgery extensive, interfering with normal function of eyelids or lips, or postoperative infections), finding complete response after 3 months in 92% of superficial BCC and 87% of nodular BCC. The cosmetic outcome was evaluated as excellent or good by investigators in 76% of the lesion after 3 months follow-up, increasing to 85% at 12 months and 94% at 24 months follow-up [29].

A recent study comparing CO_2 laser ablation *versus* PDT in immunocompetent patients with multiple AK concluded that both treatments were effective in reduction of AK, but PDT seems to be superior in terms of reduction of the affected area and overall satisfaction by patients and clinicians [30].

Foley et al., (2009), conducted a double-blind and placebo-controlled study in primary lesion of nodular BCC (up to 5 mm in depth) in two medical centers. MAL was used at concentration of 160 mg/g cream or placebo cream, with three hours of occlusion. The light source applied was in the range of 570-670 nm, with an irradiance of 50-200 mW/cm^2 and dose of 75 J/cm^2. In total, 131 patients with 150 lesions were included in the study, 66 patients with 75 lesions were treated with MAL cream and 65 patients with 75 lesions with placebo cream. The treatment was developed in cycles. The first cycle was conducted in two sessions, with one week interval between sessions. If the response was partial (≤50% reduction in greatest diameter) after 3 months follow-up, the second cycle was initiated with two more sessions with one week interval, and monitoring the patient for six months. If the answer was not complete, the responsible medical team indicated the patient for surgical procedure. The complete response after 6 months follow-up, with MAL was of 73% (55/75 lesions) versus 27% (20/75 lesions) with placebo. The response decreases in larger lesion (≥ 10mm in diameter and ≥ 1mm of baseline depth). The cosmetic outcome of the lesions treated with MAL-PDT was good or excellent in 98% of the cases [24].

Caekelberg et al., (2009), observed the PDT result after 6 months in 90 patients with superficial BCC of approximately diameter 10 mm. The complete response rate was of 88.1% with cosmetic outcome qualified as excellent in 96.25% of patients [25].

Interesting results were achieved in the study of Surrenti et al., (2008), where they evaluated the PDT response in nodular and superficial BCC. In this study, 118 lesions were treated in 69 patients, located at the chest, face, head, neck and limbs. Superficial BCC were diagnosed in 94 lesions and 24 showed nodular BCC lesions, confirmed by histology. Complete response was obtained in 84/94 (89.4%) at superficial BCC, and in 12/23 (52.2%) at nodular BCC, when evaluated at 30 days after the second session. The cosmetic outcome was evaluated as excellent in 83% of cases and good in the remaining 17% of the cases [28].

Szeimies et al., (2008), compared PDT with surgery to treat superficial BCC between 8-20 mm size, in 196 patients with 234 lesions. The lesions treated with MAL 160 mg/g, in two sessions, showed a curative rate of 92.2% compared to 99.2% of the lesions treated with surgery, when assessed after 3 months of treatment. After 12 months, the cosmetic outcome was considered by the investigator as good or excellent in 92.8% of patients treated with PDT versus 51.2% of patients treated with surgery. The recurrence was 9.3% in comparison with 0% for lesions treated with PDT and surgery, respectively [26]. In nodular BCC treatment curative rates, after three months, of 91% with PDT versus 98% with surgery were obtained. After 12 months, 96% of lesions treated with surgery showed complete response compared to the 83% of the lesions treated with PDT. This study was performed on 97 patients with 105 lesions, all confirmed by histopathology [31].

In a recent study, (2012), was compared PDT with surgery, in 72 patients with 94 lesions superficial and nodular BCC with a maximum 3 mm thick. The patients were separated into two groups according to their choice of treatment, being 48 lesions treated with PDT and 46 with surgery. After 3 months, the curative rate was 95.83 % with PDT versus 95.65% with surgery. The recurrence rate was, after 12 months, 4.16% for PDT compared to 4.34% for surgery [32].

Basset-Seguin et al., (2008) presented results comparing PDT with cryotherapy in 118 patients. The authors used PDT protocol with MAL and two sessions separated by 7 days. The complete clinical response, after 3 months of treatment, was of 97% with cryotherapy versus 95% with PDT. Comparing the cosmetic outcome, they obtained excellent and good response in 54% versus 93% with cryotherapy and PDT, respectively [33].

Another multicenter study made by Aguilar et al., (2010), compared imiquimod and PDT with surgery in the treatment of 54 Bowen's disease lesions (63%) and 32 superficial BCC lesions (37%). After 24 months, the curative rate was of 97.5% for surgery, 89.5% for PDT, and 87.5% for imiquimod. The surgery cost was approximately twice the value when compared to PDT [34].

The differences between the curative results obtained in the different studies is mainly due to the distinct treament protocols: a) different lesion selection criteria (diameter, length, thickness, site, previous treatment); b) no standardization of the pre-PDT procedures (shaving, curettage, scarification); c) distinct drugs (ALA, MAL); d) different cream incubation times (2, 3 and 4 hours); e) distinct irradiation parameters; f) number of sessions; g) different treatment evaluation times (1, 3 or 6 months) and time to evaluate recurrence (6 months, 1, 3, 5 or 10 years) [35]. However, thicker lesions and nodular BCC present lower curative rates when compared to superficial BCC [26, 28, 33, 35]. Furthermore, pretreatment procedures as shaving or curettage [29], and multiple sessions [15, 36] can increase positive response to PDT [35].

PDT may present some adverse reactions such as photosensitivity, infection, erythema, edema, pain, among others [24, 37]. In topical PDT, the photosensitive drug is localized in lesion and consumed after irradiation. Reports of local photosensitivity after treatment are scarce, and when present, are present in the following 24 hours after irradiation. The systemic PDT, on the other hand, has a longer photosensitivity time [23]. Infection is a complication that almost does not occur due to the proven action of PDT for microbiological control [37]. However, some factors may predispose to this occurrence, such as, diabetes, peripheral vascular disease, and others. In a study by Wolfe et al., (2007), 700 AK lesions were treated with PDT and only 4 cases of cellulitis were reported, but easily controled by antibiotic therapy [38]. Changes in pigmentation, hyper and hypopigmentations, are reported in literature as approximately 1% of all adverse reactions [37]. The pain may be present during irradiation or within 7 days after treatment. In the study by Morton et al., (2001), only one third of patients treated had pain qualified between moderate and severe [39]. In the experiment by Ibbotson et al., (2011), during 9 years, different lesions were trated with topical PDT, 16% of patients showed severe pain and 50% moderate pain [37]. In a multicenter, randomized, controlled and open study, comparing PDT with surgery it was found that for PDT, 37/100 (37%) of patients had an adverse reaction versus 14/96 (14,6%) of patients treated with surgery. For PDT, photosensitivity reaction, which includes sensations of discomfort, burning and erythema was the most frequent, these reactions were of mild to moderate intensity and easily treated. For surgery, the more expected reaction was infection, that occured in 5 of the 14 patients and requiring the use of systemic antibiotics for two weeks [26].

PDT can be associated with other treatment techniques, such as surgery, as described by Willey et al., (2009). In this study, surgical ressection was associated with PDT with 20% ALA for recurrence prevention. The PDT protocol consisted of an hour of inoculation and illumination with a light source with wavelength at 417 nm during 1000 seconds (irradiance of 10 mW/cm^2). The PDT cycles were repeated every 1-2 months for two years. In the first year after first PDT session, average reduction of lesions appearance was around 80%, reaching values of 95% reduction by the end of the second year [40].

The recurrence of BCC lesions when treated with traditional techniques has been estimated of 36% after one year of treatment, 61% after two years and 18% after 6 to 10 years of treatment [41]. For PDT, several studies have been published assessing the lesion recurrence after 1 to 5 [7, 15, 33, 42-43], 6 and 10 years of treatment [44].

In the clinical study done by Souza et al., (2009), the treated patients were monitored (or followed) for 60 months. The lesion recurrence was presented in 11/26 lesions (42.3%), the recurrence depending on the lesion types were of 2/5 for nodular BCC, 2/6 for superficial BCC and 7/15 to Bowen's disease [7].

According to Basset-Seguin et al., (2008), recurrence after 5 years of PDT in 103 superficial BCC, using MAL, was of 22%, all present in the first three years after treatment. This rate is comparable with the one obtained in patients treated with cryotherapy [33]. In the study by Mosterd et al., (2008), 83 nodular BCC were treated with 20% ALA-PDT and fractionated irradiation with a total dose of 150J/cm². A recurrence rate of 30.3% were obatined after 3 years. In this study, the thicknesses of 78 lesions were measured and an increased failure risk was present in thicker lesions, over 1.3 mm (42.2%), when compared to the thinner ones (15.5%) [42]. In a study by Rhodes et al., (2004), 53 nodular BCC, treated with MAL-PDT, a recurrence rate of 14% was observed after 5 years of treatment. A recurrence in 5/40 lesions treated with one PDT session and 2/9 treated with two PDT sessions, occuring especially in the first two years of treatment. When compared with surgery, the recurrence rate decreases to 4% [31]. Similar results were reported in a study of Szeimies et al., (2008), with recurrence rates for PDT of 9.3% and 0% for surgery, in a follow-up of 12 months [24].

Another study evaluating 157 BCC lesions (111 superficial BCC, 40 nodular BCC and 6 histology missing) in 90 patients treated with two sessions of MAL-PDT, recurrence rates estimated of 7% in the first 3 months, 19% in 6 months, 27% in 12 months and 31% in 24 months after treatment were obtained. When comparing recurrence rates at 12 months of nodular and superficial BCC the rates were of 28% versus 13%, respectively [43].

Christensen et al, (2009), classified 60 BCC (24 nodular BCC e 36 superficial BCC), according to size, as smaller than 1 cm, between 1-2 cm and larger than 2 cm. All lesions were curetted and DMSO was applied at the site for 5 min, then 20% ALA cream was applied and kept in position for 3 hours. PDT procedure was performed in one or two sessions. After 6 years follow up, 43/53 (81%) of lesions still showed complete response. Five patients were excluded for presenting partial response to treatment in the first three months and two patients died at the onset of follow-up period from causes unrelated to study. The recurrences were present before three years, with two thirds of these presented in the first 12 months. The average age of the patients with recurrence was of 76 y.o. for men and 77 for women. Considering lesion size, no statistical difference was observed because only one lesion measured more than 2cm [45]. The follow up of 10 years, showed an overall curative rate of 75%, 60% for lesions treated with one session and 81% for two sessions, all recurrence cases were presented in the first three years [44].

Multiple factors have been associated with recurrence in the different studies. Few sessions are associated with high recurrence rates. One PDT session is the major factor for treatment failure [33, 44, 46]. In the study by Soler et al., (2001), 33 lesions presented recurrence, 29 of them treated with a single session and four treated with two sessions [46]. Similar data were found by Christensen et.al., (2009), where 43/53 lesions remained disease-free; 63% after one treatment session and 91% after two treatment session [45].

Size and thickness are factors that also affect lesion recurrence. The study by Mosterd et al., (2008), presented recurrence rates of 42% in the lesions with ≥ 1,3 mm thickness, and of 15.5% for lesions ≤ 1,3 mm. Horn et al., (2003), showed an increased recurrence associated with lesion size when evaluated 24 months after treatment. Lesions of 0-15 mm presented 4% recurrence, increasing to 16% in lesions of 16-30mm and greater than 30mm, 33% [29].

Author and type of study	Treatment Procedure	Study size	Result
Soler et al., (2001) Retrospective study [46]	MAL 160 mg/g Preparation prior PDT: Debulking procedure was performed on all nodular.	Total: 310 lesion 131 sBCC 82 nBCC ≤ 2mm thickness 86 nBCC ≥2mm thickness	3 mo, Complete Response 91% sBCC 93% nBCC thin 86% nBCC thick 11% Recurrence at 35 mo
Horn et al., (2003) Open-label study [29]	MAL 160 mg/g cream Pre-PDT procedure in nodular lesions: Shaving.	Total:108 lesions 49 sBCC 52 nBCC 7 mixed BCC	3 mo, Complete Response 92% sBCC 87% nBCC 57% mixed BCC 9% Recurrence at 12 mo 18% Recurrence at 24 mo
Basset –Seguin et al., (2008) Randomized, comparative, multicenter study [33]	MAL cream Preparation pre-PDT: Surface debridement	Total 201 lesions 103 sBCC with PDT 98 sBCC with cryotherapy	3 mo, Complete response 97% PDT 95% Cryotherapy Recurrence at 5 years 22% PDT 20% Cryotherapy
Szeimies et al., (2008) multicentre, randomised, controlled, open study [26]	MAL 160 mg/g cream Preparation pre-PDT: remove scales and crust of lesion surface	Total 196 lesions 100 sBCC with PDT 96 sBCC with surgery.	3 mo Complete response 92.2% PDT 99.2% Surgery Recurrence at 12 mo 9.3% PDT 0% Surgery
Christensen et al., (2009) and (2012) Prospective study study [44-45]	ALA 20% DMSO 99% Preparation pre-PDT: curettage	Total:60 lesion 24 sBCC 36 nBCC	3 mo, Complete response 92% total lesion 72 mo, Complete response 81% total lesion 120mo, Complete response 75% total lesion
Lindberg-Larsen et al., (2012) Retrospective study [43]	MAL 160 mg/g Preparation pre-PDT: Superficial lesions were debrided. Nodular lesions were curetted	Total: 157 lesion 111 sBCC 40 nBCC 6 unknown	3 mo Complete response 93% lesion Recurrence at 12 mo: nBCC 28% sBCC 13%
Cosgarea et al., (2012) prospective, comparative, controlled, clinical study [32]	ALA 20% cream Preparation pre-PDT: remove scales and crusts of lesion surface	Total 94 sBCC 48 lesions with PDT 46 lesions with Surgery	3 mo Complete response 95.83% PDT 95.65% Surgery

http://dx.doi.org/10.5772/55242

Author and type of study	Treatment Procedure	Study size	Result
			Recurrence at 12 mo 4.16% PDT 4.34% Surgery

Table 1. Study results of topical PDT for non melanoma skin cancer

A higher recurrence rate is also present at nodular BCC, when compared to the superficial BCC [43, 46]. Age can be a factor that increases the lesion recurrence treated with PDT, other potential factors are gender and lesion site [43].

6. Non-oncological and off-label pdt applications in dermatology

PDT is already approved for the treatment of actinic keratosis and basal cell carcinoma. Off-label uses for PDT have been indicated for several dermatological conditions such as photo-damaged skin, scleroderma, warts, cutaneous leishmaniosis, psoriasis, cutaneous T-cell lymphoma and acne [20, 47]. Infectious disease has the potential to become one of the main indications of PDT in Dermatology. The microbiological control of bacteria, fungi and protozoa in infected lesions has been presented [48-51]. Onychomicosis is one of the new indications, where PDT presents good results even in cases where the antifungal systemic therapy failured (Paula-da-Silva, A. et al., Fast elimination of onychomycosis by hematoporphyrin derivative-photodynamic therapy. Accepted by Photodiagnosis and Photodynamic Therapy on December2012).

7. Final considerations

PDT is a noninvasive technique, with few potential adverse reactions, that presents good curative rates and excellent cosmetic outcome. It may be chosen as a first option for patients with small lesions of nonmelanoma skin cancer, especially the ones in complex sites for surgical ressection or in high risk patients.

PDT protocols and customized dosimetry for each target skin lesion still need to be defined. The development of new PDT drugs and delivery systems has the potential of increasing the curative rates of the present protocols. Instrumentation of light sources designed to adapt the emission geometry to the anatomical site characteristics is also important to improve PDT performance in cancer treatment.

The local treatment of infected lesions and cosmetics are PDT indications that have been fastly increasing. New protocols and drugs have been investigated, as well as new light devices developed, making PDT in Dermatology an exciting and growing field.

Author details

Cintia Teles de Andrade[1*], Natalia Mayumi Inada[1], Dora Patricia Ramirez[1,2], Vanderlei Salvador Bagnato[1] and Cristina Kurachi[1]

*Address all correspondence to: cintya_teles@yahoo.com.br

1 Biophotonics Laboratory, Institute of Physics of São Carlos – University of São Paulo (USP), São Paulo, Brazil

2 PPGBiotec, Federal University of São Carlos (UFSCAR), São Paulo, Brazil

References

[1] Braathen, L. R, Szeimies, R. M, Basset-seguin, N, Bissonnette, R, Foley, P, Pariser, D, et al. Guidelines on the use of photodynamic therapy for nonmelanoma skin cancer: An international consensus. J Am Acad Dermatol. (2007). Jan;, 56(1), 125-43.

[2] Lehmann, P. Methyl aminolaevulinate-photodynamic therapy: a review of clinical trials in the treatment of actinic keratoses and nonmelanoma skin cancer. Brit J Dermatol. (2007). May;, 156(5), 793-801.

[3] Braakhuis BJMTabor MP, Kummer JA, Leemans CR, Brakenhoff RH. A genetic explanation of Slaughter's concept of field cancerization: Evidence and clinical implications. Cancer Res. (2003). Apr 15;, 63(8), 1727-30.

[4] Inada, N. M. da Costa MM, Guimaraes OCC, Ribeiro ED, Kurachi C, Quintana SM, et al. Photodiagnosis and treatment of condyloma acuminatum using 5-aminolevulinic acid and homemade devices. Photodiagn Photodyn. (2012). Mar;, 9(1), 60-8.

[5] Bagnato, V. S, Kurachi, C, Ferreira, J, Sankarankutty, A. K, & Zucoloto, S. de Castro e Silva O. New photonic technologies for the treatment and diagnosis of hepatic diseases: an overview of the experimental work performed in collaboration, between Physics Institute of Sao Carlos and Ribeirao Preto Faculty of Medicine of the University of Sao Paulo. Acta Cir Bras. (2006). Suppl , 1, 3-11.

[6] Souza, C. S, Felicio, L. B, Arruda, D, Ferreira, J, Kurachi, C, & Bagnato, V. S. Systemic photodynamic therapy as an option for keratoacanthoma centrifugum marginatum treatment. J Eur Acad Dermatol Venereol. (2009). Jan;, 23(1), 101-2.

[7] Souza, C. S. Felicio LBA, Ferreira J, Kurachi C, Bentley MVB, Tedesco AC, et al. Long-term follow-up of topical aminolaevulinic acid photodynamic therapy diode laser single session for non-melanoma skin cancer. Photodiagn Photodyn. (2009). Sep-Dec;6(3-4):207-13., 5.

[8] Halliwell, B. Protection against tissue damage in vivo by desferrioxamine: what is its mechanism of action? Free Radic Biol Med. (1989). , 7(6), 645-51.

[9] Foote, C. S. Mechanisms of Photosensitized Oxidation- There Are Several Different Types of Photosensitized Oxidation Which May Be Important in Biological Systems. Science. (1968). , 162(3857), 963.

[10] Lam, M, Oleinick, N. L, & Nieminen, A. L. Photodynamic therapy-induced apoptosis in epidermoid carcinoma cells- Reactive oxygen species and mitochondrial inner membrane permeabilization. J Biol Chem. (2001). Dec 14;, 276(50), 47379-86.

[11] Oleinick, N. L, Morris, R. L, & Belichenko, T. The role of apoptosis in response to photodynamic therapy: what, where, why, and how. Photoch Photobio Sci. (2002). Jan;, 1(1), 1-21.

[12] Henderson, B. W, & Dougherty, T. J. How Does Photodynamic Therapy Work. Photochem Photobiol. (1992). Jan;, 55(1), 145-57.

[13] Morton, C. A, Brown, S. B, Collins, S, Ibbotson, S, Jenkinson, H, Kurwa, H, et al. Guidelines for topical photodynamic therapy: report of a workshop of the British Photodermatology Group. Brit J Dermatol. (2002). Apr;, 146(4), 552-67.

[14] Fotinos, N, Campo, M. A, Popowycz, F, Gurny, R, & Lange, N. aminolevulinic acid derivatives in photomedicine: Characteristics, application and perspectives. Photochem Photobiol. (2006). Jul-Aug;, 82(4), 994-1015.

[15] Rhodes, L. E, De Rie, M. A, Leifsdottir, R, Yu, R. C, Bachmann, I, Goulden, V, et al. Five-year follow-up of a randomized, prospective trial of topical methyl aminolevulinate photodynamic therapy vs surgery for nodular basal cell carcinoma. Arch Dermatol. (2007). Sep;, 143(9), 1131-6.

[16] Taber, S. W, Fingar, V. H, Coots, C. T, & Wieman, T. J. Photodynamic therapy using mono-L-aspartyl chlorin e(6) (Npe6) for the treatment of cutaneous disease: A phase I clinical study. Clin Cancer Res. (1998). Nov;, 4(11), 2741-6.

[17] De Oliveira, K. T. Silva AMS, Tome AC, Neves MGPMS, Neri CR, Garcia VS, et al. Synthesis of new amphiphilic chlorin derivatives from protoporphyrin-IX dimethyl ester. Tetrahedron. (2008). Sep 8;, 64(37), 8709-15.

[18] Babilas, P, Schreml, S, Landthaler, M, & Szeimies, R. M. Photodynamic therapy in dermatology: state-of-the-art. Photodermatol Photo. (2010). Jun;, 26(3), 118-32.

[19] Pottler, R, Krammer, B, Baumgartiner, R, & Stepp, H. Phodynamic Therapy with ALA: A clinical handbook. first ed. Europa: RCS Publishing; (2006).

[20] Issa MCAManela-Azulay M. Photodynamic therapy: a review of the literature and image documentation. An Bras Dermatol. (2010). Jul-Aug;, 85(4), 501-11.

[21] Svaasand, L. O, Wyss, P, Wyss, M. T, Tadir, Y, Tromberg, B. J, & Berns, M. W. Dosimetry model for photodynamic therapy with topically administered photosensitizers. Laser Surg Med. (1996). , 18(2), 139-49.

[22] Wilson, B. C, Patterson, M. S, & Lilge, L. Implicit and explicit dosimetry in photodynamic therapy: a new paradigm. Laser Med Sci. (1997). Fal;, 12(3), 182-99.

[23] Wolf, P, Rieger, E, & Kerl, H. Topical Photodynamic Therapy with Endogenous Porphyrins after Application of 5-Aminolevulinic Acid- an Alternative Treatment Modality for Solar Keratoses, Superficial Squamous-Cell Carcinomas, and Basal-Cell Carcinomas. J Am Acad Dermatol. (1993). Jan;, 28(1), 17-21.

[24] Foley, P, Freeman, M, Menter, A, Siller, G, Azhary, R. A, Gebauer, K, et al. Photodynamic therapy with methyl aminolevulinate for primary nodular basal cell carcinoma: results of two randomized studies. Int J Dermatol. (2009). Nov;, 48(11), 1236-45.

[25] Caekelbergh, K, Nikkels, A. F, Leroy, B, Verhaeghe, E, Lamotte, M, & Rives, V. Photodynamic Therapy Using Methyl Aminolevulinate in the Management of Primary Superficial Basal Cell Carcinoma: Clinical and Health Economic Outcomes. J Drugs Dermatol. (2009). Nov;, 8(11), 992-6.

[26] Szeimies, R. M, Ibbotson, S, Murrell, D. F, Rubel, D, Frambach, Y, De Berker, D, et al. A clinical study comparing methyl aminolevulinate photodynamic therapy and surgery in small superficial basal cell carcinoma (8-20 mm), with a 12-month follow-up. J Eur Acad Dermatol. (2008). Nov;, 22(11), 1302-11.

[27] Calzavarapinton, P. G. Repetitive Photodynamic Therapy with Topical Delta-Aminolevulinic-Acid as an Appropriate Approach to the Routine Treatment of Superficial Nonmelanoma Skin Tumors. J Photoch Photobio B. (1995). Jul;, 29(1), 53-7.

[28] Surrenti, T, & De Angelis, L. Di Cesare A, Fargnoli MC, Peris K. Efficacy of photodynamic therapy with methyl aminolevulinate in the treatment of superficial and nodular basal cell carcinoma: an open-label trial. Eur J Dermatol. (2007). Sep-Oct;, 17(5), 412-5.

[29] Horn, M, Wolf, P, Wulf, H. C, Warloe, T, Fritsch, C, Rhodes, L. E, et al. Topical methyl aminolaevulinate photodynamic therapy in patients with basal cell carcinoma prone to complications and poor cosmetic outcome with conventional treatment. Brit J Dermatol. (2003). Dec;, 149(6), 1242-9.

[30] Scola, N, Terras, S, Georgas, D, Othlinghaus, N, Matip, R, Pantelaki, I, et al. A randomized, half-side comparative study of aminolevulinate photodynamic therapy versus CO(2) laser ablation in immunocompetent patients with multiple actinic keratoses. Br J Dermatol. (2012). Jun 18.

[31] Rhodes, L. E, De Rie, M, Enstrom, Y, Groves, R, Morken, T, Goulden, V, et al. Photodynamic therapy using topical methyl aminolevulinate vs surgery for nodular basal

cell carcinoma- Results of a multicenter randomized prospective trial. Arch Dermatol. (2004). Jan;, 140(1), 17-23.

[32] Cosgarea, R, Susan, M, Crisan, M, & Senila, S. Photodynamic therapy using topical aminolaevulinic acid vs. surgery for basal cell carcinoma. J Eur Acad Dermatol. (2012). no-no., 5.

[33] Basset-seguin, N, Ibbotson, S. H, Emtestam, L, Tarstedt, M, Morton, C, Maroti, M, et al. Topical methyl aminolaevulinate photodynamic therapy versus cryotherapy for superficial basal cell carcinoma: a 5 year randomized trial. Eur J Dermatol. (2008). Sep-Oct;, 18(5), 547-53.

[34] Aguilar, M, De Troya, M, Martin, L, Benitez, N, & Gonzalez, M. A cost analysis of photodynamic therapy with methyl aminolevulinate and imiquimod compared with conventional surgery for the treatment of superficial basal cell carcinoma and Bowen's disease of the lower extremities. J Eur Acad Dermatol. (2010). Dec;, 24(12), 1431-6.

[35] Fantini, F, & Greco, A. Del Giovane C, Cesinaro AM, Venturini M, Zane C, et al. Photodynamic therapy for basal cell carcinoma: clinical and pathological determinants of response. J Eur Acad Dermatol. (2011). Aug;, 25(8), 896-901.

[36] Haller, J. C, Cairnduff, F, Slack, G, Schofield, J, Whitehurst, C, Tunstall, R, et al. Routine double treatments of superficial basal cell carcinomas using aminolaevulinic acid-based photodynamic therapy. Brit J Dermatol. (2000). Dec;, 143(6), 1270-4.

[37] Ibbotson, S. H. Adverse effects of topical photodynamic therapy. Photodermatol Photo. (2011). Jun;, 27(3), 116-30.

[38] Wolfe, C. M, Hatfield, K, & Cognetta, A. B. Jr. Cellulitis as a postprocedural complication of topical 5-aminolevulinic acid photodynamic therapy in the treatment of actinic keratosis. J Drugs Dermatol. (2007). May;, 6(5), 544-8.

[39] Morton, C. A, Whitehurst, C, Mccoll, J. H, & Moore, J. V. MacKie RM. Photodynamic therapy for large or multiple patches of Bowen disease and basal cell carcinoma. Arch Dermatol. (2001). Mar;, 137(3), 319-24.

[40] Willey, A, Mehta, S, & Lee, P. K. Reduction in the Incidence of Squamous Cell Carcinoma in Solid Organ Transplant Recipients Treated with Cyclic Photodynamic Therapy. Dermatol Surg. (2010). May;, 36(5), 652-8.

[41] Rowe, D. E, Carroll, R. J, & Day, C. L. Long-Term Recurrence Rates in Previously Untreated (Primary) Basal-Cell Carcinoma- Implications for Patient Follow-Up. J Dermatol Surg Onc. (1989). Mar;, 15(3), 315-28.

[42] Mosterd, K. Thissen MRTM, Nelemans P, Kelleners-Smeets NWJ, Janssen RLLT, Broekhof KGME, et al. Fractionated 5-aminolaevulinic acid-photodynamic therapy vs. surgical excision in the treatment of nodular basal cell carcinoma: results of a randomized controlled trial. Brit J Dermatol. (2008). Oct;, 159(4), 864-70.

[43] Lindberg-larsen, R, Solvsten, H, & Kragballe, K. Evaluation of Recurrence After Photodynamic Therapy with Topical Methylaminolaevulinate for 157 Basal Cell Carcinomas in 90 Patients. Acta Derm-Venereol. (2012). , 92(2), 144-7.

[44] Christensen, E, Mork, C, & Skogvoll, E. High and sustained efficacy after two sessions of topical 5-aminolaevulinic acid photodynamic therapy for basal cell carcinoma: a prospective, clinical and histological 10-year follow-up study. Brit J Dermatol. (2012). Jun;, 166(6), 1342-8.

[45] Christensen, E, Skogvoll, E, Viset, T, Warloe, T, & Sundstrom, S. Photodynamic therapy with 5-aminolaevulinic acid, dimethylsulfoxide and curettage in basal cell carcinoma: a 6-year clinical and histological follow-up. J Eur Acad Dermatol. (2009). Jan;, 23(1), 58-66.

[46] Soler, A. M, Warloe, T, Berner, A, & Giercksky, K. E. A follow-up study of recurrence and cosmesis in completely responding superficial and nodular basal cell carcinomas treated with methyl 5-aminolaevulinate-based photodynamic therapy alone and with prior curettage. Brit J Dermatol. (2001). Sep;, 145(3), 467-71.

[47] Garcia-zuazaga, J, Cooper, K. D, & Baron, E. D. Photodynamic therapy in dermatology: current concepts in the treatment of skin cancer. Expert Rev Anticanc. (2005). Oct;, 5(5), 791-800.

[48] Jori, G, Fabris, C, Soncin, M, Ferro, S, Coppellotti, O, Dei, D, et al. Photodynamic therapy in the treatment of microbial infections: Basic principles and perspective applications. Laser Surg Med. (2006). Jun;, 38(5), 468-81.

[49] Jori, G. Photodynamic therapy of microbial infections: State of the art and perspectives. J Environ Pathol Tox. (2006).

[50] Maisch, T, Szeimies, R. M, Jori, G, & Abels, C. Antibacterial photodynamic therapy in dermatology. Photoch Photobio Sci. (2004). , 3(10), 907-17.

[51] Zeina, B, Greenman, J, Purcell, W. M, & Das, B. Killing of cutaneous microbial species by photodynamic therapy. Brit J Dermatol. (2001). Feb;, 144(2), 274-8.

Chapter 9

Skin Cancer Screening

Carolyn J. Heckman, Susan Darlow, Teja Munshi and Clifford Perlis

Additional information is available at the end of the chapter

http://dx.doi.org/10.5772/55243

1. Introduction

This chapter reviews 1) the incidence, mortality, and risk factors for skin cancer, 2) the efficacy, cost-effectiveness, and frequency of skin cancer screening, 3) behavioral interventions to improve engagement in skin cancer screening, and 4) issues related to screening of special populations.

2. Melanoma and non-melanoma incidence, mortality and risk factors

Skin cancer is the most common cancer in the US, with almost three million individuals being diagnosed annually [1]. Both melanoma and non-melanoma (or keratinocyte) skin cancer (NMSC) incidence rates have been increasing in recent decades [2]-[4]. In 2012, melanoma is predicted to be the fifth most common cancer among US men and the sixth most common cancer among women [2]. Risk factors for melanoma and NMSC include male sex, age over 50 years, personal or family history of melanoma or NMSC, red hair, blue or green eyes, Fitzpatrick skin type I (very fair skin sensitive to ultraviolet radiation [UV]) with freckles, actinic keratosis on the head, familial atypical mole-melanoma syndrome, or numerous (i.e., > 100) moles [2], [5]-[15]. Additionally, many melanomas and NMSCs can be attributed to UV exposure such as via outdoor occupations, one blistering sunburn prior to age 18, multiple sunburns at any age, or indoor tanning [15]-[21].

3. Efficacy of skin cancer screening

During a total cutaneous examination (TCE), the healthcare professional uses observation by sight, sometimes augmented by serial photography and/or dermoscopy to detect not only skin cancer but also risk factors for skin cancer (e.g., actinic keratoses) [22]. Suspicious lesions may then be biopsied and examined histologically. TCE also allows the healthcare professional the opportunity to educate the patient regarding their risk of skin cancer [22]-[24]. Screening of those at high risk for skin cancer detects tumors at an earlier stage when tumors are thinner, resulting in lower mortality rates [25]-[31]. Due to their clinical training and expertise, dermatologists are able to detect melanoma tumors during an early stage of growth, whereas patients may not notice a tumor until it is noticeably thick [32]-[34]. To date there are no major randomized controlled trials assessing the efficacy of TCE, but a case-control study found that melanoma patients who had a TCE in the three years prior to their diagnosis were 14% less likely to have thick melanoma, resulting in 26% fewer deaths [25]. Specificity for detection of melanoma through TCE is comparable to that of other cancer screening tests [35]. Most professional organizations recommend total cutaneous examination (TCE) for high risk individuals [1], [36]-[38], and some recommend population screening [39]; although, in 2009 the US Preventive Services Task Force concluded that there was insufficient evidence to recommend skin cancer screening for the general adult population [40].

Patients and their family/friends are the first to spot half to three quarters of all melanomas [41]-[45]. To perform SSE, individuals are instructed to carefully examine all of their skin for abnormal spots following the "ABCDE" criteria: asymmetry, irregular borders, variation in color, large diameter (i.e., >6mm or a pencil eraser), and evolving (i.e., a changing spot) [46]. Skin self-examination (SSE) is associated with thinner tumors [47], may shorten the time to diagnosis [48], and may reduce melanoma mortality by up to 63% [49]. Both the National Cancer Institute [38] and the American Cancer Society [36] recommend monthly SSE.

4. Cost-effectiveness and frequency of skin cancer screening

Because of its high prevalence, NMSC is among the mostly costly cancers to treat among the Medicare population [50]. SSEs are cost-effective in that people can perform them on their own; however, there is the potential for otherwise unnecessary medical visits. Screening programs with cost ratios less than $50K per year of life saved are said to be cost-effective [51]-[54]. Two studies found that dermatologist skin cancer screening for individuals 50 years of age or older is cost-effective with costs of $10-$16K per quality-adjusted life year [QALY] saved overall and $35K per QALY for biennial screening of siblings of melanoma patients; whereas, annual screening of the general population is not cost-effective [52], [53]. A 1996 Australian study of the cost-effectiveness of every five-year screenings by family practice physicians of men over 50 years of age found a cost-effectiveness of $6.9K per QALY [55]. In comparison, the cost-effectiveness ratios for biennial mammography for women ages 50-69 years and for colorectal cancer screening every five years after age 50 are $30.5K and $47.4K per QALY saved,

http://dx.doi.org/10.5772/55243

respectively [51], [54]. With the introduction of the Patient Protection and Affordable Care Act, those previously without health insurance will have access to medical care [56]. In addition, this law will increase the focus on prevention of chronic illnesses such as cancer [57].

Although efficacious and cost-effective, rates of *ever* having had a TCE are low at approximately 15-17% among US adults [58], [59]. Despite the recommendation from some organizations for monthly SSE, SSE rates are also suboptimal. US and Australian studies conducted from 1991 to 2004 found that only 23-61% of individuals performed SSE at least annually [60]-[66]. A study of Scottish patients also noted that approximately one third of patients did not seek medical attention until more than three months after noticing a worrisome pigmented lesion, potentially contributing to thicker melanomas [67]. Due to the relatively low rates of skin cancer screening, it is important to identify efficacious and cost-effective interventions to increase engagement in screening behavior, particularly among high risk groups such as men 50 years of age and older.

5. Psychosocial barriers to skin cancer screening

Several psychosocial variables have been found to be associated with skin cancer screening. Dermatologists' main reason for not conducting TCE is patients' perceived embarrassment or reluctance [68]. An Australian study found that having a TCE in the past three years was associated with having a positive attitude toward skin cancer screening [69]. TCE intentions were higher among first-degree relatives of melanoma patients reporting greater physician and family support and perceiving greater benefits (e.g., to prevent cancer) of and lesser barriers (e.g., not enough time, anxiety) to TCE [70]. Barriers to TCE reported by Australian employees included fear of being diagnosed and difficulty attending appointments during work hours [71]. SSE has been found to be associated with higher SSE self-efficacy (i.e., SSE-related confidence) [72] and perceived benefits of and barriers to SSE [73] among melanoma patients/survivors. Intentions to receive SSE were higher among individuals with higher family support and higher benefits and lower barriers to self-examination [70]. SSE-related benefits were the strongest predictor of SSE among individuals from families with familial atypical multiple mole melanoma [74]. Other barriers to self-detection include limited ability to recall the skin's appearance and undercounting the number of moles on the skin [75]. Physicians, family, and media may serve as cues to action in skin cancer prevention and detection [76].

6. Prior interventions to increase skin cancer screening

Community and mass media campaigns (e.g., SkinWatch) that have increased TCE have been conducted mostly in Australia [35], [77]. For example, SkinWatch, a three-year Australian rural and regional community-based randomized controlled trial, involved community education ("self-help guide" to skin examination and melanoma risk factors, available in physicians' waiting rooms), a media campaign (press regarding the program and advertisements), and volunteer recruitment and activities (training of a "Volunteer SkinWatch Coordinator" in each community to serve as liaison between the community and research team). More than 16,000 people attended SkinWatch screening clinics conducted by general practitioners and special screening services [78], [79]. By two years, screening rates almost tripled in intervention communities [35]. Screening attendance was associated with age 40-49 years, fair skin, personal history of skin cancer, concern about a spot or mole, and not having had a recent TCE [80]. Reasons endorsed for failing to attend screening services included a lack of knowledge regarding services, not having time to attend services, and having had a TCE recently [80]. A few studies assessing interventions to increase TCE have found low (2-19%) uptake rates even among high risk populations [28], [81]. On the other hand, a more recent Australian study found that 71% of employees attended a free workplace skin cancer screening [71]. Finally, Manne and colleagues [82] found that a tailored print intervention increased TCE intentions and performance among first degree relatives of melanoma patients.

Interventions that have increased SSE through 1-year follow up among the general population have included in person and telephone approaches, videos, pamphlets, and free TCE [83]-[87]. For high risk populations such as melanoma patients and their family members, two UK and US groups have found success at 3-6 months using Skinsafe, an interactive multimedia intervention including characteristics of skin at risk, early signs of melanoma, personalized risk feedback, and SSE instruction [88], [89]. Other interventions have included the approaches used for general populations as well as personalized risk feedback, diaries and body maps, tailored recommendations and reminders, workbooks, a couple-based approach, guided imagery, and the use of photos of moles [75], [88], [90]-[99]. In general, interventions that have significantly increased skin cancer screening have tended to target high risk populations and be interactive and individually tailored based on personal characteristics, attitudes, and behaviors [92], [94].

7. Special populations

7.1. Older men

It is well-documented that men, particularly those aged 50 years and older, have higher incidence of, as well as morbidity and mortality from melanoma than other demographic groups [1], [100]-[103]. During the past decade, the incidence of thick melanomas (i.e., 4 mm) in the US increased significantly only in men 60 years of age and older [1]. A recent analysis of four phase III trials found that women had a consistent 30% advantage in all aspects of localized melanoma progression, which they attribute to a variety of potential tumor- and host-related biologic sex difference [100]. Studies have found that women are also more likely than men to do SSE [48], [60], [61], [63], [65], [66], [104-[107], intend to do TCE [108], and detect melanomas [42], [44]. Figure 1 shows US TCE rates in 2005 among various demographic groups.

http://dx.doi.org/10.5772/55243

Health interventions targeted specifically to men may benefit from a consideration of masculinity [109]-[117]. For example, one study found that more masculine college students were more likely to intend to do SSE if they received a worry control versus a response-efficacy (i.e., screening can detect skin cancer when it's most treatable) message [115]. Studies have found barriers to healthcare utilization and prevention among men that may be related to a stereotypical masculine identity including discomfort with communication, feelings of vulnerability or invincibility, and even homophobia [111]. Thus, interventions for men should emphasize "masculine norms" such as self-reliance, emotional control, and power [109]. A few European and Australian interventions targeting middle-aged and older men included male celebrity modeling, use of photos, a website, free exams, and education and were successful in increasing SSE [114], [118], [119] and TCE [120]-[122]. Geller and colleagues (2006) also recommend a national survey to assess men for risk factors, perceived susceptibility, attitudes toward TCE and SSE, perceived barriers, and potential social supports [113].

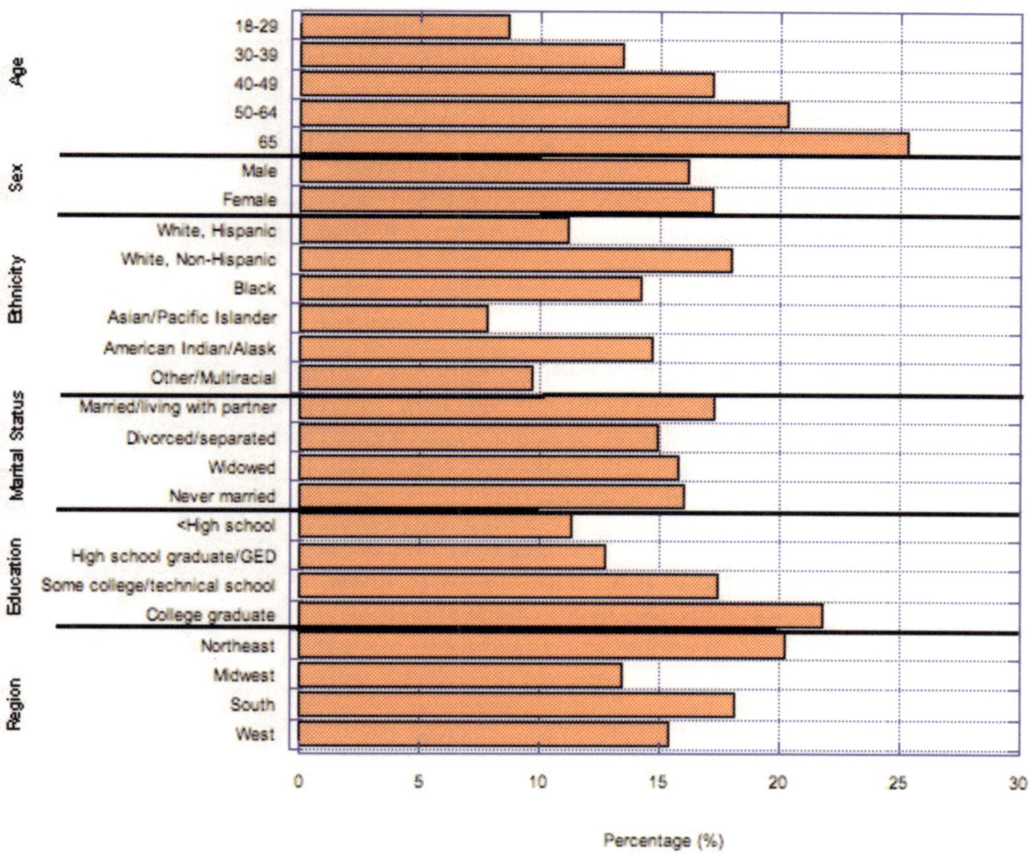

Adapted from [59]

Figure 1. Adjusted predicted value (%) for having total-body skin examination among US adults, National Health Interview Survey, 2005

7.2. Young adults

Melanoma is the second most common cancer (after lymphomas) in adolescents and adults younger than age 30 in the US [123]. The high rates of melanoma in this age group can likely be explained by high ultraviolet (UV) radiation exposure and low sun protection rates early in life [124], [125]. About one in three adolescents and young adults report intentional sunbathing [126]-[128], and 40-60% of college students have used indoor tanning booths, with higher rates among women [129]-[131]. In addition, sunscreen use is poor in this age group, with 50-85% failing to routinely wear sunscreen when outdoors [132], [133].

Some organizations recommend regular skin cancer screening beginning at 20 years of age [36], [38]. However, results of the 2000 National Health Interview Surveys showed that only 7% of young adults aged 18-29 years had ever received a TCE, down from 11% in 1998 [134]. Physicians tend to neglect young adults as a group that does not need skin cancer detection counseling [135], [136]. In addition, few studies have examined skin exam rates in young adults. Routine skin exams are largely recommended for those at high risk of skin cancer (usually older adults) [8], but the increasing rates of skin cancer in young adults indicates a potential need for culturally-appropriate interventions to increase skin exams in this age group, particularly among high risk populations such as individuals with a family history of skin cancer or indoor tanners. Skin cancer prevention interventions for young adults benefit from a focus on the negative effects on appearance stemming from UV exposure [137], [138]. Similar appearance-oriented interventions to increase skin cancer screening could focus on the effects of biopsies and skin surgeries if skin cancer is not detected early.

7.3. Racial and ethnic minorities

While white individuals are at higher risk for melanoma, non-white individuals tend to be diagnosed at later stages and have poorer survival [139], [140]. Specifically, ethnic minorities are 1.96 to 3.01 times more likely to die of melanoma, as compared to Whites of the same age and sex [139], [141], [142]. There are likely biological factors that play a role in this disparity [140]. However, another reason for later detection may be that race/ethnicity may be a proxy for some other demographic factors such as poorer SES, lower education, poorer access to healthcare, linguistic barriers, medical distrust, and occupational hazards such as UV exposure [140]. Though skin cancer rates are lower in racial and ethnic minority groups, they are not immune from this disease. Therefore, efforts should be made by healthcare professionals to educate these groups regarding their risk and signs of skin cancer.

Few studies have been conducted to determine the prevalence of TCE and SSE among racial and ethnic minority groups. One study found the rate for ever having had a TCE in Hispanic Whites was 3.7%, compared to 8.9% in non-Hispanic Whites [134]. Another study found rates of 16.2% in Blacks and 17.1% in Hispanics for regularly receiving TCE, compared to 25.5% of Whites [14[13]. A study of US university students found that 7.7% of Asian, 12.5% of Black, and 14.3% of Hispanic students reported ever having performed SSE (compared to 39.5% of White students) [144]. A study conducted by Pipitone and colleagues (2002) compared SSE in 27 Hispanic and 113 White individuals, finding that none of the 27 Hispanics reported ever being taught SSE [145]. In addition, the Hispanics reported not being told to perform SSE as often as non-Hispanics were.

7.4. Other underserved populations

Particular attention to underserved populations (e.g., based on education, older age, rural/urban status, etc.) is needed. Demographic variables found to increase prevalence and/or severity of melanoma include urban residence in some cases, lower educational level, not being married, and being retired [31], [47], [146], [147]. TCE rates have been found to be lower among some demographic groups such as non-whites [59], individuals with high occupational UV exposure or lack of health insurance [148], lower educational levels [70], [148], unmarried men [70], and men living in metropolitan areas [114]. Rates of SSE have also been found to be higher among dermatology clinic patients and in younger adults as opposed to adults older than 50 [48], [60], [106]. Skin examination behaviors are influenced by factors such as skin cancer awareness, socio-economic status, and sociocultural values. Perceived risk for and knowledge regarding skin cancer is poor, especially among blacks and those with lower education levels [149]-[153]. Analysis of results from the Health Information National Trends Survey also showed that Blacks, the elderly, and people with less education all perceived themselves as being at reduced risk for skin cancer [149]. Furthermore, these groups, along with Hispanics, tended to believe that they could not reduce their skin cancer risk or that recommendations for risk reduction were too unclear for them to adopt appropriate strategies [149]. Interventions designed to address health disparities should be culturally appropriate, inexpensive, easy to use, be appropriate for low health literacy levels, easily disseminated, address access to care, utilize tailoring, and involve the community when possible [113], [154]-[158]. Additionally, when developing interventions for an older population, it is important to keep in mind declines in cognitive abilities and a reliance on affective decision making as a result of such declines [159], [160].

8. Conclusion

Skin cancer is common and increasing in incidence. Skin cancer screening is efficacious and cost-effective in detecting more curable skin cancers. However, engagement in skin cancer screening is relatively low, even among high risk populations. Thus, research indicates a need for improved skin cancer screening interventions especially among high risk populations such as individuals with a personal or family history of skin cancer and older men. Several behavioral interventions have been developed and have demonstrated some promise in increasing skin cancer exams. However, health disparities in melanoma incidence, morbidity, and mortality exist as well as disparities in engagement in skin cancer detection. These disparities indicate a need for sensitive and culturally-appropriate behavioral interventions. Researchers should attend to individuals with low health literacy levels when designing these interventions. Young adults should also be educated regarding their risk for skin cancer and how to do skin exams, given the increasing rates of skin cancer in this age group. Future research on skin exams might benefit from the incorporation of new technology, such as use of smartphones and other wireless devices. Such approaches might enhance needed dissemination of efficacious interventions to the public.

Acknowledgements

The authors would like to thank Ms. Jeanne Pomenti, BS and Ms. Alexa Steuer for their assistance with the preparation of this chapter.

Author details

Carolyn J. Heckman*, Susan Darlow, Teja Munshi and Clifford Perlis

*Address all correspondence to: carolyn.heckman@fccc.edu

Cancer Prevention and Control Program, Fox Chase Cancer Center, Philadelphia, USA

References

[1] Rogers HW, Weinstock MA, Harris AR, Hinckley MR, Feldman SR, Fleischer AB, et al. Incidence Estimate of Nonmelanoma Skin Cancer in the United States, 2006. Archives of Dermatology 2010; 146(3) 283-287.

[2] American Cancer Society. Skin Cancer:Basal and Squamous Cell. 2012 [cited 2012 August 1]; Available from: http://www.cancer.org/Cancer/SkinCancer-BasalandSquamousCell/DetailedGuide/skin-cancer-basal-and-squamous-cell-what-is-basal-and-squamous-cell

[3] Donaldson MR, Coldiron BM. No End in Sight: The Skin Cancer Epidemic Continues. Seminars in Cutaneous Medicine and Surgery 2011; 30(1) 3-5.

[4] Linos E, Swetter SM, Cockburn MG, Colditz GA, Clarke CA. Increasing Burden of Melanoma in the United States. Journal of Investigative Dermatology 2009; 129(7) 1666-1674.

[5] Baxter AJ, Hughes MC, Kvaskoff M, Siskind V, Shekar S, Aitken JF, et al. The Queensland Study of Melanoma: Environmental and Genetic Associations (Q-Mega); Study Design, Baseline Characteristics, and Repeatability of Phenotype and Sun Exposure Measures. Twin Research and Human Genetics 2008; 11(2) 183-196.

[6] Centers for Disease Control and Prevention. Skin Cancer: Risk Factors. 2011 [cited 2012 July 30]; Available from: http://www.cdc.gov/cancer/skin/basic_info/risk_factors.htm

[7] Chuang TY, Brashear R. Risk Factors of Non-Melanoma Skin Cancer in United States Veterans Patients: A Pilot Study and Review of Literature. Journal of the European Academy of Dermatology and Venereology 1999; 12(2) 126-132.

[8] Goldberg MS, Doucette JT, Lim HW, Spencer J, Carucci JA, Rigel DS. Risk Factors for Presumptive Melanoma in Skin Cancer Screening: American Academy of Dermatology National Melanoma/Skin Cancer Screening Program Experience 2001-2005. Journal of the American Academy of Dermatology 2007; 57(1) 60-66.

[9] Grulich AE, Bataille V, Swerdlow AJ, Newton-Bishop JA, Cuzick J, Hersey P, et al. Naevi and Pigmentary Characteristics as Risk Factors for Melanoma in a High-Risk Population: A Case-Control Study in New South Wales, Australia. International Journal of Cancer 1996; 67(4) 485-491.

[10] Markovic SN, Erickson LA, Rao RD, Weenig RH, Pockaj BA, Bardia A, et al. Malignant Melanoma in the 21st Century, Part 1: Epidemiology, Risk Factors, Screening, Prevention, and Diagnosis. Mayo Clinic Proceedings 2007; 82(3) 364-380.

[11] Oberyszyn TM. Non-Melanoma Skin Cancer: Importance of Gender, Immunosuppressive Status and Vitamin D. Cancer Letters 2008; 261(2) 127-136.

[12] Perkins JL, Liu Y, Mitby PA, Neglia JP, Hammond S, Stovall M, et al. Nonmelanoma Skin Cancer in Survivors of Childhood and Adolescent Cancer: A Report from the Childhood Cancer Survivor Study. Journal of Clinical Oncology 2005; 23(16) 3733-3741.

[13] Psaty EL, Scope A, Halpern AC, Marghoob AA. Defining the Patient at High Risk for Melanoma. International Journal of Dermatology 2010; 49(4) 362-376.

[14] Qureshi AA, Zhang M, Han J. Heterogeneity in Host Risk Factors for Incident Melanoma and Non-Melanoma Skin Cancer in a Cohort of Us Women. Journal of Epidemiology 2011; 21(3) 197-203.

[15] Siskind V, Aitken J, Green A, Martin N. Sun Exposure and Interaction with Family History in Risk of Melanoma, Queensland, Australia. International Journal of Cancer 2002; 97(1) 90-95.

[16] Armstrong BK, Kricker A. How Much Melanoma Is Caused by Sun Exposure? Melanoma Research 1993; 3(6) 395-401.

[17] Dusza SW, Halpern AC, Satagopan JM, Oliveria SA, Weinstock MA, Scope A, et al. Prospective Study of Sunburn and Sun Behavior Patterns During Adolescence. Pediatrics 2012; 129(2) 309-317.

[18] Lazovich D, Vogel RI, Berwick M, Weinstock M, Anderson KE, Warshaw EM. Indoor Tanning and Risk of Melanoma: A Case-Control Study in a Highly Exposed Population. Cancer Epidemiology, Biomarkers and Prevention 2010; 19(6) 1557-1568.

[19] Skin Cancer Foundation. Preventing Skin Cancer. 2012 [cited 2012 July 31]; Available from: http://www.skincancer.org/prevention/sun-protection/prevention-guidelines/preventing-skin-cancer

[20] Swerdlow AJ, Weinstock MA. Do Tanning Lamps Cause Melanoma? An Epidemiologic Assessment. Journal of the American Academy of Dermatology 1998; 38(1) 89-98.

[21] Vishvakarman D, Wong JC. Description of the Use of a Risk Estimation Model to Assess the Increased Risk of Non-Melanoma Skin Cancer among Outdoor Workers in Central Queensland, Australia. Photodermatology, Photoimmunology & Photomedicine 2003; 19(2) 81-88.

[22] Bruce AJ, Brodland DG. Overview of Skin Cancer Detection and Prevention for the Primary Care Physician. Mayo Clinic Proceedings 2000; 75(5) 491-500.

[23] Kittler H, Pehamberger H, Wolff K, Binder M. Diagnostic Accuracy of Dermoscopy. Lancet Oncology 2002; 3(3) 159-165.

[24] Rigel DS. Is the Ounce of Screening and Prevention for Skin Cancer Worth the Pound of Cure? CA: A Cancer Journal for Clinicians 1998; 48(4) 236-238.

[25] Aitken JF, Elwood M, Baade PD, Youl P, English D. Clinical Whole-Body Skin Examination Reduces the Incidence of Thick Melanomas. International Journal of Cancer 2010; 126(2) 450-458.

[26] Masri GD, Clark Jr WH, Guerry D, Halpern A, Thompson CJ, Elder DE. Screening and Surveillance of Patients at High Risk for Malignant Melanoma Result in Detection of Earlier Disease. Journal of the American Academy of Dermatology 1990; 22(6, Part 1) 1042-1048.

[27] Pollitt RA, Geller AC, Brooks DR, Johnson TM, Park ER, Swetter SM. Efficacy of Skin Self-Examination Practices for Early Melanoma Detection. Cancer Epidemiology, Biomarkers and Prevention 2009; 18(11) 3018-3023.

[28] Rossi CR, Vecchiato A, Bezze G, Mastrangelo G, Montesco MC, Mocellin S, et al. Early Detection of Melanoma: An Educational Campaign in Padova, Italy. Melanoma Research 2000; 10(2) 181-187.

[29] Schneider JS, Moore DH, 2nd, Mendelsohn ML. Screening Program Reduced Melanoma Mortality at the Lawrence Livermore National Laboratory, 1984 to 1996. Journal of the American Academy of Dermatology 2008; 58(5) 741-749.

[30] Shore RN, Shore P, Monahan NM, Sundeen J. Serial Screening for Melanoma: Measures and Strategies That Have Consistently Achieved Early Detection and Cure. Journal of Drugs in Dermatology : JDD 2011; 10(3) 244-252.

[31] Youl PH, Baade PD, Parekh S, English D, Elwood M, Aitken JF. Association between Melanoma Thickness, Clinical Skin Examination and Socioeconomic Status: Results of a Large Population-Based Study. International Journal of Cancer 2011; 128(9) 2158-2165.

[32] Epstein DS, Lange JR, Gruber SB, Mofid M, Koch SE. Is Physician Detection Associated with Thinner Melanomas? Journal of the American Medical Association 1999; 281(7) 640-643.

[33] Fisher NM, Schaffer JV, Berwick M, Bolognia JL. Breslow Depth of Cutaneous Melanoma: Impact of Factors Related to Surveillance of the Skin, Including Prior Skin Biopsies and Family History of Melanoma. Journal of the American Academy of Dermatology 2005; 53(3) 393-406.

[34] Kantor J, Kantor DE. Routine Dermatologist-Performed Full-Body Skin Examination and Early Melanoma Detection. Archives of Dermatology 2009; 145(8) 873-876.

[35] Aitken JF, Janda M, Elwood M, Youl PH, Ring IT, Lowe JB. Clinical Outcomes from Skin Screening Clinics within a Community-Based Melanoma Screening Program. Journal of the American Academy of Dermatology 2006; 54(1) 105-114.

[36] American Cancer Society. Cancer Prevention & Early Detection Facts & Figures 2011. Atlanta, GA: American Cancer Society; 2011.

[37] American College of Obstetricians and Gynecologists. Acog Committee Opinion. Primary and Preventive Care: Periodic Assessments. Obstetrics and Gynecology 2003; 102(5 Pt 1)) 1117-1124.

[38] National Cancer Institute. Skin Cancer Screening. 2005 [cited 2012 July 31]; Available from: http://www.cancer.gov/cancertopics/pdq/screening/skin/healthprofessional

[39] American Academy of Dermatology. Be Sun Smart 2010 [cited 2010 April 20,]; Available from: http://www.aad.org/public/sun/smart.html.

[40] U.S. Preventive Services Task Force. Screening for Skin Cancer: Recommendation Statement. 2009 [cited 2012 July 30]; Available from: http://www.uspreventiveservicestaskforce.org/uspstf09/skincancer/skincanrs.htm

[41] Balch CM, Gershenwald JE, Soong SJ, Thompson JF, Ding S, Byrd DR, et al. Multivariate Analysis of Prognostic Factors among 2,313 Patients with Stage Iii Melanoma: Comparison of Nodal Micrometastases Versus Macrometastases. Journal of Clinical Oncology 2010; 28(14) 2452-2459.

[42] Brady MS, Oliveria SA, Christos PJ, Berwick M, Coit DG, Katz J, et al. Patterns of Detection in Patients with Cutaneous Melanoma. Cancer 2000; 89(2) 342-347.

[43] Francken AB, Bastiaannet E, Hoekstra HJ. Follow-up in Patients with Localised Primary Cutaneous Melanoma. Lancet Oncology 2005; 6(8) 608-621.

[44] Francken AB, Shaw HM, Accortt NA, Soong SJ, Hoekstra HJ, Thompson JF. Detection of First Relapse in Cutaneous Melanoma Patients: Implications for the Formulation of Evidence-Based Follow-up Guidelines. Annals of Surgical Oncology 2007; 14(6) 1924-1933.

[45] Koh HK, Miller DR, Geller AC, Clapp RW, Mercer MB, Lew RA. Who Discovers Melanoma? Patterns from a Population-Based Survey. Journal of the American Academy of Dermatology 1992; 26(6) 914-919.

[46] Rigel DS, Friedman RJ, Kopf AW, Polsky D. ABCDE--an Evolving Concept in the Early Detection of Melanoma. Archives of Dermatology 2005; 141(8) 1032-1034.

[47] Geller AC, Swetter SM. Reporting and Registering Nonmelanoma Skin Cancers: A Compelling Public Health Need. British Journal of Dermatology 2012; 166(5) 913-915.

[48] Oliveria SA, Christos PJ, Halpern AC, Fine JA, Barnhill RL, Berwick M. Evaluation of Factors Associated with Skin Self-Examination. Cancer Epidemiology, Biomarkers and Prevention 1999; 8(11) 971-978.

[49] Berwick M, Begg CB, Fine JA, Roush GC, Barnhill RL. Screening for Cutaneous Melanoma by Skin Self-Examination. Journal of the National Cancer Institute 1996; 88(1) 17-23.

[50] Housman TS, Williford PM, Feldman SR, Teuschler HV, Fleischer AB, Jr., Goldman ND, et al. Nonmelanoma Skin Cancer: An Episode of Care Management Approach. Dermatologic Surgery 2003; 29(7) 700-711.

[51] Frazier AL, Colditz GA, Fuchs CS, Kuntz KM. Cost-Effectiveness of Screening for Colorectal Cancer in the General Population. Journal of the American Medical Association 2000; 284(15) 1954-1961.

[52] Freedberg KA, Geller AC, Miller DR, Lew RA, Koh HK. Screening for Malignant Melanoma: A Cost-Effectiveness Analysis. Journal of the American Academy of Dermatology 1999; 41(5) 738-745.

[53] Losina E, Walensky RP, Geller A, Beddingfield FC, III, Wolf LL, Gilchrest BA, et al. Visual Screening for Malignant Melanoma: A Cost-Effectiveness Analysis. Archives of Dermatology 2007; 143(1) 21-28.

[54] Salzmann P, Kerlikowske K, Phillips K. Cost-Effectiveness of Extending Screening Mammography Guidelines to Include Women 40 to 49 Years of Age. Annals of Internal Medicine 1997; 127(11) 955-965.

[55] Girgis A, Clarke P, Burton RC, Sanson-Fisher RW. Screening for Melanoma by Primary Health Care Physicians: A Cost-Effectiveness Analysis. Journal of Medical Screening 1996; 3(1) 47-53.

http://dx.doi.org/10.5772/55243

[56] Beland D, Waddan A. The Obama Presidency and Health Insurance Reform: Assessing Continuity and Change. Social Policy and Society 2012; 11(3) 319-330.

[57] Albright HW, Moreno M, Feeley TW, Walters R, Samuels M, Pereira A, et al. The Implications of the 2010 Patient Protection and Affordable Care Act and the Health Care and Education Reconciliation Act on Cancer Care Delivery. Cancer 2011; 117(8) 1564-1574.

[58] Coups EJ, Geller AC, Weinstock MA, Heckman CJ, Manne SL. Prevalence and Correlates of Skin Cancer Screening among Middle-Aged and Older White Adults in the United States. American Journal of Medicine 2010; 123(5) 439-445.

[59] Lakhani NA, Shaw KM, Thompson T, Yaroch AL, Glanz K, Hartman AM, et al. Prevalence and Predictors of Total-Body Skin Examination among Us Adults: 2005 National Health Interview Survey. Journal of the American Academy of Dermatology 2011; 65(3) 645-648.

[60] Aitken JF, Youl PH, Janda M, Elwood M, Ring IT, Lowe JB, et al. Validity of Self-Reported Skin Screening Histories. American Journal of Epidemiology 2004; 159(11) 1098-1105.

[61] Douglass HM, McGee R, Williams S. Are Young Adults Checking Their Skin for Melanoma? Australian and New Zealand Journal of Public Health 1998; 22(5) 562-567.

[62] Friedman LC, Bruce S, Webb JA, Weinberg AD, Cooper HP. Skin Self-Examination in a Population at Increased Risk for Skin Cancer. American Journal of Preventive Medicine 1993; 9(6) 359-364.

[63] Girgis A, Campbell EM, Redman S, Sanson-Fisher RW. Screening for Melanoma: A Community Survey of Prevalence and Predictors. Medical Journal of Australia 1991; 154(5) 338-343.

[64] Kasparian NA, McLoone JK, Meiser B. Skin Cancer-Related Prevention and Screening Behaviors: A Review of the Literature. Journal of Behavioral Medicine 2009; 32(5) 406-428.

[65] Robinson JK, Rigel DS, Amonette RA. What Promotes Skin Self-Examination? Journal of the American Academy of Dermatology 1998; 39752-757.

[66] Weinstock MA, Martin RA, Risica PM, Berwick M, Lasater T, Rakowski W, et al. Thorough Skin Examination for the Early Detection of Melanoma. American Journal of Preventive Medicine 1999; 17(3) 169-175.

[67] MacKie RM, Bray CA, Leman JA. Effect of Public Education Aimed at Early Diagnosis of Malignant Melanoma: Cohort Comparison Study. British Medical Journal 2003; 326(7385) 367.

[68] Oliveria SA, Heneghan MK, Cushman LF, Ughetta EA, Halpern AC. Skin Cancer Screening by Dermatologists, Family Practitioners, and Internists: Barriers and Facilitating Factors. Archives of Dermatology 2011; 147(1) 39-44.

[69] Janda M, Elwood M, Ring IT, Firman DW, Lowe JB, Youl PH, et al. Prevalence of Skin Screening by General Practitioners in Regional Queensland. Medical Journal of Australia 2004; 180(1) 10-15.

[70] Coups EJ, Manne SL, Jacobsen PB, Ming ME, Heckman CJ, Lessin SR. Skin Surveillance Intentions among Family Members of Patients with Melanoma. BMC Public Health 2011; 11866-891.

[71] Douglas NC, Baillie L, Soyer HP. Skin Cancer Screening of Outdoor Workers in Queensland. Medical Journal of Australia 2011; 195(2) 100-101.

[72] Mujumdar UJ, Hay JL, Monroe-Hinds YC, Hummer AJ, Begg CB, Wilcox HB, et al. Sun Protection and Skin Self-Examination in Melanoma Survivors. Psycho-Oncology 2009; 18(10) 1106-1115.

[73] Manne S, Lessin S. Prevalence and Correlates of Sun Protection and Skin Self-Examination Practices among Cutaneous Malignant Melanoma Survivors. Journal of Behavioral Medicine 2006; 29(5) 419-434.

[74] Mesters I, Jonkman L, Vasen H, de Vries H. Skin Self-Examination of Persons from Families with Familial Atypical Multiple Mole Melanoma (Fammm). Patient Education and Counseling 2009; 75(2) 251-255.

[75] Phelan DL, Oliveria SA, Christos PJ, Dusza SW, Halpern AC. Skin Self-Examination in Patients at High Risk for Melanoma: A Pilot Study. Oncology Nursing Forum 2003; 30(6) 1029-1036.

[76] Garside R, Pearson M, Moxham T. What Influences the Uptake of Information to Prevent Skin Cancer? A Systematic Review and Synthesis of Qualitative Research. Health Education Research 2010; 25(1) 162-182.

[77] Geller AC, Swetter SM, Brooks K, Demierre M-F, Yaroch AL. Screening, Early Detection, and Trends for Melanoma: Current Status (2000-2006) and Future Directions. Journal of the American Academy of Dermatology 2007; 57(4) 555-572.

[78] Aitken JF, Elwood JM, Lowe JB, Firman DW, Balanda KP, Ring IT. A Randomised Trial of Population Screening for Melanoma. Journal of Medical Screening 2002; 9(1) 33-37.

[79] Lowe JB, Ball J, Lynch BM, Baldwin L, Janda M, Stanton WR, et al. Acceptability and Feasibility of a Community-Based Screening Programme for Melanoma in Australia. Health Promotion International 2004; 19(4) 437-444.

[80] Youl PH, Janda M, Elwood M, Lowe JB, Ring IT, Aitken JF. Who Attends Skin Cancer Clinics within a Randomized Melanoma Screening Program? Cancer Detection and Prevention 2006; 30(1) 44-51.

[81] Friedman LC, Webb JA, Bruce S, Weinberg AD, Cooper HP. Skin Cancer Prevention and Early Detection Intentions and Behavior. American Journal of Preventive Medicine 1995; 11(1) 59-65.

[82] Manne S, Jacobsen PB, Ming ME, Winkel G, Dessureault S, Lessin SR. Tailored Versus Generic Interventions for Skin Cancer Risk Reduction for Family Members of Melanoma Patients. Health Psychology 2010; 29(6) 583-593.

[83] Carmel S, Shani E, Rosenberg L. The Role of Age and an Expanded Health Belief Model in Predicting Skin Cancer Protective Behavior. Health Education Research 1994; 9(4) 433-447.

[84] Kundu RV, Kamaria M, Ortiz S, West DP, Rademaker AW, Robinson JK. Effectiveness of a Knowledge-Based Intervention for Melanoma among Those with Ethnic Skin. Journal of the American Academy of Dermatology 2010; 62(5) 777-784.

[85] Lee KB, Weinstock MA, Risica PM. Components of a Successful Intervention for Monthly Skin Self-Examination for Early Detection of Melanoma: The "Check It out" Trial. Journal of the American Academy of Dermatology 2008; 58(6) 1006-1012.

[86] Weinstock MA, Risica PM, Martin RA, Rakowski W, Dube C, Berwick M, et al. Melanoma Early Detection with Thorough Skin Self-Examination: The "Check It out" Randomized Trial. American Journal of Preventive Medicine 2007; 32(6) 517-524.

[87] Mickler TJ, Rodrigue JR, Lescano C. A Comparison of Three Methods of Teaching Skin Self-Examinations. Journal of Clinical Psychology in Medical Settings 1999; 6(3) 273-286.

[88] Aneja S, Brimhall AK, Kast DR, Carlson D, Cooper KD, Bordeaux JS. Improvement in Patient Performance of Skin Self-Examinations after Intervention with Interactive Education and Telecommunication Reminders: A Randomized Controlled Study. Archives of Dermatology 2012; 1-7.

[89] Glazebrook C, Garrud P, Avery A, Coupland C, Williams H. Impact of a Multimedia Intervention "Skinsafe" on Patients' Knowledge and Protective Behaviors. Preventive medicine 2006; 42(6) 449-454.

[90] Berwick M, Oliveria S, Luo ST, Headley A, Bolognia JL. A Pilot Study Using Nurse Education as an Intervention to Increase Skin Self-Examination for Melanoma. Journal of Cancer Education 2000; 15(1) 38-40.

[91] Edmondson PC, Curley RK, Marsden RA, Robinson D, Allaway SL, Willson CD. Screening for Malignant Melanoma Using Instant Photography. Journal of Medical Screening 1999; 6(1) 42-46.

[92] Glanz K, Schoenfeld ER, Steffen A. A Randomized Trial of Tailored Skin Cancer Prevention Messages for Adults: Project Scape. American Journal of Public Health 2010; 100(4) 735-741.

[93] Loescher LJ, Hibler E, Hiscox H, Quale L, Harris R. An Internet-Delivered Video Intervention for Skin Self-Examination by Patients with Melanoma. Archives of Dermatology 2010; 146(8) 922-923.

[94] Oliveria SA, Dusza SW, Phelan DL, Ostroff JS, Berwick M, Halpern AC. Patient Adherence to Skin Self-Examination. Effect of Nurse Intervention with Photographs. American Journal of Preventive Medicine 2004; 26(2) 152-155.

[95] Weinstock MA, Nguyen FQ, Martin RA. Enhancing Skin Self-Examination with Imaging: Evaluation of a Mole-Mapping Program. Journal of Cutaneous Medicine and Surgery 2004; 8(1) 1-5.

[96] Robinson JK, Turrisi R, Stapleton J. Efficacy of a Partner Assistance Intervention Designed to Increase Skin Self-Examination Performance. Archives of Dermatology 2007a; 143(1) 37-41.

[97] Robinson JK, Turrisi R, Stapleton J. Examination of Mediating Variables in a Partner Assistance Intervention Designed to Increase Performance of Skin Self-Examination. Journal of the American Academy of Dermatology 2007b; 56(3) 391-397.

[98] Boone SL, Stapleton J, Turrisi R, Ortiz S, Robinson JK, Mallett KA. Thoroughness of Skin Examination by Melanoma Patients: Influence of Age, Sex and Partner. Australasian Journal of Dermatology 2009; 50(3) 176-180.

[99] Robinson JK, Turrisi R, Mallett K, Stapleton J, Boone SL, Kim N, et al. Efficacy of an Educational Intervention with Kidney Transplant Recipients to Promote Skin Self-Examination for Squamous Cell Carcinoma Detection. Archives of Dermatology 2011; 147(6) 689-695.

[100] Joosse A, Collette S, Suciu S, Nijsten T, Lejeune F, Kleeberg UR, et al. Superior Outcome of Women with Stage I/Ii Cutaneous Melanoma: Pooled Analysis of Four European Organisation for Research and Treatment of Cancer Phase Iii Trials. Journal of Clinical Oncology 2012; 30(18) 2240-2247.

[101] Joosse A, de Vries E, Eckel R, Nijsten T, Eggermont AM, Holzel D, et al. Gender Differences in Melanoma Survival: Female Patients Have a Decreased Risk of Metastasis. Journal of Investigative Dermatology 2011; 131(3) 719-726.

[102] iegel R, Ward E, Brawley O, Jemal A. Cancer Statistics, 2011: The Impact of Eliminating Socioeconomic and Racial Disparities on Premature Cancer Deaths. CA: A Cancer Journal for Clinicians 2011; 61(4) 212-236.

[103] Tuong W, Cheng LS, Armstrong AW. Melanoma: Epidemiology, Diagnosis, Treatment, and Outcomes. Dermatologic Clinics 2012; 30(1) 113-124, ix.

[104] Balanda KP, Lowe JB, Stanton WR, Gillespie AM. Enhancing the Early Detection of Melanoma within Current Guidelines. Australian Journal of Public Health 1994; 18(4) 420-423.

[105] Federman DG, Kravetz JD, Ma F, Kirsner RS. Patient Gender Affects Skin Cancer Screening Practices and Attitudes among Veterans. Southern Medical Journal 2008; 101(5) 513-518.

[106] Robinson JK, Fisher SG, Turrisi RJ. Predictors of Skin Self-Examination Performance. Cancer 2002; 95(1) 135-146.

[107] Swetter SM, Layton CJ, Johnson TM, Brooks KR, Miller DR, Geller AC. Gender Differences in Melanoma Awareness and Detection Practices between Middle-Aged and Older Men with Melanoma and Their Female Spouses. Archives of Dermatology 2009; 145(4) 488-490.

[108] Janda M, Youl PH, Lowe JB, Elwood M, Ring IT, Aitken JF. Attitudes and Intentions in Relation to Skin Checks for Early Signs of Skin Cancer. Preventive Medicine 2004; 39(1) 11-18.

[109] Addis ME, Mahalik JR. Men, Masculinity, and the Contexts of Help Seeking. American Psychologist 2003; 58(1) 5-14.

[110] Conway M, Dube L. Humor in Persuasion on Threatening Topics: Effectiveness Is a Function of Audience Sex Role Orientation. Personality and Social Psychology Bulletin 2002; 28(7) 863-873.

[111] Galdas PM, Cheater F, Marshall P. Men and Health Help-Seeking Behaviour: Literature Review. Journal of Advanced Nursing 2005; 49(6) 616-623.

[112] Geller AC, Sober AJ, Zhang Z, Brooks DR, Miller DR, Halpern A, et al. Strategies for Improving Melanoma Education and Screening for Men Age >or= 50 Years: Findings from the American Academy of Dermatological National Skin Cancer Sreening Program. Cancer 2002; 95(7) 1554-1561.

[113] Geller J, Swetter SM, Leyson J, Miller DR, Brooks K, Geller AC. Crafting a Melanoma Educational Campaign to Reach Middle-Aged and Older Men. Journal of Cutaneous Medicine and Surgery 2006; 10(6) 259-268.

[114] Janda M, Baade PD, Youl PH, Aitken JF, Whiteman DC, Gordon L, et al. The Skin Awareness Study: Promoting Thorough Skin Self-Examination for Skin Cancer among Men 50 Years or Older. Contemporary Clinical Trials 2010; 31(1) 119-130.

[115] Millar MG, Houska JA. Masculinity and Intentions to Perform Health Behaviors: The Effectiveness of Fear Control Arguments. Journal of Behavioral Medicine 2007; 30(5) 403-409.

[116] Sabinsky MS, Toft U, Raben A, Holm L. Overweight Men's Motivations and Perceived Barriers Towards Weight Loss. European Journal of Clinical Nutrition 2007; 61(4) 526-531.

[117] Walsh LA, Stock ML. Uv Photography, Masculinity, and College Men's Sun Protection Cognitions. Journal of Behavioral Medicine 2012; 35(4) 431-442.

[118] Barysch MJ, Cozzio A, Kolm I, Hrdlicka SR, Brand C, Hunger R, et al. Internet Based Health Promotion Campaign against Skin Cancer - Results of Www.Skincheck.Ch in Switzerland. European Journal of Dermatology 2010; 20(1) 109-114.

[119] Janda M, Neale RE, Youl P, Whiteman DC, Gordon L, Baade PD. Impact of a Video-Based Intervention to Improve the Prevalence of Skin Self-Examination in Men 50 Years or Older: The Randomized Skin Awareness Trial. Archives of Dermatology 2011; 147(7) 799-806.

[120] Del Marmol V, de Vries E, Roseeuw D, Pirard C, van der Endt J, Trakatelli M, et al. A Prime Minister Managed to Attract Elderly Men in a Belgian Euromelanoma Campaign. European Journal of Cancer 2009; 45(9) 1532-1534.

[121] Hanrahan PF, D'Este CA, Menzies SW, Plummer T, Hersey P. A Randomised Trial of Skin Photography as an Aid to Screening Skin Lesions in Older Males. Journal of Medical Screening 2002; 9(3) 128-132.

[122] Hanrahan PF, Menzies SW, D'Este CA, Plummer T, Hersey P. Participation of Older Males in a Study on Photography as an Aid to Early Detection of Melanoma. Australian and New Zealand Journal of Public Health 2000; 24(6) 615-618.

[123] Bleyer A, Viny A, Barr R. Cancer in 15- to 29-Year-Olds by Primary Site. Oncologist 2006; 11(6) 590-601.

[124] Olson AL, Starr P. The Challenge of Intentional Tanning in Teens and Young Adults. Dermatologic Clinics 2006; 24(2) 131-136.

[125] Stanton WR, Janda M, Baade PD, Anderson P. Primary Prevention of Skin Cancer: A Review of Sun Protection in Australia and Internationally. Health Promotion International 2004; 19(3) 369-378.

[126] Cokkinides VE, Weinstock MA, O'Connell MC, Thun MJ. Use of Indoor Tanning Sunlamps by Us Youth, Ages 11-18 Years, and by Their Parent or Guardian Caregivers: Prevalence and Correlates. Pediatrics 2002; 109(6) 1124-1130.

[127] Dennis LK, Kancherla V, Snetselaar L. Adolescent Attitudes Towards Tanning: Does Age Matter? Pediatric Health 2009; 3(6) 565-578.

[128] Stryker JE, Lazovich D, Forster JL, Emmons KM, Sorensen G, Demierre MF. Maternal/Female Caregiver Influences on Adolescent Indoor Tanning. Journal of Adolescent Health 2004; 35(6) 528 e521-529.

[129] Gibbons FX, Gerrard M, Lane DJ, Mahler HI, Kulik JA. Using Uv Photography to Reduce Use of Tanning Booths: A Test of Cognitive Mediation. Health Psychology 2005; 24(4) 358-363.

[130] Hillhouse J, Stapleton J, Turrisi R. Association of Frequent Indoor Uv Tanning with Seasonal Affective Disorder. Archives of Dermatology 2005; 141(11) 1465.

[131] Poorsattar SP, Hornung RL. Uv Light Abuse and High-Risk Tanning Behavior among Undergraduate College Students. Journal of the American Academy of Dermatology 2007; 56(3) 375-379.

[132] Cokkinides V, Weinstock M, Lazovich D, Ward E, Thun M. Indoor Tanning Use among Adolescents in the Us, 1998 to 2004. Cancer 2009; 115(1) 190-198.

[133] Jones SE, Saraiya M, Miyamoto J, Berkowitz Z. Trends in Sunscreen Use among U.S. High School Students: 1999-2009. Journal of Adolescent Health 2012; 50(3) 304-307.

[134] Saraiya M, Hall HI, Thompson T, Hartman A, Glanz K, Rimer BK, et al. Skin Cancer Screening among U.S. Adults from 1992, 1998, and 2000 National Health Interview Surveys. Preventive Medicine 2004; 39(2) 308-314.

[135] Feldman SR, Fleischer AB, Jr. Skin Examinations and Skin Cancer Prevention Counseling by Us Physicians: A Long Way to Go. Journal of the American Academy of Dermatology 2000; 43(2 Pt 1) 234-237.

[136] Gritz ER, Tripp MK, de Moor CA, Eicher SA, Mueller NH, Spedale JE. Skin Cancer Prevention Counseling and Clinical Practices of Pediatricians. Pediatric Dermatology 2003; 20(1) 16-24.

[137] Hillhouse J, Turrisi R, Stapleton J, Robinson J. A Randomized Controlled Trial of an Appearance-Focused Intervention to Prevent Skin Cancer. Cancer 2008; 113(11) 3257-3266.

[138] Mahler HI, Kulik JA, Gibbons FX, Gerrard M, Harrell J. Effects of Appearance-Based Interventions on Sun Protection Intentions and Self-Reported Behaviors. Health Psychology 2003; 22(2) 199-209.

[139] Cormier JN, Xing Y, Ding M, Lee JE, Mansfield PF, Gershenwald JE, et al. Ethnic Differences among Patients with Cutaneous Melanoma. Archives of Internal Medicine 2006; 166(17) 1907-1914.

[140] Hernandez C, Mermelstein RJ. A Conceptual Framework for Advancing Melanoma Health Disparities Research. Archives of Dermatology 2009; 145(12) 1442-1446.

[141] Byrd-Miles K, Toombs EL, Peck GL. Skin Cancer in Individuals of African, Asian, Latin-American, and American-Indian Descent: Differences in Incidence, Clinical Presentation, and Survival Compared to Caucasians. Journal of Drugs in Dermatology 2007; 6(1) 10-16.

[142] Rouhani P, Hu S, Kirsner RS. Melanoma in Hispanic and Black Americans. Cancer Control 2008; 15(3) 248-253.

[143] Rodriguez GL, Ma F, Federman DG, Rouhani P, Chimento S, Multach M, et al. Predictors of Skin Cancer Screening Practice and Attitudes in Primary Care. Journal of the American Academy of Dermatology 2007; 57(5) 775-781.

[144] Arnold MR, DeJong W. Skin Self-Examination Practices in a Convenience Sample of U.S. University Students. Preventive Medicine 2005; 40(3) 268-273.

[145] Pipitone M, Robinson JK, Camara C, Chittineni B, Fisher SG. Skin Cancer Awareness in Suburban Employees: A Hispanic Perspective. Journal of the American Academy of Dermatology 2002; 47(1) 118-123.

[146] Coory M, Smithers M, Aitken J, Baade P, Ring I. Urban-Rural Differences in Survival from Cutaneous Melanoma in Queensland. Australian and New Zealand Journal of Public Health 2006; 30(1) 71-74.

[147] Perez-Gomez B, Aragones N, Gustavsson P, Lope V, Lopez-Abente G, Pollan M. Socio-Economic Class, Rurality and Risk of Cutaneous Melanoma by Site and Gender in Sweden. BMC Public Health 2008; 833.

[148] LeBlanc WG, Vidal L, Kirsner RS, Lee DJ, Caban-Martinez AJ, McCollister KE, et al. Reported Skin Cancer Screening of Us Adult Workers. Journal of the American Academy of Dermatology 2008; 59(1) 55-63.

[149] Buster KJ, You Z, Fouad M, Elmets C. Skin Cancer Risk Perceptions: A Comparison across Ethnicity, Age, Education, Gender, and Income. Journal of the American Academy of Dermatology 2012; 66(5) 771-779.

[150] Han PK, Moser RP, Klein WM, Beckjord EB, Dunlavy AC, Hesse BW. Predictors of Perceived Ambiguity About Cancer Prevention Recommendations: Sociodemographic Factors and Mass Media Exposures. Health Communication 2009; 24(8) 764-772.

[151] Hay J, Coups EJ, Ford J, DiBonaventura M. Exposure to Mass Media Health Information, Skin Cancer Beliefs, and Sun Protection Behaviors in a United States Probability Sample. Journal of the American Academy of Dermatology 2009; 61(5) 783-792.

[152] Rutten LF, Hesse BW, Moser RP, McCaul KD, Rothman AJ. Public Perceptions of Cancer Prevention, Screening, and Survival: Comparison with State-of-Science Evidence for Colon, Skin, and Lung Cancer. Journal of Cancer Education 2009; 24(1) 40-48.

[153] Viswanath K, Breen N, Meissner H, Moser RP, Hesse B, Steele WR, et al. Cancer Knowledge and Disparities in the Information Age. Journal of Health Communication 2006; 11 Suppl 11-17.

[154] Allen JD, Kennedy M, Wilson-Glover A, Gilligan TD. African-American Men's Perceptions About Prostate Cancer: Implications for Designing Educational Interventions. Social Science & Medicine 2007; 64(11) 2189-2200.

[155] Artinian NT, Fletcher GF, Mozaffarian D, Kris-Etherton P, Van Horn L, Lichtenstein AH, et al. Interventions to Promote Physical Activity and Dietary Lifestyle Changes for Cardiovascular Risk Factor Reduction in Adults: A Scientific Statement from the American Heart Association. Circulation 2010; 122(4) 406-441.

[156] Cooper LA, Hill MN, Powe NR. Designing and Evaluating Interventions to Eliminate Racial and Ethnic Disparities in Health Care. Journal of General Internal Medicine 2002; 17(6) 477-486.

[157] Friedman DB, Kao EK. A Comprehensive Assessment of the Difficulty Level and Cultural Sensitivity of Online Cancer Prevention Resources for Older Minority Men. Preventing Chronic Disease 2008; 5(1) A07.

[158] Taylor KL, Turner RO, Davis JL, 3rd, Johnson L, Schwartz MD, Kerner J, et al. Improving Knowledge of the Prostate Cancer Screening Dilemma among African American Men: An Academic-Community Partnership in Washington, Dc. Public Health Reports 2001; 116(6) 590-598.

[159] Finucane TE. More Promotional Rhetoric in Research: The Maryland Assisted Living Study. Journal of the American Geriatrics Society 2008; 56(1) 185; author reply 1185-1186.

[160] Isaacowitz DM, Choi Y. Looking, Feeling, and Doing: Are There Age Differences in Attention, Mood, and Behavioral Responses to Skin Cancer Information? Health Psychology 2012; 31(5) 650-659.

Chapter 10

The Role of Furin in the Development of Skin Cancer

Rethika Ravi and Terrence J Piva

Additional information is available at the end of the chapter

http://dx.doi.org/10.5772/55569

1. Introduction

Skin cancer represents a major, and growing, public health problem, and is the most common type of cancer observed in Caucasians [1-3]. The three most common forms of skin cancer are basal cell carcinoma (BCC), squamous cell carcinoma (SCC) and melanoma. BCC and SCC are together known as non-melanoma skin cancers (NMSC), and are both derived from keratinocytes whereas melanomas are derived from melanocytes [3-6]. SCCs can undergo metastasis; BCCs rarely do, while melanomas can be highly metastatic [5, 6].

The ultraviolet (UV) radiation component of sunlight is acknowledged to be the main carcinogen implicated in the formation of skin cancer. UV radiation can be divided into three components: UVC (100-280 nm), UVB (280-320 nm) and UVA (320-400 nm). Ozone depletion, seasonal and weather variations affect the amount of UV radiation reaching the Earth's surface [7]. UVC and most of the UVB radiation emitted from the sun is blocked from reaching the Earth's surface by the ozone layer. The component of UV light that reaches the Earth's surface consists of 90-95% UVA and 5-10% UVB [3, 8]. The penetration of shorter-wavelength UVB radiation is predominantly confined to the epidermis while UVA penetrates into the dermis because of its longer wavelength [9].

UVB can cause sunburn, inflammation, DNA mutations and membrane damage as well as skin cancer [8, 10, 11]. It is known that UVB directly damages DNA and can induce Reactive Oxygen Species (ROS) by interactions with chromophores in the skin [12]. The DNA damage caused by UVB irradiation typically results in the formation of cyclobutane pyrimidine dimers (CPD) and pyrimidine (6-4) photoproducts. The mutations are frequently found in the p53, p16, PTCH and INK4α/CDKN2A genes of skin cancer patients [13, 14]. Inflammation plays a significant role in creating an environment where cells possessing mutated DNA can become carcinogenic. UVA can cause premature skin ageing, wrinkle formation, blotching and induces sunburn cell formation in the epidermis, as well as skin cancer [8, 10, 15]. It affects keratinocytes at a transcriptional level by altering the expression of genes involved in apoptosis, cell cycle, DNA repair, signal transduction, RNA processing and translation, and metabolism [9]. UVA can cause DNA damage by generating ROS [12] resulting in genomic damage e.g. single-stranded breaks, protein-DNA crosslinks, and oxidative base damage (i.e. 8-oxo-7,8-dihydroxyguanine) [16]. It can also initiate signal transduction pathways [13, 17] as well as inducing the expression of cytokines such as Interleukin (IL)-6, heme oxygenase-1, and cyclo-oxygenase [18] as well as inflammatory mediators such as tumor necrosis factor-α (TNFα) [15, 19].

While UVB has been thought to be the main contributor toward skin cancers, based largely on the DNA action spectrum of UV radiation, UVA has more recently been acknowledged as playing an important role in this process [9, 11, 20]. While UVA does not produce an inflammatory response like that of UVB, it produces ROS and as such activates many of the same signalling pathways [13]. It is clear that doses of UVB, UVA and solar stimulated UV that are too low to cause inflammation can induce mutations in epidermal cells. However, this does not exclude a role for ROS from inflammatory cells contributing to skin carcinogenesis, but it may be important for tumour progression [20]. UV-induced inflammation seen in the skin involves the action of many molecules. Of these inflammatory molecules TNFα plays a major role in UV-irradiated inflammation in the skin [15, 19]. TNFα is cleaved from its membrane-bound precursor by the action of the metalloprotease, Tumour Necrosis Factor-α Converting Enzyme (TACE) [21, 22]. While UVB radiation increases the release of TNFα from skin cells, it is not known whether this is due to increased TACE activity and/or expression. However, before TACE is activated it is cleaved from its proform by the action of furin, a proprotein convertase [23, 24]. Furin can cleave other proteases such as matrix metalloproteases (MMPs) [23, 24]. Exposure to UVB radiation also increases MMP activity in skin cells [25]. While furin is expressed in skin cells, the effect UV radiation has on its expression and/or activity and that of the proteases it activates is not fully known. As a result of elevated furin levels in a mutated cell, enhanced TACE activity would see an increase in the secretion of TNFα thereby sustaining a localised inflammatory environment allowing for the development of carcinogenic cells. As furin activates MMP activity, these carcinogenic cells have the potential to become metastatic. This review investigates the role that furin plays in the activation of TACE and MMPs and the effect that this has on a skin cells exposed to UV radiation, as well as that its role in cancer cells which undergoes metastasis, and how an understanding of the role played by this proprotein convertase, may assist in the design of new inhibitors which have therapeutic potential.

2. UV-induced inflammation

High doses of UV can induce inflammation in the skin that results in the appearance of macrophages and other leucocytes [15, 26]. Along with the activation of these cells, many mediators of inflammation are also seen including; prostaglandins [18], nitric oxide (NO) [27] and ROS [12, 17], and cytokines such as interleukin (IL)-1, interferon (IFN)-γ, and TNFα [14, 19, 28, 29]. ROS can cause DNA strand breaks as well as lipid peroxidation, membrane and protein damage [12, 30]. The effects of UV radiation on the levels of these proinflammatory molecules in skin cells are seen in Table 1 [8, 15, 31-33].

http://dx.doi.org/10.5772/55569

Inflammatory mediators such as IL-1, TNFα and IL-6 have been postulated to play a major role in both melanoma [34] and NMSC formation [26,35,36]. Male mice are known to be more sensitive to UVB-induced skin carcinogenesis than female mice [4], which is consistent with human studies showing men having a higher incidence of skin cancer than women [20]. Damian *et al.* [20] found that while women developed a larger inflammatory response to UVB radiation, men had lower antioxidant levels in the skin resulting in a higher level of oxidative damage to DNA, and were more sensitive to UV immunosuppression. This suggests that UV-induced immunosuppression and DNA damage plays a greater role in the formation of skin cancers in men compared to women [20]. IL-1α and IL-1β are both induced in keratinocytes exposed to UVB radiation [31, 37]. IL-1α has been shown to enhance the expression and release of TNFα from UVB-irradiated keratinocytes [38,39], while IL-1β enhances the expression of matrix metalloprotease (MMP)-9 in these irradiated cells [40]. Apart from IL-1β, UVB can stimulate MMP-9 expression in human skin via the induction of Activator protein-1 (AP-1) and NFκB activities [41].

Mediator	Produced By	Function	References
TNFα	Keratinocytes Mast cells Dermal fibroblasts Langerhans cells	Langerhans cell migration, sunburn cell information, stimulates prostaglandin (PG) synthesis, changes in adhesion molecule expression	[15, 31, 33]
IL-1α	Keratinocytes Langerhans cells	Simulates PG synthesis, increases TNFα and IL-6, inhibited by IL-1 receptor antagonist	[15, 33]
IL-1β	Keratinocytes Langerhans cells	Langerhans cell migration	[15, 31, 33]
IL-6	Keratinocytes, Langerhans cells	Fever Severe sunburn	[8, 15, 33]
IL-10	Macrophages Melanocytes	Blocks cytokine production by T cells, macrophages and NK cells Decreases antigen presentation, Increases IL-1 receptor antagonist	[33] [8, 15, 32, 33]
IL-l2p40 (not bioactive)	Keratinocytes, Dendritic cell, Langerhans cells	Decreases Th1 response Decreases antigen presentation	[33]
IFNγ	T cells	Triggers apoptosis T-cell mediated tumour cell destruction	[33]
PGE_2	Keratinocytes, Mast cells	Erythema Decreases antigen presentation Increases IL-4, decreases IL-12	[15, 33]
Histamine	Mast Cells	Increases release of PG Inhibit lymphocyte functions like IL-2 and IFNγ	[3, 15, 33]

Table 1. Effect of UV radiation on the expression of bioactive molecules in human skin cells

UVB radiation can increase cyclo-oxygenase (COX)-2 expression and activity in keratinocytes [20, 28, 42]. High levels of COX-2 activity have been observed in human epithelial skin cancers [43]. Nonsteroidal anti-inflammatory drugs can inhibit COX-2 activity and subsequent PGE formation in the skin, and have been used in the treatment of actinic keratosis (AK) [44], BCC, SCC and melanoma [45]. This suggests a role for COX-2 in the formation of skin cancers, and high levels of activity have been observed in many of these tumours [46].

Upregulation of TNFα is a key early response observed in keratinocytes exposed to UVB radiation [8, 38, 47] and represents an important component of the inflammatory cascade in skin. The expression of TNFα mRNA was enhanced a few hours post-UVB irradiation in both keratinocytes and dermal fibroblasts [38, 47]. IL-1α was shown to stimulate TNFα expression in UVB-irradiated keratinocytes [47] and melanocytes [48]. While Bashir *et al.* [38] observed that TNFα expression in keratinocytes was only induced by UVB irradiation, others have shown that UVA can also induce expression in these cells [49, 50]. This increase in TNFα released by the cells is due to elevated gene transcription [38, 49]. The IL-1α formed in the skin, can in turn, induce mast cells to express inflammatory cytokines (e.g. TNFα and IL-1α), as well as prostaglandins which can enhance the inflammation caused by direct UV exposure on the epidermis [15, 20, 28, 51]. Histamine released from the mast cells can induce vasodilation of the surrounding blood vessels, which assists leucocytes in undergoing diapedesis and entering this region [20, 51]. UVB radiation can induce the synthesis and release of IL-6 and IL-8 from irradiated keratinocytes and fibroblasts [33, 36, 37, 51]. IL-8 assists in the homing of leucocytes, primarily neutrophils, from surrounding blood vessels into the inflamed region, while IL-6 can trigger the activation of monocytes and other infiltrating leucocytes to secrete cytokines and chemokines [51]. Figure 1 shows the complex interaction that occurs between different bioactive molecules in the skin following exposure to UV radiation.

TNFα can induce the expression of adhesion molecules and chemokines in surrounding epithelial cells, resulting in the recruitment of inflammatory leucocytes from surrounding blood vessels via diapedesis [15, 20, 51, 52]. These inflammatory cells in turn can express additional cytokines that form a positive feedback loop that further upregulates TNFα as well as downstream TNF⟨− induced chemokines, cytokines, and other pro-inflammatory mediators in irradiated skin [8, 38, 53]. The effects elicited by these infiltrating inflammatory cells occur some hours following exposure to UV irradiation, thereby prolonging the inflammatory response. UVB radiation also induces inducible nitric oxide synthase (iNOS) activity in dermal endothelial cells, through a TNFα-dependent pathway [38, 54].

TNFα plays a pro-inflammatory role in the skin due to; (a) the direct effects of UV radiation and (b) the indirect effects of inflammatory cells that chemotax to the skin. UV- and inflammatory cell-derived cytokines further enhance TNFα gene transcription in human skin cells [38], which can again increase its production by epidermal cells. In contrast, clustering and internalization of the TNF receptors may lessen the cell's response to TNFα, which may account for why the upregulation of TNFα mRNA is not sustained over time in culture [20]. For further information on the complex interplay of cytokines, chemokines and other mediators in UV-induced inflammation please refer to the following reviews [15, 20, 41, 42].

http://dx.doi.org/10.5772/55569

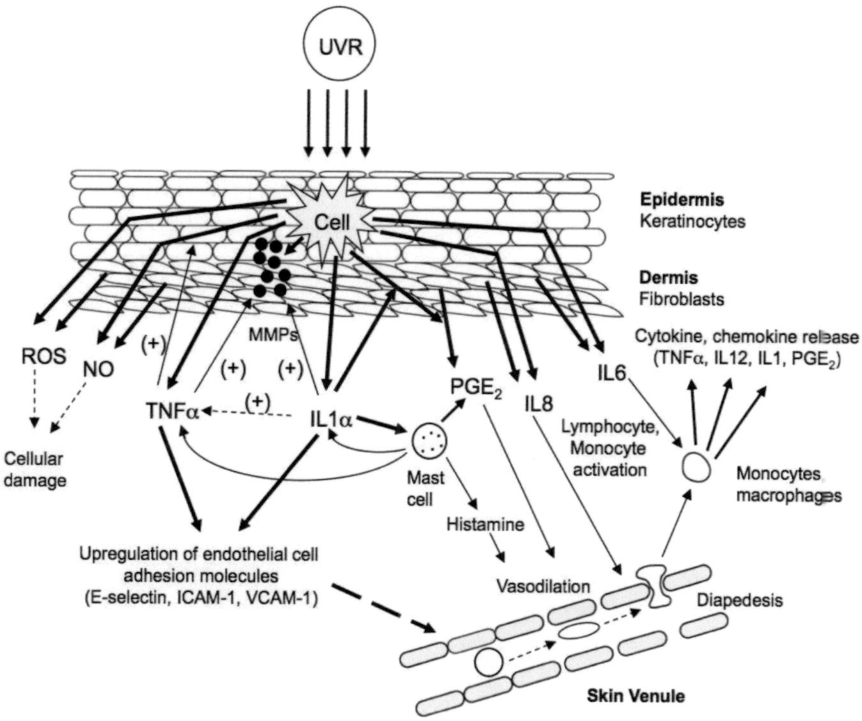

Figure 1. The inflammatory response seen in the skin following exposure to UV radiation. Inflammation can be induced as a direct result of UV exposure on epidermal cells, or due to the release of secreted molecules, which in turn induce the release of inflammatory mediators from the dermis, as well as attracting inflammatory cells from circulation into this region of the skin. The infiltrating monocytes and macrophages, which enter the irradiated skin tissue in turn, secrete mediators that prolong the inflammatory response. See text for details and references.

3. Tumor necrosis factor α

TNFα, is a member of the TNF ligand superfamily, and is a type II transmembrane glycoprotein of 234 amino acids possessing an extracellular carboxy-terminus and a cytoplasmic amino group [53, 55, 56]. It can exist in one of two forms; a 26 kDa membrane-bound form (mTNFα) and a 17 kDa soluble form (sTNFα). sTNFα is cleaved from its membrane bound precursor between Ala^{76} - Val^{77} by the action of the metalloprotease TACE [22, 55].

Numerous cells produce TNFα, including macrophages, leucocytes, dendritic cells, keratinocytes, melanocytes and fibroblasts [8, 47, 57, 58]. It plays a role in apoptosis, cellular proliferation, differentiation, inflammation, tumorigenesis, viral replication, immune response to extracellular stimuli, as well as in local and systemic inflammation [21, 53, 55-57, 59]. Most of the cellular actions described for TNFα correspond to its secreted, mature soluble form. There is increasing evidence that mTNFα is also biologically active [58]. Both forms of TNFα can specifically bind to one of two receptors: TNF-R1 (CD120a receptor), a 55 kDa protein; TNF-R2 (CD120b receptor), a 75 kDa protein [57]. The receptors are both transmembrane glycoproteins, and display a high degree of structural homology and are expressed on most cell types [60].

TNF-R1 is expressed on a wide range of cell types and its signalling mediates cytotoxicity, cell proliferation, antiviral activity and many of the proinflammatory actions of TNFα [58, 61]. TNF-R2 is expressed on a limited range of cells, including leucocytes, endothelial cells, Langerhans cells (LC) and epithelial cells but its actions are less clear [58, 61]. Membrane-bound TNF-R1 and TNF-R2 can be cleaved by TACE to release the soluble forms of these receptors and this process is activated by IL-10 [58]. The soluble forms of TNF-R may act as (a) an antagonist to the surface receptors by competing for sTNFα or (b) an agonist by stabilizing the TNF trimer; therefore maintaining saturating concentrations in extracellular fluids [58, 62].

When TNFα is bound to the TNF-R1 receptor it plays a role in UVB-induced apoptosis in keratinocytes [54, 63]. Transgenic mice deficient for either TNF-R1 and/or TNF-R2 have been shown to be less susceptible to UVB-induced skin tumours than were wild type controls [64]. Through the use of TNF-R1 [65, 66] and TNF-R2 [65] gene-targeted mutant mice, it has been shown that TNF-R1 plays a decisive role in the host's defence against microorganisms, while TNF-R2 plays a role in the induction of tissue necrosis. Through the use of agonist and antagonist antibodies, TNF-RI was shown to be the main mediator of TNFα action in the cell [67].

Dermal injection of TNFα resulted in the accumulation of dendritic cells in draining lymph nodes as well as in impairment of contact hypersensitivity (CHS) in the skin [60, 68]. This suggests that TNFα induces the migration of LC from the skin to the surrounding regional lymph nodes. Streilein and colleagues [69, 70] observed that UVB indirectly induced TNFα, which then caused morphologic and functional changes on LC resulting in the impairment of CHS, suggesting that TNFα plays a role in this process.

Studies using TNF-R1(-) mutant mice have shown that TNFα was not involved in UVB-induced immunosuppression [71]. UVB-induced immunosuppression is implicated in the pathogenesis of skin cancers, and is mediated in part by *cis*-urocanic acid (*cis*-UCA) [72, 73]. *trans*-Urocanic acid, a deamination product of histidine, is a major chromophore present at high concentrations in the stratum corneum [73]. Upon exposure to UV radiation, *trans*-UCA undergoes a photoisomerization to its *cis*-isomer until equilibrium is reached. In humans, this occurs after one minimal erythemal dose of UV radiation, which is the lowest dose that can induce a visibly perceptible erythema [72, 73]. *cis*-UCA does not exert its immunosuppressive effects via TNFα, but through other factors such as prostaglandin E_2 [72]. Amerio *et al.* [71] showed that in TNF-R1 and TNF-R2 double knockout mice, TNFα played a minimal role in UVB-induced immunosuppression and therefore cannot be considered as a major mediator of *cis*-UCA-induced immunosuppression. While TNFα does not play a major role in UV-induced immunosuppression [60, 71] it does play a significant role in UV-induced inflammation [20] as well as in other inflammatory diseases such as rheumatoid arthritis, psoriasis, systemic lupus erythematosus and cancer [21, 38, 46, 74].

4. TACE

TNFα is cleaved from its proform by the action of the metalloprotease TACE [75]. This enzyme is a member of the disintegrin and metalloprotease (ADAM) family of proteases, and is

http://dx.doi.org/10.5772/55569

also known as ADAM 17 [22, 75-77]. ADAM proteases belong to the adamalysin/reprolysin subfamily of the metzincin superfamily, and contain a Zn^{2+}-dependent catalytic domain [75, 77].

TACE was first purified, characterized and cloned in 1997 and is a multi-domain type I transmembrane protein of 824 amino acids in length [22, 76, 78]. While its amino acid sequence shows relatively low homology to other ADAM family members, its structure contains all the domain regions, which are characteristic for this family of metalloproteases [22, 76, 79]. Structurally TACE consists of a signal peptide followed by a pro, catalytic, disintegrin, cysteine-rich, transmembrane and cytoplasmic domain [55, 80]. The catalytic domain contains the zinc-binding consensus motif HEXGHXXGXXHD involved in coordinating Zn^{2+} with His residues and creating the active site of the enzyme [79, 81]. The cysteine-rich domain may play a role in enzyme maturation or substrate recognition [75, 76].

TACE is synthesized as an inactive zymogen, which is subsequently proteolytically processed to the catalytically active form. In order for TACE to be activated its prodomain is removed at the furin cleavage site RVKR (Arg-Val-Lys-Arg) localized between the pro- and the catalytic domain, and is due to the action of a furin-type proprotein convertase [24, 77, 82-84]. In mammalian cells, proTACE is located in the endoplasmic reticulum and the proximal Golgi body whereas the mature form is located both intracellularly and on the cell membrane [83, 85]. TACE maturation is closely linked to the transport of proTACE through the medial Golgi, where upon exit, prodomain removal occurs before the enzyme reaches the cell's surface [77].

Apart from TNFα, TACE cleaves a wide range of molecules including transforming growth factor α (TGFα), amphiregulin, neuregulin, growth hormone receptor, TNF-R1, TNF-R2, L-selectin, amyloid precursor protein and IL-6R [77, 86-89]. TACE-knockout mice are far less efficient at processing TNFα on the cell membrane compared to wild type controls [75, 86]. This suggests that TACE is the main protease responsible for the processing of TNFα in the cell. Although some matrix metalloproteases (MMP) can cleave TNFα, the cleaved products are inactive due to hydrolysis occurring at different sites within the molecule [75, 81, 89].

Some metalloproteases are activated in epidermal cells following UV radiation [90-93]. Piva and co-workers found that there were a number of proteases whose activity was upregulated in UVC- or UVB-irradiated HeLa cells [91-93]. These enzymes included aminopeptidases and a "TGFαase" [91, 92]. On re-evaluation of their data, the TGFαase in questions is most likely TACE, because (a) the later enzyme is known to cleave TGFα among other growth factors [81, 88] and (b) the substrate used in these studies was a nonapeptide based on the N-terminal cleavage site of TGFα [90-93]. In cells undergoing UV-induced apoptosis, the level of cell surface protease activity (aminopeptidase and "TGFαase") was shown to be higher than that seen in viable or necrotic cells [91, 93]. The results of these studies were the first to show that TACE activity was elevated in cells exposed to UV radiation. Recently Skiba *et al.* [29] reported that UVA and UVB irradiation increased TACE mRNA levels in HaCaT cells, with higher induction induced by UVA. The expression patterns for both UVA- and UVB-irradiated cells in general appeared to be constant, although mRNA levels were significantly higher than controls throughout the 48 h post-exposure period [29].

In UV-irradiated HaCaT cells, TACE was responsible for the increased cleavage of EGF family members [28, 94]. Inhibition of TACE by metalloprotease inhibitors reduced the release of these growth factors, resulting in an increase in apoptotic cell death [28, 94]. It appears that TACE mediates a EGF receptor/AKT signalling pathway in these cells that is activated as a result of its cleavage of EGF family members. In HaCaT cells exposed to UVA-radiation TACE mediated EGF receptor activation and cell cycle progression, which suggests that UVA, at non-lethal doses, has the potential to be a skin cancer promoter [28, 94]. TACE has also shown to be overexpressed in some tumours [21, 46, 56], as well in a large number of skin cancer cells lines compared to their non tumorous counterparts [28, 94]. It is also known that members of the EGF family are overexpressed in skin cancers [95], and this could be a mechanism by which skin cancer growth is stimulated by autogenic growth factors. The results of these recent studies suggest that inhibition of TACE following UV radiation may prevent the stimulation of surviving irradiated cells. This has the potential in reducing the incidence of skin cancer that may arise from prolonged sun exposure. It is not clear if the increase in TACE activity seen in UV-irradiated skin cells is due to increased numbers or a higher level of activity. Furin is known to activate TACE [83, 85, 96] as well as matrix metalloproteases (MMP) [97, 98] and may indirectly play a role in this process.

5. Furin

Furin, also known as PACE, is a 94 kDa, type I transmembrane, Ca^{2+}-dependant serine protease. It is a member of the proprotein convertase (PC) family which is related to the bacterial subtisilin enzyme [23, 97-99]. The PC family consists of seven distinct members (furin and PC1-PC7) that vary in regards to their tissue and subcellular distribution as well as enzymatic and biochemical properties [23, 24, 97, 100]. Furin, PACE 4, PC5/6 and PC7/8 are widely expressed in the epidermis whereas PC2 and PC1/3 are limited to neuroendocrine tissues and PC4 is restricted to the testis [23, 24, 98]. The PC enzymes recognize basic motifs, cleaving after paired basic residues (PC2 and PC1/3); or after a canonical Rx (R/K) R (Arg-x-(Arg/Lys)-Arg) motif (furin and PACE4) [24, 97, 98, 100-102]. Both PC7 and furin share cleave similar substrates and the selectivity of which depends on their cellular localization. As their cytosolic domains regulate intracellular trafficking it is likely that the cellular localization of PC7 differs to that for furin [85].

Structurally furin and other PCs consist of a signal peptide followed by pro, catalytic, middle, and cytoplasmic domains, respectively [24]. The signal peptide directs the translocation of the peptide chain to the endoplasmic reticulum and the secretory pathway [82, 97, 103]. The pro-region is cleaved in the endoplasmic reticulum, where it then associates with the catalytic domain and helps to guide the protein through this region to the Golgi apparatus where it becomes catalytically active [97, 103]. The trans-membrane region anchors the enzyme in the membrane of the trans Golgi network (TGN) or on the cell membrane. The cytosolic tail contains the information necessary for furin's sorting to various intracellular compartments [82, 97, 103]. In the epidermis, furin can exist either as: (a) a mature 97 kDa membrane bound enzyme or (b) a smaller 75 kDa form that lacks the transmembrane domain [97]. This suggests that post-translational cleavage at the C-terminus occurs within in the cell [97, 98, 103]. Furin and other PC family members process inactive precursor proteins to their functional or mature form, and these include growth factor receptors, growth factors, hormones, plasma proteins, and MMPs [23, 24, 97, 98, 103] as seen in Table 2. PC family members play crucial roles in a variety of physiological processes and are involved in the pathology of diseases such as cancer and viral infection [23, 101, 103-106].

Functional group	Substrate	References
Serum proteins	Von Willebrand Factor	[107]
	Coagulation factor IX	[108]
Signalling peptides	Endothelin-1	[103, 109]
Growth factors	TGFβ	[103, 110]
	Vascular endothelial growth factor (VEGF)	[111]
	β-Nerve growth factor	[112]
Membrane proteins	MT1-MMP	[86, 113, 114]
	TACE	[72, 99, 115]
Transmembrane receptors	Notch1 Receptor	[98, 116]
	Insulin growth factor 1 receptor	[117]
Extracellular matrix proteins	N-Cadherin	[113, 118]
	Integrin α-chain subunits	[119]
Viral proteins	Ebola virus glycoprotein	[103, 120]
	Papillomavirus minor capsid protein L2	[121]
Bacterial toxins	Anthrax toxin	[122]
	Clostridium septicum alpha-toxin	[103, 123]

Table 2. Some biological molecules cleaved by furin

As a result of the role furin plays in many disease states, considerable effort has been directed at designing specific inhibitors that may have therapeutic applications. The first furin inhibitors that were synthesised where peptidyl chloromethyl ketones [124]. The next major furin inhibitor that was developed, decanoyl-Arg-Val-Lys-Arg-chloromethylketone (dec-RVKR-cmk, or CMK) was less cytotoxic and is cell permeable and has been used in many experimental studies [86, 106, 125]. It was recently shown to reduce the incidence of skin cancer in transgenic mice by inhibiting PACE4 as well as other PCs [126]. However a limitation of CMK's use is that it is not furin specific, and is also known to inhibit other proprotein convertases [86, 102, 127]. Zhu *et al.* [127] has recently developed an antibody-based single domain nanobody which is a furin specific inhibitor. Through the use of this and other furin-specific inhibitors, it will be possible to delineate the role furin plays in the processing of specific substrates within in the cell. This will help in development of specific inhibitors, which will have therapeutic potential in the treatment of a variety of diseases.

Furin and other PCs have been shown to be involved in the maturation of both TACE and MMP within skin cells. ProTACE is processed by both furin and PC7 to its mature form thereby increasing its proteolytic activity [83, 85]. The maturation of TACE occurs as it transits through the Golgi compartment where the prodomain was removed by a furin-type proprotein convertase [77, 84, 85]. As increased amounts of mature TACE are detected in furin overexpressing cells, it appears that proTACE is a better substrate for furin than it is for PC7 [85]. A similar observation has been seen in cells overexpressing TACE [58, 83, 99] where furin was shown to be responsible for its cleavage [83, 99]. This finding was confirmed using cell permeable furin inhibitors CMK and PDX in Cos7 cells [83] and keratinocytes [98] where reduced levels of mature TACE were formed.

Furin mRNA, protein and enzyme activity has been observed in human epidermal keratinocytes [29, 98, 111, 128, 129]. Skiba *et al.* [29] found that UVA and UVB radiation immediately increased furin mRNA levels in HaCaT cells. UVB irradiation induced higher levels of furin mRNA expression [29]. The time course for furin mRNA levels in cells irradiated with low dose of UVA or high dose of UVB was similar to that for TNFα, whereas maximal mRNA induction of both genes were detected 8 h post-irradiation [29]. Although UV irradiation does appear to have an effect on furin gene expression, no direct relationship was apparent between TACE and furin mRNA induction. A recent study has shown that following exposure to UVA and UVB, furin levels in HaCaT cells fell with respect to time [49, 129]. However, it was unknown whether this was due to the loss of the pro or mature form of the enzyme. Through its effect on stimulating MMPs, as well as activating TACE and the resultant effect this has on TNFα released by the cell, furin activity has an influence on the inflammation seen in the skin following exposure to UV radiation as seen in Figure 2.

Furin/PC processing of substrates has been shown to also contribute to tumour progression, aggressiveness, metastasis, and angiogenesis [23, 24, 104-106]. Tumour invasion and metastasis represent a multistep process that depends on the activity of many proteins [46, 101, 104, 130]. Proteolytic degradation of the ECM components is a central event of this process. Several classes of proteases, including MMPs, serine proteases and cysteine proteases have been implicated in the tumour cell invasive process [104, 130, 131]. Of these, MMPs appear to be primarily responsible for much of the ECM degradation observed during invasive processes [111, 130, 132-134]. They can contribute to tumour growth not only by degradation of the ECM but by the release of sequestered growth factors or the generation of bioactive fragments VEGF, bFGF or TGFβ, the suppression of tumour cell apoptosis and the destruction of immune-modulating chemokine gradients [131, 132, 135]. Furin also cleaves a number of MMPs from their proform, and activating them as a result [23, 86, 102, 105].

6. MMPs

MMPs belong to the family of zinc-dependent endopeptidases collectively referred to as metzincins. The metzincins can be subdivided into four families: seralysins, astacins, ADAMs/adamalysins, and MMPs [130, 136]. So far to date, 28 members of the MMP family have been identified [130, 135, 136] which are primarily responsible for most of the ECM degradation observed during the invasive processes. MMPs are produced by skin cells (fibroblasts, keratinocytes, melanocytes) as well as macrophages, endothelial cells and mast cells [10, 25, 81, 137].

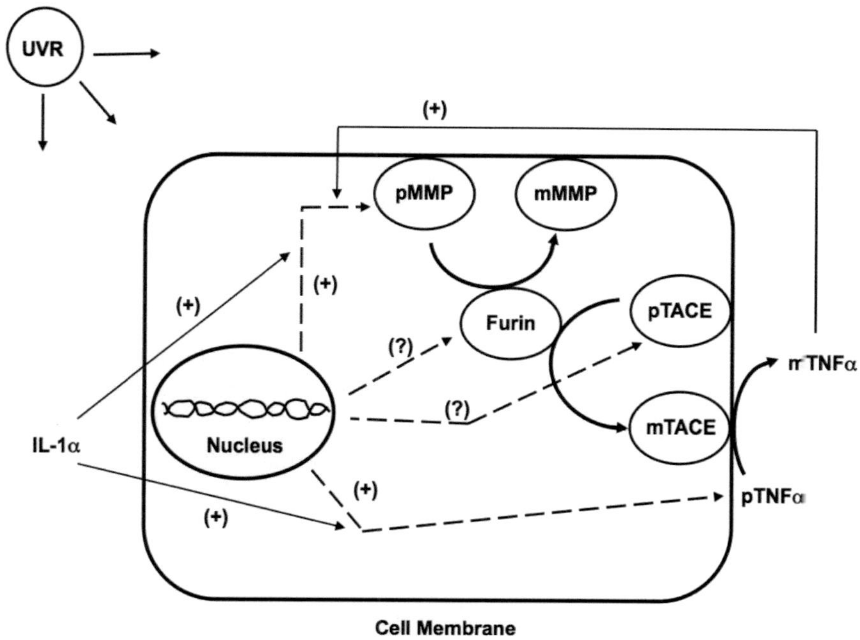

Figure 2. The role furin plays in the maturation of TACE and MMPs in skin cells. Furin cleaves and activates TACE, which in turn can process TNFα from its proform. Keratinocytes secrete TNFα following exposure to UVB radiation, and this is enhanced if IL-1α is present. Furin also cleaves MMPs from their respective proforms, and the expression and activity of these proteases are elevated when the cells have been exposed to UVB radiation, and they are enhanced if either IL-1α (MMP-9) or TNFα (MMP-2) is present. The effect of UVB radiation on the expression of the enzymes and pTNFα in the cell is represented by dashed lines, if it is enhanced it is represented by (+), and if it is unknown (?)

MMPs are also implicated in cell migration, proliferation, and tissue remodelling and thereby may also play a role in growth and development, angiogenesis, and atherosclerosis [138, 139].

Structurally MMPs consist of a signal peptide followed by pro, catalytic, hemopexin and cytoplasmic domains, respectively [130]. MMPs cleave peptides and proteins, which have a myriad of functions that are independent of their proteolytic activity [140]. They have distinct but often overlapping substrate specificities, hence leading to the absence of distinct phenotypes in most genetically-engineered mice with knockdown of specific MMPs [140].

MMPs are generally expressed in very low amounts and their transcription is tightly regulated either positively or negatively by cytokines and growth factors such as IL-1, IL-4, IL-6, TGFβ, or TNFα [130, 135, 141, 142]. Some of these regulatory molecules can be proteolytically activated or inactivated by MMPs (via a feedback loop). MMPs are synthesized as latent proenzymes, which are converted into mature, catalytically active forms in the TGN by PCs [111, 139]. Activation of MMPs following secretion from the cell depends on disruption of the prodomain interaction with the catalytic site, which may occur either by conformational changes or proteolytic removal of the prodomain. With the exception of MMP-2, the mechanism for *in vivo* activation of secreted MMPs is not well understood [135].

In normal skin, MMPs are not constitutively expressed but can be induced temporarily in response to exogenous signals such as UVR [10, 25, 143]. Elevated levels of MMP activity in human skin, as a result of prolonged periods of sun exposure, confirm that it plays a major role in photoageing [10, 25, 28]. Onoue *et al.* [144] suggested that MMP-9 secreted from keratinocytes after UVB irradiation might result from apoptotic events. UV radiation is known to elevate the expression of MMP-1, MMP-3 (stromelysin-1) and MMP-9 in human skin *in vivo* [25]. All three MMPs (1, 3 and 9) can degrade most of the proteins found in the extracellular matrix [25]. MMP-1, which is produced by both dermal fibroblasts and epidermal keratinocytes, cleaves type 1 collagen into specific fragments. These fragments can then be further hydrolysed by MMP-2 and MMP-9 [137, 145]. Steinbrenner *et al.* [137] found that UVA irradiation dose-dependently decreased the steady-state mRNA levels of MMP-2 and MMP-9 and lowered the gelatinolytic activity of both enzymes in cell culture supernatants. Of interest is that *in vivo*, following exposure to UV radiation only keratinocytes express large levels of MMP on the cell membrane [146], but when fibroblasts grown in culture are irradiated they express higher levels of MMP on their plasma membrane [147]. The reasons for the discrepancies between the responses of human skin cells under *in vivo* and *in vitro* conditions are not known.

TNFα has been shown to induce proMMP-2 in human dermal fibroblasts [8], while IL-1α induced proMMP-9 levels in fibroblasts and keratinocytes [148]. In mesenchymal cells TNFα was shown to stimulate MMP-2 activity by activating a proteolytic cascade involving furin and MT1-MMP [139]. It is not known if TNFα activates MMP activity in epidermal cells via a similar mechanism. MMP-9 [144], has been shown to play an important role in the pathophysiologies of many skin conditions such as wound healing [145], and angiogenesis [87]. Activation of pro-MMP2 takes place at the cell surface and involves interactions with active MT1-MMP, which is itself activated through rapid trafficking to the cell surface and proteolytic processing [139]. Maquoi *et al.* [114] demonstrated that furin-inhibitor reduces the level of mature MT1-MMP, which is paralleled by a decrease in pro-MMP-2 activation as well as in cell invasiveness, confirming the furin plays a role in this process. Direct cleavage of proMMP-2 by furin in the TGN has shown to inactivate this matrix metalloprotease [149]. Therefore changes to the level of MMP-2 activity on the surface of the cell can be directly or indirectly regulated by furin either through cleavage in the TGN to reduce activity or indirectly via MT1-MMP, which increases activity. The mechanism by which this is regulated is not clear.

7. Role of furin in skin cancer

Low doses of UV radiation while they are not inflammatory, can cause mutations in skin tissue [9, 19, 30] or in cultured fibroblasts [150]. Constant exposure to UV radiation will not only result in mutations in p53 [150, 151] but in other genes including p16, PTCH, B-Raf, which will result in these cells becoming carcinogenic [6, 152, 153]. Apart from causing these mutations, UV radiation enhances the release of inflammatory molecules (e.g. TNFα, IL-1α, ROS, chemokines) from the skin (see section 2 for details). The result of which is the creation of an environment that allows for these mutated skin cells to become cancerous over time [15, 19, 21, 46, 56]. As a result of increased levels of MMP activity on the cell membrane, either as a

http://dx.doi.org/10.5772/55569

result of UV exposure or other factors, these skin cancer cells may become metastatic as a result of epithelial to mesenchymal transition (EMT) [154].

In the progression of a mutated cell to that of a tumorigenic or metastatic cell, PCs have been shown to cleave a range of precursors of growth factors, their receptors, adhesion molecules, proteases and MMPs. Some of these molecules include cadherins, TGFβ, platelet derived growth factor as well as insulin-like growth factor 1 and its receptor [23, 101, 106, 117, 155]. Tumour progression and metastasis may enhanced by a number of factors such as (a) hypoxia-induced upregulation of furin activity within the solid tumour mass [105], (b) changes in cell adhesion through PC cleavage and activation of integrins and related adhesion molecules [156], (c) furin processing of vascular endothelial growth factor resulting in increased angiogenic activity [157], and (d) furin enhanced expression of MMPs [84, 158].

Furin/PC expression and processing can increase the incidence and severity of the cancer phenotype [104, 111]. Aberrant furin expression has been observed in a number of tumours including those from the breast [159], ovary [160], liver [125], brain [161], skin [111, 132] and from other tissues [23, 128, 162, 163]. Bassi *et al.* [101] observed that PACE4 transgenic mice were more susceptible to epidermal carcinogenesis and tumour progression compared to controls. These transgenic keratinocytes had higher rates of processing of MT1-MMP and MT2-MMP resulting in increased collagen degradation.

MMP-2 (gelatinase A) and MMP-9 (gelatinase B) have been frequently associated with the invasive and metastatic potential of tumour cells [10, 104, 111, 130, 132, 133, 137]. The expression of MMP-2, is regulated independently of MMP-9 [144]. The close correlation observed between MMP-2 activation and metastatic progression in various tumours suggests that it may act as a "master switch" triggering tumour spread [114]. The expression of MMP is low in keratinocytes but elevated in BCC and SCC [49, 164, 165]. In SCC, MMP proteins (1, 2, 3 and MT1-MMP) are expressed both in tumorous and stromal cells [165], while MMP proteins (1, 2, 3 and 9) are observed in BCCs and melanomas [165, 166]. This expression correlates with the progression and the metastatic potentials of these tumours [106, 135, 165, 167]. UVR can participate to the development of skin cancer by the activation of MMPs. Two molecular mechanisms contribute to the UV-induced MMPs expression. First, the activation of cell-surface receptors with subsequent activation of mitogen activated protein kinase (MAPK) cascade that in turn contributes to the transcriptional up-regulation of MMPs [168]. Second, through the expression of pro-inflammatory cytokines, which induce the expression of MMPs [46, 133, 142, 143]. The role of UV in the induction of MMPs is supported by two experimental findings. First, UV-irradiation of SCC cell lines results in an increased secretion of MMPs [49, 132]. Second, UV-induced phosphorylation of extracellular signal-regulated kinase (ERK) and stress kinases precedes the rapid stimulation of MMPs in SCC cells [10]. If there are cells in the skin which become cancerous as a result of DNA damage, some may go onto become metastatic due to increased MMP activity [111]. This increase in levels of activated MMPs on the surface of the cell could be due to either increased expression of proMMP protein and/or increased furin activity. The role furin plays in the development of skin cancer suggests that it could be significant, and as such the development of specific inhibitors may offer a new therapy to treat such tumours.

Recently, Fu *et al.* [106] showed that in transgenic mice overexpressing furin, exposed to chemical carcinogens formed more and larger tumours than did control mice. This suggests that furin enhances skin cancer growth. Of interest was that these tumours were induced by chemical carcinogens and not by UV radiation. While enhanced furin levels were shown to enhance skin tumour development, in studies using cultured melanoma and glioma cells, furin inhibition was shown to reduce the processing of the pro-N-cadherin adhesion molecule, enhancing their migratory and aggressive nature [118]. The result of this study suggests that high furin levels may not enhance the metastasis of some tumours. Huang *et al.* [125] when investigating the expression of furin in hepatocellular carcinoma and surrounding tissue in humans, observed that if this ratio was >3.5 this resulted in higher patient survival rates compared to those who had ratios <3.5. This suggests that furin may play a dual role in cancer development, though the exact nature of which is not clear at this stage. Further study on this is warranted, and may result in a better understanding of its role in cancer development, and from which it may be possible to develop specific furin inhibitors which could be used clinically to treat these tumours.

8. Conclusion

While it has been shown that UVA and UVB radiation cause different effects on the immune response this could be related to the activity of cell surface metalloproteases found on skin cells. Although the effect of TNFα in UV-induced inflammation has been well documented, little is known if the changes in TACE activity are due to increased protein levels or changes in enzyme activity. The inflammatory environment, seen in the skin, following exposure to UV radiation is known to stimulate the development of mutated cells which possess DNA damage caused directly by UV radiation or indirectly through the generation of ROS. Apart from processing TNFα, TACE also cleaves EGF family members, which would stimulate the growth of these mutated cells, which over time may become cancerous. As TNFα is a powerful inflammatory cytokine, considerable research has been under taken to develop specific TACE inhibitors [55, 56, 80]. Such inhibitors may play an important role in preventing the development of UV-induced skin cancers. An increased knowledge of the roles played by metalloproteases in tumour progression, combined with the use of more selective inhibitors, could lead to effective use of these compounds in cancer therapies [55].

Similar to that of TACE, MMPs are also activated by UV radiation and also play a crucial role in skin tumour cell development and metastasis. Furin and other PCs have been shown to play an important role in activating both TACE and many MMPs in skin cells. Whereas the overexpression and activity of furin exacerbates the cancer phenotype, inhibition of its activity decreases or nullifies its effects, and thus, the development and use of specific inhibitors may also be a viable route to cancer therapy [23, 86, 102, 127].

It is known that UV induces furin mRNA in skin cells, though protein levels do not appear to change with respect to time, which suggests a rapid turnover of the enzyme. Further study is needed on how UV radiation activates furin, TACE and MMPs in skin cells. These proteases play an important role in the changes observed in those epidermal cells exposed to UV radiation. The development of specific furin inhibitors has the potential to reduce the carcinogenic effects of sunlight by preventing the activation of TACE and MMPs and their subsequent downstream effects. Such compounds may have the potential to offer new therapies both in the prevention and treatment of skin cancer.

Acknowledgements

We would like to that the School of Medical Sciences, RMIT University, Bundoora, Australia for supporting this study, and for the awarding of a School of Medical Science's Postgraduate Research Scholarship to RR.

Author details

Rethika Ravi[1] and Terrence J Piva[2*]

*Address all correspondence to: terry.piva@rmit.edu.au

1 Endeavour College of Natural Health, Melbourne, Australia

2 School of Medical Sciences, RMIT University, Melbourne, Australia

References

[1] Guy GP, Ekwueme DU. Years of potential life lost and indirect costs of melanoma and non-melanoma skin cancer: a systematic review of the literature. Pharmacoeconomics. 2011;29(10) 863-874.

[2] Qureshi AA, Laden F, Colditz GA, Hunter DJ. Geographic variation and risk of skin cancer in US women. Differences between melanoma, squamous cell carcinoma, and basal cell carcinoma. Archives of Internal Medicine. 2008;168(5) 501-507.

[3] Narayanan DL, Saladi RN, Fox JL. Ultraviolet radiation and skin cancer. International Journal of Dermatology. 2010;49(9) 978-986.

[4] Thomas-Ahner JM, Wulff BC, Tober KL, Kusewitt DF, Riggenbach JA. Oberyszyn TM. Gender differences in UVB-induced skin carcinogenesis, inflammation, and DNA damage. Cancer Research. 2007;67(7) 3468-3474.

[5] Erb P, Ji J, Kump E, Mielgo A, Wernli M. Apoptosis and pathogenesis of melanoma and nonmelanoma skin cancer. Advances in Experimental Medicine and Biology. 2008;624 283-295.

[6] Rass K, Reichrath J. UV damage and DNA repair in malignant melanoma and nonmelanoma skin cancer. Advances in Experimental Medicine and Biology. 2008;624 162-178.

[7] Maverakis E, Miyamura Y, Bowen MP, Correa G, Ono Y, Goodarzi H. Light, including ultraviolet. Journal of Autoimmunity. 2010;34(3) J247-257.

[8] Clydesdale GJ, Dandie GW, Muller HK. Ultraviolet light induced injury: immunological and inflammatory effects. Immunology and Cell Biology. 2001;79(6) 547-568.

[9] Agar NS, Halliday GM, Barnetson RS, Ananthaswamy HN, Wheeler M, Jones AM. The basal layer in human squamous tumors harbors more UVA than UVB fingerprint mutations: a role for UVA in human skin carcinogenesis. Proceedings of the National Academy of Sciences of the United States of America. 2004;101(14) 4954-4959.

[10] Dong KK, Damaghi N, Picart SD, Markova NG, Obayashi K, Okano Y, Masaki H, Grether-Beck S, Krutmann J, Smiles KA, Yarosh DB. UV-induced DNA damage initiates release of MMP-1 in human skin. Experimental Dermatology. 2008;17(12) 1037-1044.

[11] Pfeifer GP, Besaratinia A. UV wavelength-dependent DNA damage and human nonmelanoma and melanoma skin cancer. Photochemical and Photobiological Sciences. 2012;11(1) 90-97.

[12] Sander CS, Chang H, Hamm F, Elsner P, Thiele JJ. Role of oxidative stress and the antioxidant network in cutaneous carcinogenesis. International Journal of Dermatology. 2004;43(5) 326-335.

[13] Muthusamy V, Piva TJ. The UV response of the skin: a review of the MAPK, NFκB and TNFα signal transduction pathways. Archives for Dermatological Research (Archiv fur Dermatologische Forschung). 2010;302(1) 5-17.

[14] Rangwala S, Tsai KY. Roles of the immune system in skin cancer. British Journal of Dermatology. 2011;165(5) 953-965.

[15] Ullrich SE, Byrne SN. The immunologic revolution: photoimmunology. Journal of Investigative Dermatology. 2012;132(3 Pt 2) 896-905.

[16] Shorrocks J, Paul ND, McMillan TJ. The dose rate of UVA treatment influences the cellular response of HaCaT keratinocytes. Journal of Investigative Dermatology. 2008;128(3) 685-693.

[17] Valencia A, Kochevar IE. Nox1-based NADPH oxidase is the major source of UVA-induced reactive oxygen species in human keratinocytes. Journal of Investigative Dermatology. 2008;128(1) 214-222.

[18] Mahns A, Wolber R, Stab F, Klotz LO, Sies H. Contribution of UVB and UVA to UV-dependent stimulation of cyclooxygenase-2 expression in artificial epidermis. Photochemical and Photobiological Sciences. 2004;3(3) 257-262.

[19] Halliday GM, Lyons JG. Inflammatory doses of UV may not be necessary for skin carcinogenesis. Photochemistry and Photobiology. 2008;84(2) 272-283.

[20] Damian DL, Patterson CR, Stapelberg M, Park J, Barnetson RS, Halliday GM. UV radiation-induced immunosuppression is greater in men and prevented by topical nicotinamide. Journal of Investigative Dermatology. 2008;128(2) 447-454.

[21] Balkwill F. Tumour necrosis factor and cancer. Nature Reviews Cancer. 2009;9(5) 361-371.

[22] Black RA, Rauch CT, Kozlosky CJ, Peschon JJ, Slack JL, Wolfson MF, Castner BJ, Stocking KL, Reddy P, Srinivasan S, Nelson N, Boiani N, Schooley KA, Gerhart M, Davis R, Fitzner JN, Johnson RS, Paxton RJ, March CJ, Cerretti DP. A metalloproteinase disintegrin that releases tumour-necrosis factor-α from cells. Nature. 1997;385(6618) 729-733.

[23] Artenstein AW, Opal SM. Proprotein convertases in health and disease. New England Journal of Medicine. 2011;365(26) 2507-2518.

[24] Seidah NG. The proprotein convertases, 20 years later. Methods in Molecular Biology. 2011;768 23-57.

[25] Quan T, Qin Z, Xia W, Shao Y, Voorhees JJ, Fisher GJ. Matrix-degrading metalloproteinases in photoaging. Journal of Investigative Dermatology Symposium Proceedings. 2009;14(1) 20-24.

[26] Sluyter R, Halliday GM. Infiltration by inflammatory cells required for solar-simulated ultraviolet radiation enhancement of skin tumor growth. Cancer Immunology, Immunotherapy. 2001;50(3) 151-156.

[27] Weller R. Nitric oxide: a key mediator in cutaneous physiology. Clinical and Experimental Dermatology. 2003;28(5) 511-514.

[28] Bennett MF, Robinson MK, Baron ED, Cooper KD. Skin immune systems and inflammation: protector of the skin or promoter of aging? Journal of Investigative Dermatology Symposium Proceedings. 2008;13(1) 15-19.

[29] Skiba B, Neill B, Piva TJ. Gene expression profiles of TNF-α, TACE, furin, IL-1β and matrilysin in UVA- and UVB-irradiated HaCat cells. Photodermatology, Photoimmunology and Photomedicine. 2005;21(4) 173-182.

[30] Halliday GM. Inflammation, gene mutation and photoimmunosuppression in response to UVR-induced oxidative damage contributes to photocarcinogenesis. Mutation Research. 2005;571(1-2) 107-120.

[31] Barr RM, Walker SL, Tsang W, Harrison GI, Ettehadi P, Greaves MW, Young AR. Suppressed alloantigen presentation, increased TNF-α, IL-1, IL-1Ra, IL-10, and modulation of TNF-R in UV-irradiated human skin. Journal of Investigative Dermatology. 1999;112(5) 692-698.

[32] Byrne SN, Limon-Flores AY, Ullrich SE. Mast cell migration from the skin to the draining lymph nodes upon ultraviolet irradiation represents a key step in the induction of immune suppression. Journal of Immunology. 2008;180(7) 4648-4655.

[33] Norval M. Effects of solar radiation on the human immune system. Journal of Photochemistry and Photobiology B, Biology. 2001;63(1-3) 28-40.

[34] Morelli JG, Norris DA. Influence of inflammatory mediators and cytokines on human melanocyte function. Journal of Investigative Dermatology. 1993;100(2 Suppl) 191S-195S.

[35] Berhane T, Halliday GM, Cooke B, Barnetson RS. Inflammation is associated with progression of actinic keratoses to squamous cell carcinomas in humans. British Journal of Dermatology. 2002;146(5) 810-815.

[36] Meeran SM, Punathil T, Katiyar SK. IL-12 deficiency exacerbates inflammatory responses in UV-irradiated skin and skin tumors. Journal of Investigative Dermatology. 2008;128(11) 2716-2727.

[37] Yoshizumi M, Nakamura T, Kato M, Ishioka T, Kozawa K, Wakamatsu K, Kimura H. Release of cytokines/chemokines and cell death in UVB-irradiated human keratinocytes, HaCaT. Cell Biology International. 2008;32(11) 1405-1411.

[38] Bashir MM, Sharma MR, Werth VP. UVB and proinflammatory cytokines synergistically activate TNF-α production in keratinocytes through enhanced gene transcription. Journal of Investigative Dermatology. 2009;129(4) 994-1001.

[39] Bashir MM, Sharma MR, Werth VP. TNF-α production in the skin. Archives for Dermatological Research (Archiv fur Dermatologische Forschung). 2009;301(1) 87-91.

[40] Lyons JG, Birkedal-Hansen B, Pierson MC, Whitelock JM, Birkedal-Hansen H. Interleukin-1β and transforming growth factor-α/epidermal growth factor induce expression of M(r) 95,000 type IV collagenase/gelatinase and interstitial fibroblast-type collagenase by rat mucosal keratinocytes. Journal of Biological Chemistry. 1993;268(25) 19143-19151.

[41] Fisher GJ, Datta SC, Talwar HS, Wang ZQ, Varani J, Kang S, Voorhees JJ. Molecular basis of sun-induced premature skin ageing and retinoid antagonism. Nature. 1996;379(6563) 335-339.

[42] Rundhaug JE, Fischer SM. Cyclo-oxygenase-2 plays a critical role in UV-induced skin carcinogenesis. Photochemistry and Photobiology. 2008;84(2) 322-329.

[43] An KP, Athar M, Tang X, Katiyar SK, Russo J, Beech J, Aszterbaum M, Kopelovich L, Epstein EH, Jr., Mukhtar H, Bickers DR. Cyclooxygenase-2 expression in murine and human nonmelanoma skin cancers: implications for therapeutic approaches. Photochemistry and Photobiology. 2002;76(1) 73-80.

[44] Patel MJ, Stockfleth E. Does progression from actinic keratosis and Bowen's disease end with treatment: diclofenac 3% gel, an old drug in a new environment? British Journal of Dermatology. 2007;156 Suppl 3 53-56.

[45] Butler GJ, Neale R, Green AC, Pandeya N, Whiteman DC. Nonsteroidal anti-inflammatory drugs and the risk of actinic keratoses and squamous cell cancers of the skin. Journal of the American Academy of Dermatology. 2005;53(6) 966-972.

[46] Sethi G, Shanmugam MK, Ramachandran L, Kumar AP, Tergaonkar V. Multifaceted link between cancer and inflammation. Bioscience Reports. 2012;32(1) 1-15.

[47] Yarosh D, Both D, Kibitel J, Anderson C, Elmets C, Brash D, Brown D. Regulation of TNFα production and release in human and mouse keratinocytes and mouse skin after UV-B irradiation. Photodermatology, Photoimmunology and Photomedicine. 2000;16(6) 263-270.

[48] Muthusamy V, Hodges LD, Macrides TA, Boyle GM, Piva TJ. Effect of novel marine nutraceuticals on IL-1α-mediated TNF-α release from UVB-irradiated human melanocyte-derived cells. Oxidative Medicine and Cellular Longevity. 2011;2011 728645.

[49] Ravi R. The effect of UV radiation on furin activity in human keratinocyte cell lines [PhD Thesis]. RMIT University; Melbourne: 2010.

[50] Muthusamy V. The role cell signalling pathways play in TNFα release from UV-irradiated human skin cells [PhD Thesis]. RMIT University; Melbourne: 2010.

[51] Fuller BB, Smith DR. Topical anti-inflammatories. In: Draelos ZD, Thaman LA, editors. Cosmetic formulation of skin care products. New York: Informa Healthcare; 2002. p. 351-376.

[52] Ogilvie AL, Luftl M, Antoni C, Schuler G, Kalden JR, Lorenz HM. Leukocyte infiltration and mRNA expression of IL-20, IL-8 and TNF-R P60 in psoriatic skin is driven by TNF-alpha. Int J Immunopathol Pharmacol. 2006;19(2) 271-278.

[53] Serwin AB, Sokolowska M, Chodynicka B. Tumour necrosis factor α (TNF-α)-converting enzyme (TACE) and soluble TNF-α receptor type 1 in psoriasis patients treated with narrowband ultraviolet B. Photodermatology, Photoimmunology and Photomedicine. 2007;23(4) 130-134.

[54] Schwarz A, Bhardwaj R, Aragane Y, Mahnke K, Riemann H, Metze D, Luger TA, Schwarz T. Ultraviolet-B-induced apoptosis of keratinocytes: evidence for partial in-

volvement of tumor necrosis factor-α in the formation of sunburn cells. Journal of Investigative Dermatology. 1995;104(6) 922-927.

[55] Saftig P, Reiss K. The "A Disintegrin And Metalloproteases" ADAM10 and ADAM17: novel drug targets with therapeutic potential? European Journal of Cell Biology. 2011;90(6-7) 527-535.

[56] Scheller J, Chalaris A, Garbers C, Rose-John S. ADAM17: a molecular switch to control inflammation and tissue regeneration. Trends in Immunology. 2011;32(8) 380-387.

[57] DasGupta S, Murumkar PR, Giridhar R, Yadav MR. Current perspective of TACE inhibitors: a review. Bioorganic and Medicinal Chemistry. 2009;17(2) 444-459.

[58] Goetz FW, Planas JV, MacKenzie S. Tumor necrosis factors. Developmental and Comparative Immunology. 2004;28(5) 487-497.

[59] Bouwmeester T, Bauch A, Ruffner H, Angrand PO, Bergamini G, Croughton K, Cruciat C, Eberhard D, Gagneur J, Ghidelli S, Hopf C, Huhse B, Mangano R, Michon AM, Schirle M, Schlegl J, Schwab M, Stein MA, Bauer A, Casari G, Drewes G, Gavin AC, Jackson DB, Joberty G, Neubauer G, Rick J, Kuster B, Superti-Furga G. A physical and functional map of the human TNF-α/NF-κB signal transduction pathway. Nature Cell Biology. 2004;6(2) 97-105.

[60] Lewis M, Tartaglia LA, Lee A, Bennett GL, Rice GC, Wong GH, Chen EY, Goeddel DV. Cloning and expression of cDNAs for two distinct murine tumor necrosis factor receptors demonstrate one receptor is species specific. Proceedings of the National Academy of Sciences of the United States of America. 1991;88(7) 2830-2834.

[61] Choo-Kang BS, Hutchison S, Nickdel MB, Bundick RV, Leishman AJ, Brewer JM, McInnes IB, Garside P. TNF-blocking therapies: an alternative mode of action? Trends in Immunology. 2005;26(10) 518-522.

[62] Cumberbatch M, Kimber I. Tumour necrosis factor-α is required for accumulation of dendritic cells in draining lymph nodes and for optimal contact sensitization. Immunology. 1995;84(1) 31-35.

[63] Zhuang L, Wang B, Shinder GA, Shivji GM, Mak TW, Sauder DN. TNF receptor p55 plays a pivotal role in murine keratinocyte apoptosis induced by ultraviolet B irradiation. Journal of Immunology. 1999;162(3) 1440-1447.

[64] Starcher B. Role for tumour necrosis factor-α receptors in ultraviolet-induced skin tumours. British Journal of Dermatology. 2000;142(6) 1140-1147.

[65] Erickson SL, de Sauvage FJ, Kikly K, Carver-Moore K, Pitts-Meek S, Gillett N, Sheehan KC, Schreiber RD, Goeddel DV, Moore MW. Decreased sensitivity to tumour-necrosis factor but normal T-cell development in TNF receptor-2-deficient mice. Nature. 1994;372(6506) 560-563.

[66] Rothe J, Lesslauer W, Lotscher H, Lang Y, Koebel P, Kontgen F, Althage A, Zinkernagel R, Steinmetz M, Bluethmann H. Mice lacking the tumour necrosis factor receptor 1 are resistant to TNF-mediated toxicity but highly susceptible to infection by Listeria monocytogenes. Nature. 1993;364(6440) 798-802.

[67] Tartaglia LA, Pennica D, Goeddel DV. Ligand passing: the 75-kDa tumor necrosis factor (TNF) receptor recruits TNF for signaling by the 55-kDa TNF receptor. Journal of Biological Chemistry. 1993;268(25) 18542-18548.

[68] Cumberbatch M, Kimber I. Dermal tumour necrosis factor-α induces dendritic cell migration to draining lymph nodes, and possibly provides one stimulus for Langerhans' cell migration. Immunology. 1992;75(2) 257-263.

[69] Kurimoto I, Streilein JW. cis-urocanic acid suppression of contact hypersensitivity induction is mediated via tumor necrosis factor-α. Journal of Immunology. 1992;148(10) 3072-3078.

[70] Streilein JW. Sunlight and skin-associated lymphoid tissues (SALT): if UVB is the trigger and TNF α is its mediator, what is the message? Journal of Investigative Dermatology. 1993;100(1) 47S-52S.

[71] Amerio P, Toto P, Feliciani C, Suzuki H, Shivji G, Wang B, Sauder DN. Rethinking the role of tumour necrosis factor-α in ultraviolet (UV) B-induced immunosuppression: altered immune response in UV-irradiated TNFR1R2 gene-targeted mutant mice. British Journal of Dermatology. 2001;144(5) 952-957.

[72] Kaneko K, Smetana-Just U, Matsui M, Young AR, John S, Norval M, Walker SL. cis-Urocanic acid initiates gene transcription in primary human keratinocytes. Journal of Immunology. 2008;181(1) 217-224.

[73] Moodycliffe AM, Bucana CD, Kripke ML, Norval M, Ullrich SE. Differential effects of a monoclonal antibody to cis-urocanic acid on the suppression of delayed and contact hypersensitivity following ultraviolet irradiation. Journal of Immunology. 1996;157(7) 2891-2899.

[74] Dinarello CA. The paradox of pro-inflammatory cytokines in cancer. Cancer and Metastasis Reviews. 2006;25(3) 307-313.

[75] Black RA. Tumor necrosis factor-α converting enzyme. International Journal of Biochemistry and Cell Biology. 2002;34(1) 1-5.

[76] Moss ML, Jin SL, Milla ME, Bickett DM, Burkhart W, Carter HL, Chen WJ, Clay WC, Didsbury JR, Hassler D, Hoffman CR, Kost TA, Lambert MH, Leesnitzer MA, McCauley P, McGeehan G, Mitchell J, Moyer M, Pahel G, Rocque W, Overton LK, Schoenen F, Seaton T, Su JL, Becherer JD, et al. Cloning of a disintegrin metalloproteinase that processes precursor tumour-necrosis factor-α. Nature. 1997;385(6618) 733-736.

[77] Schlondorff J, Becherer JD, Blobel CP. Intracellular maturation and localization of the tumour necrosis factor α convertase (TACE). Biochemical Journal. 2000;347 Pt 1 131-138.

[78] Schlondorff J, Blobel CP. Metalloprotease-disintegrins: modular proteins capable of promoting cell-cell interactions and triggering signals by protein-ectodomain shedding. Journal of Cell Science. 1999;112 (Pt 21) 3603-3617.

[79] Mezyk R, Bzowska M, Bereta J. Structure and functions of tumor necrosis factor-α converting enzyme. Acta Biochimica Polonica. 2003;50(3) 625-645.

[80] Rabinowitz MH, Andrews RC, Becherer JD, Bickett DM, Bubacz DG, Conway JG, Cowan DJ, Gaul M, Glennon K, Lambert MH, Leesnitzer MA, McDougald DL, Moss ML, Musso DL, Rizzolio MC. Design of selective and soluble inhibitors of tumor necrosis factor-α converting enzyme (TACE). Journal of Medicinal Chemistry. 2001;44(24) 4252-4267.

[81] Mohan R, Chintala SK, Jung JC, Villar WV, McCabe F, Russo LA, Lee Y, McCarthy BE, Wollenberg KR, Jester JV, Wang M, Welgus HG, Shipley JM, Senior RM, Fini ME. Matrix metalloproteinase gelatinase B (MMP-9) coordinates and effects epithelial regeneration. Journal of Biological Chemistry. 2002;277(3) 2065-2072.

[82] Anderson ED, VanSlyke JK, Thulin CD, Jean F, Thomas G. Activation of the furin endoprotease is a multiple-step process: requirements for acidification and internal propeptide cleavage. EMBO Journal. 1997;16(7) 1508-1518.

[83] Peiretti F, Canault M, Deprez-Beauclair P, Berthet V, Bonardo B, Juhan-Vague I, Nalbone G. Intracellular maturation and transport of tumor necrosis factor alpha converting enzyme. Experimental Cell Research. 2003;285(2) 278-285.

[84] Komiyama T, Coppola JM, Larsen MJ, van Dort ME, Ross BD, Day R, Rehemtulla A, Fuller RS. Inhibition of furin/proprotein convertase-catalyzed surface and intracellular processing by small molecules. Journal of Biological Chemistry. 2009;284(23) 15729-15738.

[85] Endres K, Anders A, Kojro E, Gilbert S, Fahrenholz F, Postina R. Tumor necrosis factor-α converting enzyme is processed by proprotein-convertases to its mature form which is degraded upon phorbol ester stimulation. European Journal of Biochemistry. 2003;270(11) 2386-2393.

[86] de Cicco RL, Bassi DE, Benavides F, Conti CJ, Klein-Szanto AJ. Inhibition of proprotein convertases: approaches to block squamous carcinoma development and progression. Molecular Carcinogenesis. 2007;46(8) 654-659.

[87] Mohan MJ, Seaton T, Mitchell J, Howe A, Blackburn K, Burkhart W, Moyer M, Patel I, Waitt GM, Becherer JD, Moss ML, Milla ME. The tumor necrosis factor-α converting enzyme (TACE): a unique metalloproteinase with highly defined substrate selectivity. Biochemistry. 2002;41(30) 9462-9469.

[88] Peschon JJ, Slack JL, Reddy P, Stocking KL, Sunnarborg SW, Lee DC, Russell WE, Castner BJ, Johnson RS, Fitzner JN, Boyce RW, Nelson N, Kozlosky CJ, Wolfson MF, Rauch CT, Cerretti DP, Paxton RJ, March CJ, Black RA. An essential role for ectodomain shedding in mammalian development. Science. 1998;282(5392) 1281-1284.

[89] Sunnarborg SW, Hinkle CL, Stevenson M, Russell WE, Raska CS, Peschon JJ, Castner BJ, Gerhart MJ, Paxton RJ, Black RA, Lee DC. Tumor necrosis factor-α converting enzyme (TACE) regulates epidermal growth factor receptor ligand availability. Journal of Biological Chemistry. 2002;277(15) 12838-12845.

[90] Brown SB, Krause D, Ellem KA. Low fluences of ultraviolet irradiation stimulate HeLa cell surface aminopeptidase and candidate "TGFαase" activity. Journal of Cellular Biochemistry. 1993;51(1) 102-115.

[91] Piva TJ, Davern CM, Francis KG, Chojnowski GM, Hall PM, Ellem KA. Increased ecto-metallopeptidase activity in cells undergoing apoptosis. Journal of Cellular Biochemistry. 2000;76(4) 625-638.

[92] Piva TJ, Krause DR, Ellem KO. UVC activation of the HeLa cell membrane "TGFαase," a metalloenzyme. Journal of Cellular Biochemistry. 1997;64(3) 353-368.

[93] Piva TJ, Davern CM, Hall PM, Winterford CM, Ellem KA. Increased Activity of Cell Surface Peptidases in HeLa Cells Undergoing UV-Induced Apoptosis Is Not Mediated by Caspase 3. International Journal of Molecular Sciences. 2012;13(3) 2650-2675.

[94] Singh B, Schneider M, Knyazev P, Ullrich A. UV-induced EGFR signal transactivation is dependent on proligand shedding by activated metalloproteases in skin cancer cell lines. International Journal of Cancer. 2009;124(3) 531-539.

[95] Krahn G, Leiter U, Kaskel P, Udart M, Utikal J, Bezold G, Peter RU. Coexpression patterns of EGFR, HER2, HER3 and HER4 in non-melanoma skin cancer. European Journal of Cancer. 2001;37(2) 251-259.

[96] Adrain C, Zettl M, Christova Y, Taylor N, Freeman M. Tumor necrosis factor signaling requires iRhom2 to promote trafficking and activation of TACE. Science. 2012;335(6065) 225-228.

[97] Denault J, Bissonnette L, Longpre J, Charest G, Lavigne P, Leduc R. Ectodomain shedding of furin: kinetics and role of the cysteine-rich region. FEBS Letters. 2002;527(1-3) 309-314.

[98] Pearton DJ, Nirunsuksiri W, Rehemtulla A, Lewis SP, Presland RB, Dale BA. Proprotein convertase expression and localization in epidermis: evidence for multiple roles and substrates. Experimental Dermatology. 2001;10(3) 193-203.

[99] Srour N, Lebel A, McMahon S, Fournier I, Fugere M, Day R, Dubois CM. TACE/ADAM-17 maturation and activation of sheddase activity require proprotein convertase activity. FEBS Letters. 2003;554(3) 275-283.

[100] Tian S, Huang Q, Fang Y, Wu J. FurinDB: A Database of 20-Residue Furin Cleavage Site Motifs, Substrates and Their Associated Drugs. International Journal of Molecular Sciences. 2011;12(2) 1060-1065.

[101] Bassi DE, Fu J, Lopez de Cicco R, Klein-Szanto AJ. Proprotein convertases: "master switches" in the regulation of tumor growth and progression. Molecular Carcinogenesis. 2005;44(3) 151-161.

[102] Becker GL, Lu Y, Hardes K, Strehlow B, Levesque C, Lindberg I, Sandvig K, Bakowsky U, Day R, Garten W, Steinmetzer T. Highly potent inhibitors of proprotein convertase furin as potential drugs for treatment of infectious diseases. Journal of Biological Chemistry. 2012;287(26) 21992-22003.

[103] Thomas G. Furin at the cutting edge: from protein traffic to embryogenesis and disease. Nature Reviews Molecular Cell Biology. 2002;3(10) 753-766.

[104] Coppola JM, Bhojani MS, Ross BD, Rehemtulla A. A small-molecule furin inhibitor inhibits cancer cell motility and invasiveness. Neoplasia. 2008;10(4) 363-370.

[105] Arsenault D, Lucien F, Dubois CM. Hypoxia enhances cancer cell invasion through relocalization of the proprotein convertase furin from the trans-Golgi network to the cell surface. Journal of Cellular Physiology. 2012;227(2) 789-800.

[106] Fu J, Bassi DE, Zhang J, Li T, Nicolas E, Klein-Szanto AJ. Transgenic overexpression of the proprotein convertase furin enhances skin tumor growth. Neoplasia. 2012;14(4) 271-282.

[107] Wise RJ, Barr PJ, Wong PA, Kiefer MC, Brake AJ, Kaufman RJ. Expression of a human proprotein processing enzyme: correct cleavage of the von Willebrand factor precursor at a paired basic amino acid site. Proceedings of the National Academy of Sciences of the United States of America. 1990;87(23) 9378-9382.

[108] Wasley LC, Rehemtulla A, Bristol JA, Kaufman RJ. PACE/furin can process the vitamin K-dependent pro-factor IX precursor within the secretory pathway. Journal of Biological Chemistry. 1993;268(12) 8458-8465.

[109] Blais V, Fugere M, Denault JB, Klarskov K, Day R, Leduc R. Processing of proendothelin-1 by members of the subtilisin-like pro-protein convertase family. FEBS Letters. 2002;524(1-3) 43-48.

[110] Dubois CM, Blanchette F, Laprise MH, Leduc R, Grondin F, Seidah NG. Evidence that furin is an authentic transforming growth factor-β1-converting enzyme. American Journal of Pathology. 2001;158(1) 305-316.

[111] Lopez de Cicco R, Watson JC, Bassi DE, Litwin S, Klein-Szanto AJ. Simultaneous expression of furin and vascular endothelial growth factor in human oral tongue squamous cell carcinoma progression. Clinical Cancer Research. 2004;10(13) 4480-4488.

[112] Seidah NG, Benjannet S, Pareek S, Savaria D, Hamelin J, Goulet B, Laliberte J, Lazure C, Chretien M, Murphy RA. Cellular processing of the nerve growth factor precursor

by the mammalian pro-protein convertases. Biochemical Journal. 1996;314 (Pt 3) 951-960.

[113] Bassi DE, Mahloogi H, Klein-Szanto AJ. The proprotein convertases furin and PACE4 play a significant role in tumor progression. Molecular Carcinogenesis. 2000;28(2) 63-69.

[114] Maquoi E, Noel A, Frankenne F, Angliker H, Murphy G, Foidart JM. Inhibition of matrix metalloproteinase 2 maturation and HT1080 invasiveness by a synthetic furin inhibitor. FEBS Letters. 1998;424(3) 262-266.

[115] Li X, Perez L, Pan Z, Fan H. The transmembrane domain of TACE regulates protein ectodomain shedding. Cell Research. 2007;17(12) 985-998.

[116] Logeat F, Bessia C, Brou C, LeBail O, Jarriault S, Seidah NG, Israel A. The Notch1 receptor is cleaved constitutively by a furin-like convertase. Proceedings of the National Academy of Sciences of the United States of America. 1998;95(14) 8108-8112.

[117] Khatib AM, Siegfried G, Prat A, Luis J, Chretien M, Metrakos P, Seidah NG. Inhibition of proprotein convertases is associated with loss of growth and tumorigenicity of HT-29 human colon carcinoma cells: importance of insulin-like growth factor-1 (IGF-1) receptor processing in IGF-1-mediated functions. Journal of Biological Chemistry. 2001;276(33) 30686-30693.

[118] Maret D, Gruzglin E, Sadr MS, Siu V, Shan W, Koch AW, Seidah NG, Del Maestro RF, Colman DR. Surface expression of precursor N-cadherin promotes tumor cell invasion. Neoplasia. 2010;12(12) 1066-1080.

[119] Lehmann M, Rigot V, Seidah NG, Marvaldi J, Lissitzky JC. Lack of integrin alpha-chain endoproteolytic cleavage in furin-deficient human colon adenocarcinoma cells LoVo. Biochemical Journal. 1996;317 (Pt 3) 803-809.

[120] Volchkov VE, Feldmann H, Volchkova VA, Klenk HD. Processing of the Ebola virus glycoprotein by the proprotein convertase furin. Proceedings of the National Academy of Sciences of the United States of America. 1998;95(10) 5762-5767.

[121] Richards RM, Lowy DR, Schiller JT, Day PM. Cleavage of the papillomavirus minor capsid protein, L2, at a furin consensus site is necessary for infection. Proceedings of the National Academy of Sciences of the United States of America. 2006;103(5) 1522-1527.

[122] Klimpel KR, Molloy SS, Thomas G, Leppla SH. Anthrax toxin protective antigen is activated by a cell surface protease with the sequence specificity and catalytic properties of furin. Proceedings of the National Academy of Sciences of the United States of America. 1992;89(21) 10277-10281.

[123] Gordon VM, Benz R, Fujii K, Leppla SH, Tweten RK. Clostridium septicum alpha-toxin is proteolytically activated by furin. Infection and Immunity. 1997;65(10) 4130-4134.

[124] Angliker H, Wikstrom P, Shaw E, Brenner C, Fuller RS. The synthesis of inhibitors for processing proteinases and their action on the Kex2 proteinase of yeast. Biochemical Journal. 1993;293 (Pt 1) 75-81.

[125] Huang YH, Lin KH, Liao CH, Lai MW, Tseng YH, Yeh CT. Furin overexpression suppresses tumor growth and predicts a better postoperative disease-free survival in hepatocellular carcinoma. PLoS ONE. 2012;7(7) e40738.

[126] Bassi DE, Zhang J, Cenna J, Litwin S, Cukierman E, Klein-Szanto AJ. Proprotein convertase inhibition results in decreased skin cell proliferation, tumorigenesis, and metastasis. Neoplasia. 2010;12(7) 516-526.

[127] Zhu J, Declercq J, Roucourt B, Ghassabeh GH, Meulemans S, Kinne J, David G, Vermorken AJ, Van de Ven WJ, Lindberg I, Muyldermans S, Creemers JW. Generation and characterization of non-competitive furin-inhibiting nanobodies. Biochemical Journal. 2012;448(1) 73-82.

[128] Bassi DE, Lopez De Cicco R, Mahloogi H, Zucker S, Thomas G, Klein-Szanto AJ. Furin inhibition results in absent or decreased invasiveness and tumorigenicity of human cancer cells. Proceedings of the National Academy of Sciences of the United States of America. 2001;98(18) 10326-10331.

[129] Huynh TT, Chan KS, Piva TJ. Effect of ultraviolet radiation on the expression of pp38MAPK and furin in human keratinocyte-derived cell lines. Photodermatology, Photoimmunology and Photomedicine. 2009;25(1) 20-29.

[130] Hua H, Li M, Luo T, Yin Y, Jiang Y. Matrix metalloproteinases in tumorigenesis: an evolving paradigm. Cellular and Molecular Life Sciences. 2011;68(23) 3853-3868.

[131] Noel A, Jost M, Maquoi E. Matrix metalloproteinases at cancer tumor-host interface. Seminars in Cell and Developmental Biology. 2008;19(1) 52-60.

[132] Vosseler S, Lederle W, Airola K, Obermueller E, Fusenig NE, Mueller MM. Distinct progression-associated expression of tumor and stromal MMPs in HaCaT skin SCCs correlates with onset of invasion. International Journal of Cancer. 2009;125(10) 2296-2306.

[133] Rucci N, Sanita P, Angelucci A. Roles of metalloproteases in metastatic niche. Current Molecular Medicine. 2011;11(8) 609-622.

[134] Pytliak M, Vargova V, Mechirova V. Matrix metalloproteinases and their role in oncogenesis: a review. Onkologie. 2012;35(1-2) 49-53.

[135] Murphy G, Nagase H. Progress in matrix metalloproteinase research. Molecular Aspects of Medicine. 2008;29(5) 290-308.

[136] Stocker W, Bode W. Structural features of a superfamily of zinc-endopeptidases: the metzincins. Current Opinion in Structural Biology. 1995;5(3) 383-390.

[137] Steinbrenner H, Ramos MC, Stuhlmann D, Sies H, Brenneisen P. UVA-mediated downregulation of MMP-2 and MMP-9 in human epidermal keratinocytes. Biochemical and Biophysical Research Communications. 2003;308(3) 486-491.

[138] Newby AC. Dual role of matrix metalloproteinases (matrixins) in intimal thickening and atherosclerotic plaque rupture. Physiological Reviews. 2005;85(1) 1-31.

[139] Tellier E, Negre-Salvayre A, Bocquet B, Itohara S, Hannun YA, Salvayre R, Auge N. Role for furin in tumor necrosis factor alpha-induced activation of the matrix metalloproteinase/sphingolipid mitogenic pathway. Molecular and Cellular Biology. 2007;27(8) 2997-3007.

[140] Sternlicht MD, Werb Z. How matrix metalloproteinases regulate cell behavior. Annual Review of Cell and Developmental Biology. 2001;17 463-516.

[141] Han YP, Tuan TL, Wu H, Hughes M, Garner WL. TNF-α stimulates activation of pro-MMP2 in human skin through NF-κB mediated induction of MT1-MMP. Journal of Cell Science. 2001;114(Pt 1) 131-139.

[142] Wan Y, Belt A, Wang Z, Voorhees J, Fisher G. Transmodulation of epidermal growth factor receptor mediates IL-1β-induced MMP-1 expression in cultured human keratinocytes. International Journal of Molecular Medicine. 2001;7(3) 329-334.

[143] Ramos MC, Steinbrenner H, Stuhlmann D, Sies H, Brenneisen P. Induction of MMP-10 and MMP-1 in a squamous cell carcinoma cell line by ultraviolet radiation. Biological Chemistry. 2004;385(1) 75-86.

[144] Onoue S, Kobayashi T, Takemoto Y, Sasaki I, Shinkai H. Induction of matrix metalloproteinase-9 secretion from human keratinocytes in culture by ultraviolet B irradiation. Journal of Dermatological Science. 2003;33(2) 105-111.

[145] McCawley LJ, Li S, Benavidez M, Halbleib J, Wattenberg EV, Hudson LG. Elevation of intracellular cAMP inhibits growth factor-mediated matrix metalloproteinase-9 induction and keratinocyte migration. Molecular Pharmacology. 2000;58(1) 145-151.

[146] Fisher GJ, Voorhees JJ. Molecular mechanisms of photoaging and its prevention by retinoic acid: ultraviolet irradiation induces MAP kinase signal transduction cascades that induce Ap-1-regulated matrix metalloproteinases that degrade human skin in vivo. Journal of Investigative Dermatology Symposium Proceedings. 1998;3(1) 61-68.

[147] Fagot D, Asselineau D, Bernerd F. Matrix metalloproteinase-1 production observed after solar-simulated radiation exposure is assumed by dermal fibroblasts but involves a paracrine activation through epidermal keratinocytes. Photochemistry and Photobiology. 2004;79(6) 499-505.

[148] Han YP, Downey S, Garner WL. Interleukin-1α-induced proteolytic activation of metalloproteinase-9 by human skin. Surgery. 2005;138(5) 932-939.

[149] Cao J, Rehemtulla A, Pavlaki M, Kozarekar P, Chiarelli C. Furin directly cleaves proMMP-2 in the trans-Golgi network resulting in a nonfunctioning proteinase. Journal of Biological Chemistry. 2005;280(12) 10974-10980.

[150] Kappes UP, Luo D, Potter M, Schulmeister K, Runger TM. Short- and long-wave UV light (UVB and UVA) induce similar mutations in human skin cells. Journal of Investigative Dermatology. 2006;126(3) 667-675.

[151] Ratushny V, Gober MD, Hick R, Ridky TW, Seykora JT. From keratinocyte to cancer: the pathogenesis and modeling of cutaneous squamous cell carcinoma. Journal of Clinical Investigation. 2012;122(2) 464-472.

[152] Nickoloff BJ, Qin JZ, Chaturvedi V, Bacon P, Panella J, Denning MF. Life and death signaling pathways contributing to skin cancer. Journal of Investigative Dermatology Symposium Proceedings. 2002;7(1) 27-35.

[153] Besaratinia A, Pfeifer GP. Sunlight ultraviolet irradiation and BRAF V600 mutagenesis in human melanoma. Human Mutation. 2008;29(8) 983-991.

[154] Thiery JP. Epithelial-mesenchymal transitions in tumour progression. Nature Reviews Cancer. 2002;2(6) 442-454.

[155] Qi J, Chen N, Wang J, Siu CH. Transendothelial migration of melanoma cells involves N-cadherin-mediated adhesion and activation of the β-catenin signaling pathway. Molecular Biology of the Cell. 2005;16(9) 4386-4397.

[156] Berthet V, Rigot V, Champion S, Secchi J, Fouchier F, Marvaldi J, Luis J. Role of endoproteolytic processing in the adhesive and signaling functions of alphavbeta5 integrin. Journal of Biological Chemistry. 2000;275(43) 33308-33313.

[157] Siegfried G, Basak A, Cromlish JA, Benjannet S, Marcinkiewicz J, Chretien M, Seidah NG, Khatib AM. The secretory proprotein convertases furin, PC5, and PC7 activate VEGF-C to induce tumorigenesis. Journal of Clinical Investigation. 2003;111(11) 1723-1732.

[158] McMahon S, Laprise MH, Dubois CM. Alternative pathway for the role of furin in tumor cell invasion process. Enhanced MMP-2 levels through bioactive TGFβ. Experimental Cell Research. 2003;291(2) 326-339.

[159] Cheng M, Watson PH, Paterson JA, Seidah N, Chretien M, Shiu RP. Pro-protein convertase gene expression in human breast cancer. International Journal of Cancer. 1997;71(6) 966-971.

[160] Page RE, Klein-Szanto AJ, Litwin S, Nicolas E, Al-Jumaily R, Alexander P, Godwin AK, Ross EA, Schilder RJ, Bassi DE. Increased expression of the pro-protein convertase furin predicts decreased survival in ovarian cancer. Cellular Oncology. 2007;29(4) 289-299.

[161] Mercapide J, Lopez De Cicco R, Bassi DE, Castresana JS, Thomas G, Klein-Szanto AJ. Inhibition of furin-mediated processing results in suppression of astrocytoma cell growth and invasiveness. Clinical Cancer Research. 2002;8(6) 1740-1746.

[162] Bassi DE, Mahloogi H, Al-Saleem L, Lopez De Cicco R, Ridge JA, Klein-Szanto AJ. Elevated furin expression in aggressive human head and neck tumors and tumor cell lines. Molecular Carcinogenesis. 2001;31(4) 224-232.

[163] Bassi DE, Mahloogi H, Lopez De Cicco R, Klein-Szanto A. Increased furin activity enhances the malignant phenotype of human head and neck cancer cells. American Journal of Pathology. 2003;162(2) 439-447.

[164] Dumas V, Kanitakis J, Charvat S, Euvrard S, Faure M, Claudy A. Expression of basement membrane antigens and matrix metalloproteinases 2 and 9 in cutaneous basal and squamous cell carcinomas. Anticancer Research. 1999;19(4B) 2929-2938.

[165] Varani J, Hattori Y, Chi Y, Schmidt T, Perone P, Zeigler ME, Fader DJ, Johnson TM. Collagenolytic and gelatinolytic matrix metalloproteinases and their inhibitors in basal cell carcinoma of skin: comparison with normal skin. British Journal of Cancer. 2000;82(3) 657-665.

[166] Hofmann UB, Eggert AA, Blass K, Brocker EB, Becker JC. Expression of matrix metalloproteinases in the microenvironment of spontaneous and experimental melanoma metastases reflects the requirements for tumor formation. Cancer Research. 2003;63(23) 8221-8225.

[167] Hernandez-Perez M, Mahalingam M. Matrix metalloproteinases in health and disease: insights from dermatopathology. American Journal of Dermatopathology. 2012;34(6) 565-579.

[168] Wan YS, Wang ZQ, Shao Y, Voorhees JJ, Fisher GJ. Ultraviolet irradiation activates PI 3-kinase/AKT survival pathway via EGF receptors in human skin in vivo. International Journal of Oncology. 2001;18(3) 461-466.